2009

Standards for **Long Term Care**

Accreditation Policies

Standards

Elements of Performance

Scoring

SLTC

The Joint Commission
Accreditation
Long Term Care

http://www.jointcommission.org

Joint Commission Mission

The mission of The Joint Commission on Accreditation of Healthcare Organizations is to continuously improve the safety and quality of care provided to the public through the provision of health care accreditation and related services that support performance improvement in health care organizations.

Joint Commission Resources, Inc. (JCR), a not-for-profit affiliate of the Joint Commission on Accreditation of Healthcare Organizations (Joint Commission), has been designated by the Joint Commission to publish publications and multimedia products. JCR reproduces and distributes these materials under license from the Joint Commission.

JCR educational programs and publications support, but are separate from, the accreditation activities of the Joint Commission. Attendees at JCR educational programs and purchasers of JCR publications receive no special consideration or treatment in, or confidential information about, the accreditation process.

Printed in the U.S.A. 5 4 3 2 1

Requests for permission to make copies of any part of this work should be mailed to
Permissions Editor
Department of Publications
Joint Commission Resources
One Renaissance Boulevard
Oakbrook Terrace, Illinois 60181
permissions@jcrinc.com

ISBN: 978-1-59940-265-9
ISSN: 1096-0546

For more information about the Joint Commission on Accreditation of Healthcare Organizations, please visit http://www.jointcommission.org.

Contents

1.88

HB

2009

SLTC

How to Use This Book (HB)

HB

How to Use This Book

This chapter will help you understand the way this accreditation book works. "How to Use This Book" is a user's guide to the *2009 Standards for Long Term Care (SLTC)*. Not only does this chapter orient you to your accreditation book, it also highlights new features of The Joint Commission's accreditation process.

What Is This Book's Purpose?

The *SLTC* is a one-stop resource to help your organization maintain continuous compliance with The Joint Commission's requirements. The material in this book will guide your staff in developing processes to provide the highest level of care, treatment, or services.

The *SLTC* includes all the information your organization needs for continuous operational improvement: standards, rationales, elements of performance (EPs), Accreditation Participation Requirements, scoring, National Patient Safety Goals, decision rules, and accreditation policies and procedures. The standards' user-friendly format fosters understanding of each standard, its rationale (when applicable), and its EPs. Additional chapters provide guidance on how to use the standards-related information found throughout the book.

Changes to the *SLTC* are made in response to suggestions from accredited organizations and relate to important issues that clearly support quality care, treatment, or services.

What Does This Book Include?

Standards Chapter

Each standards (functional) chapter is set up as follows:

- An **overview** at the beginning of each chapter explains the chapter's purpose and the principles that support the standards in it.
- The **chapter outline** provided for some chapters shows you exactly how the chapter is laid out and provides a frame of reference for the new numbering system (explained below).
- The **standards list** that follows the Overview in some standards chapters is a handy, at-a-glance list of all standards found in that chapter.
- **Introductions** at the beginning of some standards (or cluster of standards) provide information about the standard's origin and any issues that surround it.

ACC

2009

SLTC

The Accreditation Process (ACC)

ACC

The Accreditation Process

Overview

This chapter introduces The Joint Commission's accreditation process, beginning with general information about the application process, types of surveys, the Periodic Performance Review (PPR), priority focus areas (PFAs), and clinical/service groups (CSGs). The chapter then provides details on what organizations can expect during their accreditation survey, including the survey agenda, the tracer methodology, and scoring guidelines. Finally, the chapter includes information important to organizations after the survey, including the accreditation decision, accreditation decision rules, Evidence of Standards Compliance (ESC), and the review and appeal process.

The policies and procedures described in this chapter are relevant to all health care organizations interested in Joint Commission accreditation, whether they are applying for the first time or seeking continued accreditation. You can locate the policies and procedures applicable to your organization according to where your organization is in its accreditation cycle. All organizations must follow the policies and procedures listed in this chapter to participate and continue to participate in the accreditation process. Failure to follow the policies and procedures described in this chapter can result in denial or withdrawal of accreditation. Because this information is reviewed and revised as necessary on a continuous basis, all organizations are responsible for keeping track of these policies and procedures.

Note: *The "Accreditation Participation Requirements" (APR) chapter includes specific requirements for accreditation participation. The APRs are existing policies and are currently effective for accreditation purposes. Cross-references to the APRs are noted in the applicable sections of this chapter.*

Eligibility

Organizations Eligible for Accreditation

General Eligibility Requirements

Any health care organization may apply for Joint Commission accreditation under the standards in this book* if all the following requirements are met:

- The organization is in the United States or its territories or, if outside the United States, is operated by the U.S. government, or under a charter of the U.S. Congress.
- The organization assesses and improves the quality of its services. This process includes a review of care by clinicians, when appropriate.
- The organization identifies the services it provides, indicating which services it provides directly, under contract, or through some other arrangement.
- The organization provides services addressed by The Joint Commission's standards.

---

* The Joint Commission will work with the organization to determine which standards from other accreditation books are applicable.

Policies

Scope of Accreditation Surveys

General Survey Categories

The Joint Commission surveys and accredits health care organizations, using standards from one or more of the following manuals:

- *Comprehensive Accreditation Manual for Hospitals: The Official Handbook*
- *Comprehensive Accreditation Manual for Critical Access Hospitals*
- *Comprehensive Accreditation Manual for Office-Based Surgery Practices*
- *Comprehensive Accreditation Manual for Ambulatory Care*
- *Comprehensive Accreditation Manual for Behavioral Health Care*
- *Comprehensive Accreditation Manual for Home Care* (includes standards for home health, personal/support care, hospice, home medical equipment, and pharmacies)
- *Comprehensive Accreditation Manual for Long Term Care*
- *Comprehensive Accreditation Manual for Laboratory and Point-of-Care Testing*

In addition to using standards, The Joint Commission also surveys organizations by using the standards, elements of performance (EPs), performance measurement data (when applicable), and Accreditation Participation Requirements (APRs), including The Joint Commission National Patient Safety Goals (*see* the "National Patient Safety Goals" [NPSG] chapter). Used in conjunction with the standards, these items help assess an organization's performance.

Tailored Survey Policy

The Joint Commission survey, assuming satisfactory compliance, provides one accreditation award for all the organization's services, programs, and related organizations. Another service, program, or related entity (that is, component), whether providing services directly or through a contractual arrangement, is included in the survey of the applicant organization under the following circumstances:

- There are Joint Commission standards applicable to the component.
- There is organizational and functional integration between the component and the applicant organization.

Note: *Any service, program, or related entity that is a component of an accreditation-eligible organization may independently seek accreditation if it can meet Joint Commission survey eligibility requirements. The results of such a separate accreditation survey will still apply to the overall organization's decision in accordance with applicable decision rules.*

Organizational and functional integration refers to the degree to which the component is overseen and managed by the applicant organization. *Applicant organization* refers both to an organization seeking accreditation and to an organization that is currently accredited. A *component* is a service, program, or related entity that delivers care or services and is eligible for survey under one of The Joint Commission's accreditation programs. These include the following:

- General, acute psychiatric, pediatric, critical access, surgical specialty, long term acute care, and rehabilitation hospitals

- Home care organizations, including those that provide home health services, personal care and support services, home infusion and other pharmacy services, long term care pharmacies and infusion centers, durable medical equipment services, and hospice services
- Skilled nursing facilities, nursing homes and other long term care facilities
- Behavioral health care organizations, including those that provide mental health services, substance abuse treatment services, foster care services, and services for persons with developmental disabilities of various ages and in various organized service settings
- Ambulatory care providers, including surgery centers and office-based surgery practices, rehabilitation centers, sleep labs, imaging centers, group practices, community health centers, student health centers, and others
- Clinical laboratories

Organizational integration exists when an applicant organization's governing body, either directly or ultimately, controls budgetary and resource allocation decisions for the component or, where individual corporate entities are involved, there is greater than 50% common governing board membership for the applicant organization and on the board of the component.

Functional integration exists when the entity meets at least three of the following eight criteria:

1. The applicant organization and the component do the following:
   - Use the same process for determining membership of licensed independent practitioners in practitioner panels or medical or professional staff and/or
   - Have a common organized medical or professional staff for the applicant organization and the component
2. The applicant organization's human resources function hires and assigns staff at the component and has the authority to do the following:
   - Terminate staff at the component
   - Transfer or rotate staff between the applicant organization and the component
   - Conduct performance appraisals of the staff who work in the component
3. The applicant organization's policies and procedures are applicable to the component, with few or no exceptions.
4. The applicant organization manages significant operations of the component; that is, the component has little or no management authority or autonomy independent of the applicant organization.
5. The component's resident records are integrated into the applicant organization's resident record system.
6. The applicant organization applies its performance improvement program to the component and has authority to implement actions intended to improve performance at the component.
7. The applicant organization bills for services provided by the component under the name of the applicant organization.
8. The applicant organization and/or the component portrays to the public that the component is part of the organization through the use of common names or logos; references on letterheads, brochures, telephone book listings, or Web sites; or representations in other published materials.

A checklist to assist in determining organizational and functional integration is provided in Figure 1 on page 17.

The Joint Commission evaluates all health care services provided by the organization for which The Joint Commission has standards and makes one accreditation decision and Summary of Survey Findings Report. An organization must be prepared to provide evidence of its compliance with each applicable standard. To gain accreditation, an organization must demonstrate overall compliance with the standards and their EPs.

Complex Organization Survey Process

The complex organization survey process is applied to organizations that are governed by the Tailored Survey Policy. The Joint Commission conducts a complex organization survey based on the services provided by the organization, as reported in its electronic application for accreditation (e-App). Because a complex organization survey process involves standards in more than one of the manuals listed in this chapter, The Joint Commission provides the organization with a copy of each of the manuals to be used in the survey before it is conducted.

An organization that has acquired a new component that requires a survey in an accreditation program that is new to the organization is given a 12-month grace period from the time the component is acquired before the performance of that component is factored into the organization's overall accreditation decision. The newly acquired component is usually surveyed within six months of its acquisition as an extension survey, even though the component would still be considered accredited.

Single Accreditation Award

The Joint Commission surveys and, assuming satisfactory compliance, provides one accreditation award for all of an organization's services, programs, and related organizations that are organizationally and functionally integrated to the applicant organization. If, after accreditation is rendered to an organization, the organization's structure changes whereby one or more of its services, programs, or related organizations is no longer part of the organization that was originally surveyed, the service, program, or related organization is no longer included in the organization's accreditation.

Contracted Services

The Joint Commission evaluates an organization's assessment of the quality of services provided under contractual arrangements. The Joint Commission reserves the right to evaluate, as part of its survey, services provided by another organization or provider. It may survey performance issues between the contracted organization and the applicant organization, regardless of the accreditation decision of the contracted organization. The Joint Commission also surveys services provided on-site under contract.

Checklist to Determine Organizational and Functional Integration

Organizational	Description	Check Yes or No		Comments
1. Governance	Governing body of the organization applying for accreditation controls budget and resource allocation for component	Yes	No	
2. Shared governance	If separate corporate entities, over 50% of governing body membership is shared by the organization applying for accreditation and the component	Yes	No	

Functional	Description	Check Yes or No		Comments
1. Common medical staff and/or licensed independent practitioner process	Unified process for credentialing of licensed independent practitioners	Yes	No	
2. Human resources	The organization applying for accreditation has hiring/firing/performance appraisal authority over the component's staff	Yes	No	
3. Policies and procedures	Common policies and procedures	Yes	No	
4. Management	Component is managed by the organization applying for accreditation	Yes	No	
5. Patient records	Integrated patient record system	Yes	No	
6. Performance improvement	Integrated performance improvement program, with organization authority to implement performance improvement actions at component	Yes	No	
7. Billing	Component's services are billed by applicant organization	Yes	No	

(continued on next page)

Figure 1. *Checklist to determine organizational and functional integration.*

Table 1. Minimum Requirements for Organizations/Programs Seeking Joint Commission Accreditation/Certification for the First Time and High-Risk/Critical Services That Will Be Subject to a One-Year Follow-Up Survey

Note: *It is not intended that the minimum number of patients will equate with the minimum number of tracers for all size organizations. As an organization increases in size, the required number of tracers will also increase. The minimum number of patients is only a measure of patient volume that an organization must have before seeking Joint Commission accreditation or certification.*

Program	Volume of Patients/Services; Minimum Number	High-Risk/Critical Services
Long Term Care	Five residents served, with two active residents at the time of survey	• Not applicable because of annual state surveys

3. Residents and/or the organization are being moved to a new building on the day or days of the survey

Note: *If an organization is undergoing an unannounced survey and on the day of the survey the organization experiences one of these situations, the survey may be postponed.*

Fees for Postponements for Initial Surveys

In rare circumstances, The Joint Commission may, at its discretion, approve a request to postpone a survey for an organization not meeting any of the criteria described here. In such cases, the organization may be charged a fee to defray costs. In addition, if the initial survey is of a new program or service of a complex organization already accredited, the organization may be required to undergo an extension survey. Please contact your account representative or the Pricing Unit at 630/792-5115.

Refusal of a Survey

An organization that fails to permit a survey, whether announced or unannounced, to proceed for a reason other than what is listed under the "Survey Postponement Policy for Initial Announced Surveys" section (on page 19) will be recommended for a Denial of Accreditation decision.

Information Accuracy and Truthfulness Policy

The accuracy and veracity of relevant information, whether actually used in the accreditation process or not, are essential to the integrity of The Joint Commission's

* **Requirement for Improvement** A survey finding cited in an organization's Accreditation Survey Findings Report that must be addressed in the organization's Evidence of Standards Compliance.

accreditation process. Information provided at any time by the organization must be accurate and truthful.* Such information may do the following:

- Be provided verbally or in writing
- Be obtained through direct observation or interview by Joint Commission surveyors
- Be derived from documents supplied by the organization to The Joint Commission, including, but not limited to, an organization's root cause analysis (RCA) in response to a sentinel event, an organization's request for accreditation, or a plan of correction submitted as part of the Conditional Accreditation process
- Involve data or documents transmitted electronically to The Joint Commission, including, but not limited to, data or documents provided as part of the e-App process

  or
- Involve an attestation that an organization has not knowingly used Joint Commission full-time, part-time, or intermittent surveyors to provide any accreditation-related consulting services after January 1, 2004. Examples of such services include, but are not limited to, the following:
  - Helping an organization meet Joint Commission standards
  - Helping an organization in the PPR process
  - Conducting mock surveys for an organization
  - Helping an organization in the ESC process

    or
  - Providing consultation to an organization to address Priority Focus Process (PFP) information

Falsification, as the term is used in The Joint Commission's Information Accuracy and Truthfulness Policy, applies to both commissions and omissions in sharing information with The Joint Commission.*

Policy Requirements

The Joint Commission's Information Accuracy and Truthfulness Policy includes the following:

1. An organization must never provide The Joint Commission with falsified information relevant to the accreditation process. The Joint Commission construes any effort to do so as a violation of the organization's obligation to engage in the accreditation process in good faith.
2. *Falsification* is defined for this policy as the fabrication, in whole or in part, and through commission or omission, of any information provided by an applicant or accredited organization to The Joint Commission. This includes, but is not limited to, any redrafting, reformatting, or content deletion of documents.
3. The organization may submit additional material that summarizes or otherwise explains original information submitted to The Joint Commission. These materials must be properly identified, dated, and accompanied by the original documents.
4. The Joint Commission conducts an evaluation when it has cause to believe that an accredited organization may have provided falsified information to The Joint Com-

* *See* APR.01.02.01 on page 135 in the "Accreditation Participation Requirements" (APR) chapter.

mission relevant to the accreditation process. Except as otherwise authorized by the president of The Joint Commission, the evaluation includes an unannounced on-site survey. This survey uses special protocols designed to address the alleged information falsification. It assesses the degree of actual organization compliance with the standards and EPs that are the subject of the allegation, if appropriate.

5. The Joint Commission takes action to deny accreditation to an accredited organization whenever The Joint Commission is reasonably persuaded that the organization has provided falsified information.
6. The Joint Commission notifies responsible federal and state government agencies of any organization subject to such action.
7. If an organization is denied accreditation because it provided falsified information, The Joint Commission prohibits it from participating in the accreditation process for a period of one year. The president of The Joint Commission, for good cause only, may waive all or a portion of this waiting period.

Good Faith Participation in Accreditation

The Joint Commission requires each organization seeking accreditation or reaccreditation to engage in the accreditation process in good faith. The Joint Commission may deny accreditation to any organization that fails to participate in the accreditation process in good faith.

Ways of interfering with good faith participation can fall into the following categories:

- *Deceiving The Joint Commission.* Compliance with the Information Accuracy and Truthfulness Policy requires a commitment on the part of the accredited organization not to deceive The Joint Commission in any aspect of the accreditation process, such as during the completion of an application for accreditation, during the PPR process, or during a survey.
- *Deceiving the public.* An accredited organization is not acting in good faith if it misleads the public about the meaning and limitations of accreditation. Also, an accredited organization must not inaccurately suggest to the public that its accreditation award applies to any unaccredited affiliated or otherwise related activities.
- *Reprisals.* The Joint Commission invites open communication from any accredited organization's staff and recipients of care and services about any standards compliance or other issues related to the accreditation process. An organization's good faith participation in the accreditation process is questioned if the organization does any of the following:
    - Attempts to discourage such communication—for example, by taking disciplinary steps against an employee solely because that employee provides information to The Joint Commission
    - Threatens those who communicate with The Joint Commission with a defamation lawsuit based solely on what was said to The Joint Commission
    - Allows the treatment or access to services of any individual or staff member to be adversely affected by his or her or a family member's communication with The Joint Commission
- *Standards compliance.* If an organization's conduct reflects a lack of commitment to standards compliance, issues of good faith may be raised. For example, an inten-

tional refusal to attempt to comply with a standard could suggest a cavalier view of the accreditation process.

The good faith participation requirement applies continuously throughout the accreditation cycle.

Public Information Policy*

This Public Information Policy is applicable to all organizations with an accreditation history, subject to any requirements of any applicable laws.

The Joint Commission is committed to making relevant and accurate information about health care organizations available to interested parties. Information regarding a health care organization's quality and safety of care helps organizations improve their services. This information may also help educate consumers and health care purchasers in making informed choices about health care. At the same time, it is important that confidentiality be maintained for certain information to encourage candor in the accreditation process. The Joint Commission's primary vehicles for providing this information publicly are Quality Check® and Quality Reports.

Quality Check and Quality Reports

Quality Check is The Joint Commission's Web site for making available descriptive and performance information about accredited and nonaccredited organizations. Quality Reports are publicly available and include relevant and useful information about the quality and safety of care provided in individual Joint Commission–accredited organization(s). Quality Reports are created at the organization level and contain information regarding an organization's accreditation status, its compliance with National Patient Safety Goals, and performance measurement results, as appropriate. Joint Commission Quality Reports for each accredited organization include the following information:

- The date of the most recent full on-site survey
- The accreditation decision based on the most recent full on-site survey
- The organization's current accreditation decision. If an organization has been denied accreditation, this information will be posted on Quality Check for one year.
- The date of the most recent on-site evaluation of the organization, if not a full survey
- Standards areas with Requirements for Improvement, if the organization has a decision of Provisional Accreditation, Conditional Accreditation, or Preliminary Denial of Accreditation or has been denied accreditation
- Subsequent satisfaction of Requirements for Improvement and the date(s) of resolution for specific standards areas
- Subsequent new Requirements for Improvement and the date(s) assigned
- Services included in the accreditation survey
- Joint Commission policies or rules that lead to Provisional Accreditation, Conditional Accreditation, Preliminary Denial of Accreditation, or Denial of Accreditation
- Disease-specific care certification(s) and the effective date of each certification
- The receipt of special quality recognition awards, as recognized by the Board of Commissioners (for example, the Ernest Amory Codman Award, Magnet status)

* This policy meets the requirements of the Health Insurance Portability and Accountability Act of 1996 (HIPAA).

- Compliance with National Patient Safety Goal requirements
- Performance against National Quality Improvement Goals
- Performance in relation to Patient Experience of Care Measures, as data becomes available

Each accredited organization is afforded the opportunity to prepare a commentary of up to two pages regarding its Quality Report. The commentary accompanies any organization Quality Reports distributed by The Joint Commission, whether via hard copy or The Joint Commission Web site. Each Quality Report released by The Joint Commission will also include appropriate background information. When performance measurement data are included in Quality Reports, such data must be accompanied by information regarding their source of derivation; accuracy, reliability and validity; appropriate uses; and limitations and potential misuses. An organization's Quality Report may be obtained via the Customer Service Department or through Quality Check.

Information About Health Care Organizations Not Accredited by The Joint Commission

For organizations not accredited by The Joint Commission, the following information will be provided on Quality Check:

- The organization's name and location
- The primary services provided by the organization
- If the organization is accredited by another accrediting body(ies), the name(s) of that accrediting body(ies)

Health care organizations not accredited by The Joint Commission will be responsible for maintaining the currency and accuracy of information about them. Information regarding an organization's accreditation status with another accrediting body must be provided electronically and be verified by that accrediting body and updated whenever there is a change in the accreditation status. Information about accredited health care organizations not accredited by The Joint Commission is to be accompanied with appropriate disclaimers regarding the use, accuracy, reliability, limitations, and potential misuses of such information.

In addition, Quality Check users can now locate health care providers by the types of services they provide (for example, home health care, intensive care, or respiratory services). The new search-by-service (or "Type of Care") feature is located under the "Advanced Search" option, in addition to the search by "Type of Provider" function. The inventory of services on the electronic application for accreditation (e-App) has been expanded to support the search-by-service feature. An organization can update its inventory of services at any time by accessing its secure *The Joint Commission Connect*™ extranet site.

Information That Is Publicly Disclosed on Request

In addition to information provided in Quality Reports, the following information may be obtained by writing or calling The Joint Commission:

- The organization's accreditation history
- Survey fees paid by an accredited organization

- The organization's scheduled survey date(s) once the organization has been surveyed
- Applicable standards used for an accreditation survey
- For a tailored survey, the organizational component(s) contributing to a Conditional Accreditation or Denial of Accreditation decision
- Requirements for Improvement for which The Joint Commission had no or insufficient evidence of resolution when an organization withdrew from accreditation
- The standards areas for which The Joint Commission had no or insufficient evidence of resolution of Requirements for Improvement when an organization withdrew from accreditation
- As applicable, confirmation of the occurrence of a sentinel event at an accredited organization and The Joint Commission's intent to apply its Sentinel Event Policy to that occurrence

Release of Complaint-Related Information on Request

The Joint Commission addresses all complaints that pertain to patient safety or quality of care issues within the scope of Joint Commission standards. Complaints may be forwarded by the Centers for Medicare & Medicaid Services (CMS) or other federal or state agencies having oversight responsibilities for health care organizations, or may be received directly from consumers, payers, or health care professionals. As used here, the term "complaint" includes potentially relevant reports that are received from federal or state agencies, identified in the media, or otherwise obtained by The Joint Commission. The Joint Commission has a toll-free hotline to provide patients, their families, caregivers, and others with an opportunity to share concerns regarding quality of care issues at accredited health care organizations. The toll-free number is 800/994-6610 and is available 24 hours a day, 7 days a week; however, staff members are available to answer calls only on weekdays between 8:30 A.M. and 5:00 P.M. central time.

Upon request from any party, The Joint Commission releases the following aggregate information related to complaints about an accredited organization for the three-year period prior to receipt of the request:

- The number of standards-related written complaints filed against an accredited organization that has met criteria for review
- If the inquirer submitted or knows about a specific complaint, the applicable standards areas involved in a specific complaint review
- If the inquirer submitted or knows about a specific complaint, the standards for which Requirements for Improvement were issued as a result of a specific complaint review
- If the inquirer is not seeking information in relation to a specific complaint, a summary of the standards areas that were the focus of the complaint evaluation activities
- If the inquirer is not seeking information in relation to a specific complaint, a summary of the standards areas for which Requirements for Improvement were issued as a result of complaint evaluation activities
- When an unannounced or unscheduled survey is based on information derived from a complaint or public sources, the standards areas related to the complaint

The Joint Commission also provides the following information, as appropriate, to complainants regarding their complaints:

- Any determination that the complaint is not related to Joint Commission standards
- If the complaint is related to standards, the course of action to be taken regarding the complaint, including the specific standards that will be evaluated
- Whether The Joint Commission has decided to take action regarding an organization's accreditation decision following completion of the complaint investigation. If The Joint Commission has decided to take no action, the complainant is to be so advised. If The Joint Commission has taken action, the complainant is to be advised in conformance with the guidelines for release of complaint information as set forth here.
- Any change in an organization's accreditation decision following completion of the complaint investigation, including the specific standards that were the subject of Requirements for Improvement

Release of Aggregate Performance Data

The Joint Commission reserves the right to publish or release aggregate performance data; however, no case-identifiable or protected health information is ever made publicly available. Performance data displayed on Quality Check are available to any interested party at no cost. Performance data on Quality Check may be downloaded electronically in a series of predefined report formats through a linked Web page called "Quality Data."

Data Release to Government Agencies and Organizations with Which The Joint Commission Performs Coordinated Survey Activities*

The Joint Commission makes available to federal, state, local, or other government certification or licensing agencies, and to organizations with which The Joint Commission performs survey activities, specific accreditation-related information under the following circumstances: when The Joint Commission identifies a serious situation in an organization that may jeopardize the health or safety of patients or the public and immediately takes action to deny accreditation; and, upon request, when the request involves otherwise publicly available information.

Additional information is made available when an organization is certified for participation in a federal or state program or licensed to operate by a state agency on the basis of its accreditation. In addition, The Joint Commission may make available information to organizations with which The Joint Commission performs coordinated survey activities. The Joint Commission so advises the organization's chief executive

---

* Section 92, PL 96-499, the Omnibus Budget Reconciliation Act of 1980, requires that Medicare providers include, in all their contracts for services costing $10,000 or more in any 12-month period, a clause allowing the Secretary of the U.S. Department of Health and Human Services (DHHS), the U.S. Comptroller General, or their representatives to examine the contract and the contractor's books and records. The Joint Commission herein stipulates that if its charges to any such organization amount to $10,000 or more in any 12-month period, the contract or any agreement on which such charges are based and any of The Joint Commission's books, documents, and records that may be necessary to verify the extent and nature of Joint Commission costs will be available to the Secretary of DHHS, the Comptroller General, or any of their duly authorized representatives for four years after the survey. The same conditions will apply to any subcontracts The Joint Commission has with related organizations if the payments under such contracts amount to $10,000 or more in any 12-month period.

officer and provides timely notice to local, state, and federal authorities having jurisdiction. The information available to government agencies and organizations with which The Joint Commission performs coordinated survey activities includes:

- The official accreditation decision and any subsequent change in this decision or any designation, such as Accreditation Watch.
- Complaint information requested by CMS or state agencies in accordance with deemed status or other recognition requirements, including:
  - Actual complaint if the allegation(s) results in the classification of the complaint as high priority* and the governmental entity or organization with which The Joint Commission conducts a coordinated survey has entered into a written information-sharing agreement.
  - Action taken on the complaint
  - The standards area(s) in which Requirements for Improvement were issued as a result of the complaint evaluation
  - The status of the case
- Specific information when an organization is assigned a Conditional Accreditation, Preliminary Denial of Accreditation, or Denial of Accreditation decision. This includes the following: All final Requirements for Improvement; a statement, if any, from the organization regarding its views on the validity of Joint Commission survey findings; and a copy of the approved plan of correction and the results of the plan of correction follow-up survey.
- Notification of upcoming full surveys and retrospective dates of other surveys conducted, such as random unannounced or for-cause surveys, only if the governmental agency enters into an information-sharing agreement with The Joint Commission and agrees to maintain the confidentiality of the unannounced survey dates.
- A copy of the Official Accreditation Decision Report for CMS, upon request respecting deemed status determinations, and for state agencies that have entered into specific information-sharing agreements that permit provider-authorized release of such reports to the state agency.

The Joint Commission will report to CMS or the Office of the Inspector General in the event that credible evidence of potential fraud or criminal or civil law violation has been identified, and upon notice to the health care organization.

---

* *High-priority incidents* are defined as harm that impairs mental, physical, and/or psychosocial status. This level of priority is assigned to an incident if the organization's alleged noncompliance with one or more standards may have caused harm that negatively impacts the resident's mental, physical, and/or psychosocial status. Usually, specific rather than general information factors into the assignment of this priority level. Examples include the following:

- Allegation of a sentinel event (Complaints alleging the occurrence of a sentinel event will not be shared with CMS or state agencies if the alleged event has already been self-reported to The Joint Commission.)
- Allegation of an identification of a serious situation involving the potential jeopardy to the safety of residents
- Allegation of falsification of medical records or other information presented in the accreditation process
- Allegation of resident abuse/inappropriate use of restraints
- Allegation of unethical treatment of residents/families
- Allegation of resident-dumping
- Allegation of denial of care
- Allegation of failure to obtain surgical consent

Data Release to Cooperative Accrediting Bodies

The Joint Commission makes available to accrediting bodies with which it has formal cooperative agreements relevant portions of Official Accreditation Decision Reports and complaint-related information that are pertinent to the accrediting activities of the cooperative partner. Judgments as to pertinence are made solely by The Joint Commission.

The Joint Commission Right to Clarify

The Joint Commission reserves the right to clarify information, even if the information involved would otherwise be considered confidential, when an organization disseminates inaccurate information regarding its accreditation.

Confidential Information

The Joint Commission keeps confidential the following information received or developed during the accreditation process:

- The Official Accreditation Decision Report unless its submission is required by a government agency (*see* the Data Release to Government Agencies section); is required by organizations with which The Joint Commission performs coordinating surveys; or is requested by an accrediting body with which The Joint Commission has a formal agreement (*see* the Data Release to Cooperative Accrediting Bodies section)
- Information learned from the organization before, during, or following the accreditation survey, which is used to determine compliance with specific accreditation standards
- An organization's root cause analysis prepared in response to a sentinel event or in response to other circumstances specified by The Joint Commission
- All other materials that may contribute to the accreditation decision (for example, medical records, surveyor notes)
- Written staff analyses and Accreditation Committee minutes and agenda materials
- The algorithms used in the Priority Focus Process
- The Priority Focus Process information used in an organization's survey, other than that provided to the organization's staff prior to survey
- An organization's self-assessment and related Plan(s) of Action
- The identity of any individual who files a complaint about an accredited organization, except when the complaint is shared by The Joint Commission with a governmental entity, an organization with which The Joint Commission performs coordinated surveys, or accrediting organizations with which The Joint Commission has formal complaint-sharing agreements and the receiving organization has agreed to maintain the confidentiality of the complainant. In instances in which the receiving organization cannot assure the confidentiality of the complainant, any complainant-identifying information shall be redacted by The Joint Commission prior to sharing.

Process for Responding to a Complaint About a Joint Commission–Accredited Organization

The Complaint Response Unit of The Joint Commission's Office of Quality Monitoring (OQM) triages and reviews complaints, concerns, and inquiries related to accredited health care organizations, as received from a variety of sources. These complaints may be submitted by patients, families, and health care providers, by state and federal agencies in the form of reports, or through information from the media. The term *complaint* therefore covers a broad spectrum of information received by the Complaint Response Unit.

Upon Joint Commission review of a complaint, a number of actions may result. These include recording the information for trending purposes and possible action in the future, obtaining the involved health care organization's response to the complaint, and conducting an immediate for-cause survey. If The Joint Commission determines that the organization should respond to the complaint, the organization will be so notified. The request for a response will be e-mailed to the organization's CEO and posted to the organization's secure, password protected *The Joint Commission Connect* extranet site. The organization's response to the complaint also takes place through its extranet site.

The complaint information posted on the extranet site may be either of the following:

- The complaint itself, if the complainant has given permission to do so
- A summary of the complaint, if the complainant requested anonymity

If a health care organization is required to respond to the complaint, it is required to do so usually **within 30 days of being notified**. For more serious issues, the organization may be required to respond to the complaint **within 7 days of being notified, or sooner**. When a response in a short time frame is required, the organization will be so notified.

Once a response is received, it is evaluated for compliance with The Joint Commission's standards, National Patient Safety Goals, and Accreditation Participation Requirements, as applicable. If additional information is required, the organization will be notified.

When the organization's response is complete and has been accepted, a letter indicating acceptance is e-mailed to the CEO, and the case is considered closed.

Early Survey Policy

Figure 2 on page 30 highlights the Early Survey Policy option. An organization that wants to be accredited for the first time by The Joint Commission may choose the Early Survey Policy option described here.

Early Survey Policy (Preliminary Accreditation)

A. Eligibility. The Early Survey Policy is available to any organization that is currently not accredited, except an organization that has been denied accreditation. An organization must declare during the application process that it wishes to be surveyed under this policy.

B. The First Survey. When an organization chooses to be surveyed under the Early Survey Policy, The Joint Commission conducts two on-site surveys, both of which will be announced, unless the organization is using accreditation to meet deemed status purposes. The Joint Commission can conduct the first survey as early as two months

Early Survey Policy

First Survey
- Conducted up to two months before opening
- Licensed
- Building identified, constructed, and equipped
- CEO or administrator, director of clinical or medical services (medical director), and nurse executive identified
- Identified opening date
- Limited set of standards (physical plant, policies and procedures)
- Announced (except for deemed status purposes)
- Outcome: Preliminary Accreditation

Second Survey
- Four months after the decision from the first survey
- Unannounced
- Full survey
- Outcome: Change in Preliminary Accreditation decision to Accredited, Provisional Accreditation, Conditional Accreditation, Preliminary Denial of Accreditation, or Denial of Accreditation. The effective date of the accreditation decision is the day after the *second* survey if the organization does not receive any Requirements for Improvement. If the organization receives at least one Requirement for Improvement and therefore must submit an ESC that resolves all Requirements for Improvement, the effective date of the accreditation decision is then set retroactively as the date the successful ESC is submitted.

Figure 2. *Early Survey Policy option.*

before the organization begins operating, provided that the organization meets the following criteria:

- It is licensed or has a provisional license, according to applicable law and regulation
- The building in which the services will be offered or from which the services will be coordinated is identified, constructed, and equipped to support such services
- It has identified its CEO or administrator, its director of clinical or medical services, and its nurse executive, if applicable
- It has identified the date it will begin operations

Generally, the first survey uses a limited set of standards and assesses only the organization's physical facilities, policies and procedures, plans, and related structural considerations. For this reason, organizations surveyed under this policy are not recognized by CMS to meet the requirements for Medicare certification.

C. Preliminary Accreditation. The Joint Commission grants Preliminary Accreditation to an organization that is in satisfactory compliance with a subset of the standards and their EPs assessed in the first survey. An organization that is not in satisfactory compliance must reapply and begin the accreditation process again.

The Preliminary Accreditation decision includes assignment of an additional unannounced survey against the full set of applicable standards within six months of the first survey. The survey assesses evidence of compliance with the standards for at least four months.

For an organization operating when the survey is conducted, the effective date for its Preliminary Accreditation decision is the day after the survey is conducted if the organization does not receive any Requirements for Improvement (RFIs). If the organization receives at least one RFI and therefore must submit an acceptable ESC report that resolves all RFIs, the effective date for Preliminary Accreditation is the date of the acceptable ESC submission.

For an organization not in operation at the time of the survey, the effective date for its Preliminary Accreditation decision is the day after it begins operating if the organization does not receive any requirements for improvement. If the organization receives at least one RFI and therefore must submit an acceptable ESC report that resolves all RFIs, the effective date for Preliminary Accreditation is then set retroactively as the date of the acceptable ESC submission. If the organization is not in operation at the time of survey, the organization must confirm in writing the date it begins operating.

A Preliminary Accreditation decision remains in effect until the organization has completed a second, full survey or until The Joint Commission has withdrawn the Preliminary Accreditation. The Joint Commission may withdraw Preliminary Accreditation in the following situations:

- If an organization that was not providing services at the time of the first survey does not begin providing services when expected
- If an organization does not meet the survey eligibility criteria (*see* page 13)
- If an organization fails to accept the date of the second survey

  or
- If an organization is found to be not in satisfactory compliance with the applicable standards and their EPs

In any of these cases, the organization must begin the accreditation process again.

D. The Second Survey. The second survey under the Early Survey Policy is an unannounced full accreditation survey. The Joint Commission conducts this survey at the following times:

- Approximately six months after the first survey
- At least four months after the organization begins operating

Based on survey results, the organization's accreditation decision then changes to one of the following:

- Accredited
- Provisional Accreditation
- Conditional Accreditation
- Preliminary Denial of Accreditation

  or
- Denial of Accreditation

The effective date of the accreditation decision is the day after the second survey if the organization does not receive any RFIs. If the organization receives at least one RFI and therefore must submit an acceptable ESC report that resolves all RFIs, the effective date for Preliminary Accreditation is then set retroactively as the date of the acceptable ESC submission. The organization's accreditation cycle begins the day after the second survey was conducted, unless The Joint Commission reached a decision to deny accreditation. Submission of an acceptable ESC may be required based on the survey findings of the second survey.

Before the Survey

This section provides information on the steps leading to a full accreditation survey. These steps include the application process; the assignment of an account representative; the PPR process; the PFP; the assignment of a survey team; policies regarding survey scheduling; postponements and delays; and continuous public involvement. In accordance with the requirements of the Health Insurance Portability and Accountability Act of 1996 (HIPAA), a health care organization and the Joint Commission must have a signed Business Associate agreement before the organization's survey can begin.

Application for Accreditation

An organization needs to complete its electronic application for accreditation (e-App) once, and it is required to provide updates as appropriate. The e-App can be completed via the organization's secure extranet site. When an organization notifies The Joint Commission that it wants to become accredited, The Joint Commission provides the organization with information explaining how to access and complete its application on its secure site on *The Joint Commission Connect* extranet site. After an organization completes its application, the e-App will remain valid until the organization no longer wishes to be Joint Commission accredited, as long as the organization completes and submits its updates to The Joint Commission. Initial applications are valid for six months.

Organizations that use the e-App are able to enter data directly in the application and submit the e-App to The Joint Commission electronically. The application provides essential information about the organization, including ownership, demographics, and types and volume of services provided.

The e-App does the following:

- Describes the organization seeking accreditation in terms of size and scope of services
- Requires the organization to provide The Joint Commission with all official records and reports of public or publicly recognized licensing (for example, state licenses), examining, reviewing, or planning bodies*
- Authorizes The Joint Commission to obtain any records and reports not possessed by the organization
- When accepted, establishes the terms of the relationship between the organization and the Joint Commission

* *See* APR.05.01.01 on page 138 in the "Accreditation Participation Requirements" (APR) chapter.

For an organization that chooses not to complete its application via its secure site on *The Joint Commission Connect* extranet site, the organization may request a printed copy of the application by contacting its account representative. An organization can find out who its account representative is by calling 630/792-3007.

Accreditation Contract

Organizations seeking Joint Commission accreditation for the first time or reaccreditation with The Joint Commission must sign an accreditation contract. The contract outlines the responsibilities of both the organization and The Joint Commission relative to the accreditation process. This contract is separate from the e-App.

Contracts are available for printing and approval via each organization's secure extranet site. An organization will not be scheduled for survey until a contract is in effect. Governmental organizations may enter into unique contracts with The Joint Commission in accordance with the scope of services available from The Joint Commission and the laws for contracting that bind that government entity.

An organization will not be scheduled for survey until it signs an accreditation contract. When this happens, The Joint Commission will proceed with the organization's survey plans unless the organization notifies The Joint Commission in writing of its intent to withdraw from accreditation and terminate the accreditation contract. Notification in writing is necessary to terminate the accreditation contract, cease survey scheduling, and avoid a final decision of Denial of Accreditation. If an organization fails to notify The Joint Commission in writing of its intent to withdraw from accreditation and terminate its accreditation contract before a scheduled unannounced survey, The Joint Commission's decision rules provide for a final decision of Denial of Accreditation.

Accuracy of the Application Information

The Joint Commission schedules surveys based on information provided in an organization's e-App. With the information provided, The Joint Commission determines the number of days required for a survey and the number and type of surveyors.

Inaccurate or incomplete information in the e-App may necessitate an additional survey, which could delay the processing of survey findings and rendering of an accreditation decision. It may also cause the organization to incur additional survey charges.

Handling Changes Affecting Application Information*

At any time during the accreditation process, an organization may undergo a change that modifies the information reported in its e-App. The organization must notify The Joint Commission in writing within 30 calendar days after such a change is made. Information that must be reported includes the following:

- A change in ownership
- A change in location
- A significant increase or decrease in the volume of services
- The addition of a new type of health service or site of care
- The acquisition of a new component

---

* *See* APR.01.03.01 on page 136 in the "Accreditation Participation Requirements" (APR) chapter.

- The deletion of an existing health service or site of care
  or
- The deletion of an existing component

The Joint Commission may conduct an additional survey at a later date if its surveyor or survey team arrives at the organization and discovers that a change was not reported. The Joint Commission may also survey any unreported services and sites addressed by its standards. The Joint Commission makes the final accreditation decision for the organization only after surveying all or an appropriate sample of all services, programs, and sites provided by the organization for which The Joint Commission has standards. Information reported in the e-App is subject to The Joint Commission's Information Accuracy and Truthfulness Policy (*see* page 20).

Forfeiture of Survey Deposit

A nonrefundable, nontransferable deposit toward accreditation fees is required for initial surveys only. The Joint Commission applies the deposit to the organization's accreditation fees if a survey is conducted. An organization scheduled for an initial survey forfeits its deposit if its survey is not conducted within six months of submitting its application. The organization must then reapply and submit a new deposit to begin the accreditation process again.

An Organization's Secure Site on The Joint Commission Extranet Site

A key feature of The Joint Commission's accreditation process is increased use of technology. The use of technology better enables The Joint Commission and accredited organizations to communicate accreditation-related information in a more efficient and timely manner.

To fully use technology in the accreditation process, The Joint Commission provides each organization with a secured Web site on The Joint Commission's extranet site, *The Joint Commission Connect*. Access to this site can only be accomplished through the use of the organization's password. This site permits an organization to complete its e-App and PPR electronically. In addition, shortly after an organization's survey, the organization's Accreditation Survey Findings Report and its ESC report are posted on the organization's secure extranet site.

Role of the Account Representative

The Joint Commission assigns an account representative to an organization after receiving its e-App. This person serves as the primary contact between the organization and The Joint Commission. He or she coordinates survey planning and handles policies, procedures, accreditation issues or services, and inquiries throughout the accreditation cycle. If an organization does not know who its account representative is, it can call 630/792-3007.

Survey Fees

The Joint Commission uses a subscription billing system for all programs. For all accredited programs, the subscription approach involves an annual billing at a base rate and the assessment of an add-on fee to cover survey-related costs in those years in which an on-site survey is conducted. The use of an annual fee subscription approach is more consistent with the continuous nature of The Joint Commission's current accreditation process.

The nonrefundable annual fee is assessed on each accredited program and is due each January. Electronic invoices will be posted to the organization's secure *The Joint Commission Connect*™ extranet site; paper invoices will not be sent. The annual fee level for an organization is determined based on the organization's size and complexity, just as in the previous approach. The annual fee for organizations applying for accreditation for the first time will be prorated, based upon the quarter in which the e-App and deposit is submitted.

In addition to annual fees, organizations are also billed an on-site survey fee after the survey has been performed. The on-site survey fee, which is designed to cover the costs of performing a survey, is due upon receipt. Other types of surveys such as conditional follow-up surveys and PPR surveys, will continue to be charged separately, after the event has occurred.

The annual payment will also not take into account the costs of having as part of the survey team a specialist surveyor, such as an ambulatory health care specialist, chemical dependency specialist, or a *Life Safety Code*® Specialist on a long term care organization survey. Thus, if an organization has one of these specialist surveyors, the organization will be invoiced subsequently to the event, to cover the costs of having these surveyors.

For an initial survey, an organization must send a nonrefundable deposit toward accreditation fees with its e-App.

An organization that has not paid its annual or on-site accreditation fee in full prior to issuance of the accreditation decision and report must remit the outstanding balance within 60 calendar days from receipt of the report. Failure to provide timely payment of any Joint Commission fees may result in the loss of accreditation. The Joint Commission notifies an organization with significant standards compliance problems of either a Conditional Accreditation or a Preliminary Denial of Accreditation decision as soon as possible, whether or not payment has been received.

Questions regarding fees can be directed to the Pricing Unit (pricingunit@jointcommission.org) or by calling 630/792-5115.

Periodic Performance Review*

The Periodic Performance Review (PPR) process is a key component in the more continuous accreditation process. It is designed to help organizations incorporate Joint Commission standards as part of routine operations and ongoing quality improvement efforts. An organization has access to its PPR tool on a continuous basis throughout its accreditation cycle. The PPR tool becomes available to organizations seeking accreditation for the first time after submitting their e-App and deposit. The PPR tool permits the organization to evaluate compliance with all applicable Joint Commission stan-

* The PPR is not applicable to the Medicare/Medicaid certification–based long term care accreditation option.

dards and EPs. For every noncompliant standard, the organization must identify a plan of action at the EP level, identifying how it plans to come into compliance with the requirement(s). This plan must include a Measure of Success (MOS), if applicable, for each EP within a standard that is identified as not compliant and that requires an MOS. (Not all EPs require an MOS, and an organization needs to demonstrate achievement with an MOS only for an EP that is within a noncompliant standard and that requires an MOS.) The MOS is a numeric or other quantitative measure, usually related to an audit, that can help determine whether a planned action was effective and sustained.

The PPR helps your long term care organization review applicable standards, APRs, and National Patient Safety Goals; assess compliance; develop and implement Plans of Action (POAs); and identify measures by which you will gauge your success in carrying out those plans. By participating in the PPR, your organization will be better able to incorporate Joint Commission standards into routine operations, which in turn will help to ensure the provision of safe, high-quality care on an ongoing basis.

The evaluation and plan of action must be completed electronically on the organization's secure extranet site and transmitted to The Joint Commission by its annual due date. Following receipt of the evaluation and plan of action, and if requested by the organization, staff from The Joint Commission's Standards Interpretation Group schedule a telephone call with the organization to discuss and agree upon an acceptable plan of action. The time line for the PPR is such that the organization should have sufficient time to implement the actions identified in the POA. The track record will be based on the plan of action implementation date. (The PPR submission is not required of organizations undergoing initial survey.)

An organization is required to annually submit to The Joint Commission an update to its PPR. Organizations that select Option 2 or Option 3 are required to undergo annual Option 2 or Option 3 surveys.*

Due dates for annual PPR updates will be at one-year intervals after the organization's last full survey. For example, if a long term care organization had its last full survey end on January 1, 2008, its next annual PPR update would be due January 1, 2009, and the following annual PPR updates would be due January 1, 2010. If a full survey occurs before an organization's anticipated PPR update due date, the PPR due date will reset accordingly. Each accredited organization must either submit its updated PPR to The Joint Commission or select Option 1, Option 2, or Option 3 on an annual basis. An organization may change its selection or options as often as annually. The annual update to the PPR facilitates a long term care organization's ongoing quality improvement efforts and supports a continuous accreditation process. If your long term care organization's laboratory services are accredited by The Joint Commission, the laboratory PPR will be due at the same time as the long term care organization's PPR.

Table 2 on pages 37–38 outlines some of the activities in each of these PPR options.

If an organization, through their participation in The Joint Commission's PPR process, has self-identified compliance issues that are then identified by surveyors on site, The

* *See* pages 136–137 for the full text of the PPR and its options.

Table 2. PPR Options

Full PPR

- Organization uses the automated PPR tool to assess and score compliance with EPs for each applicable standard
- Organization creates a plan of action* addressing each EP scored partial or insufficient compliance within any standards found not compliant
- Organization identifies an MOS, if required, for each EP scored partial or insufficient compliance within any standards scored not compliant
- Organization submits PPR to The Joint Commission annually
- Organization may elect to participate in a conference call with Joint Commission staff to discuss plan(s) of action, MOS, and other standards-related issue of their choosing. If a conference call is not requested, the data will be reviewed by Joint Commission staff. Should they determine a conference call is needed, your organization will be contacted to schedule a call.
- Because The Joint Commission may request a conference call even if an organization does not request one, all organizations submitting the full PPR or Option 2 second submission with not compliant standards need to enter their conference call "avoid dates" when they submit their PPR. "Avoid dates" are dates on which the organization prefers that the conference call not be scheduled.
- Joint Commission staff reviews and approves Plan(s) of Action during conference call
- Surveyors review any required MOS at full survey

Option 1

- Organization uses PPR tool to annually affirm that, for substantive reasons, legal counsel advises organization not to participate in the full PPR and instead will complete a PPR and plan of action and identify appropriate MOS
- Organizations can use the PPR tool to score compliance and can print and view standards and EPs to conduct its assessment on paper. These data are not submitted to The Joint Commission.
- Organization affirms that it has completed an assessment of its compliance with applicable EPs and developed Plans of Action and MOS, as necessary, but does not submit data to Joint Commission
- Organization can submit standards-related issues in the PPR tool for telephone discussion with Joint Commission staff, if desired, and receive design approval
- Surveyors review any required MOS at full survey

Option 2

- Organization uses PPR tool to annually attest that, after careful consideration with legal counsel, it has decided not to participate in full PPR and instead intends to undergo either a limited survey, or a full-length PPR survey. The organization may choose between either the limited survey or the full-length survey. When an organization selects a full-length PPR options 2 or 3 survey, it may independently select these options without advice of legal counsel.

* A Plan of Action details the action(s) an organization will take to come into compliance with each standard identified as not compliant.

(continued on next page)

Table 2. PPR Options *(continued)*

- The limited survey will be approximately one-third the length of the full survey; a fee will be charged
- Organizations that choose a full-length PPR survey will also be charged a fee. The full-length PPR survey can be either announced or unannounced, depending on the organization's request.
- Survey will be conducted using tracer methodology and PFP output; all standards are subject to review
- Surveyor leaves written report of findings with organization
- The organization must submit the tool again within 30 days of the survey. This submission addresses not compliant standards, choice of a conference call, and any other topics for discussion with Joint Commission staff.
- Organization creates a Plan of Action and any required MOS for each standard scored not compliant and submits data to Joint Commission via the PPR tool within 30 days of survey
- Organization may elect to participate in a conference call with Joint Commission staff to discuss the plan(s) of action and MOS. If a conference call is not requested, the data will be reviewed by Joint Commission staff. Should it determine a conference call is needed, your organization will be contacted to schedule a call.
- Joint Commission staff reviews and approves Plan(s) of Action during conference call
- Surveyors will review any required MOS at full survey

Option 3

- Organization uses the PPR tool to annually attest that after careful consideration with legal counsel, it has decided not to participate in the full PPR and instead intends to undergo either a limited survey, or a full length PPR survey. The organization may choose between either the limited survey or the full-length survey. When an organization selects a full-length PPR options 2 or 3 survey, it may independently select these options without advice of legal counsel.
- The limited survey will be approximately one-third the length of the full survey; a fee will be charged
- Organizations that choose a full-length PPR survey will also be charged a fee. The full-length PPR survey can be either announced or unannounced, depending upon the organization's request.
- Survey will be conducted using tracer methodology and PFP output; all standards are subject to review
- Unlike Option 2, however, Option 3 stipulates that no written report of findings will be left at the organization. The surveyor delivers an oral report of findings at the closing conference of the on-site survey.
- The organization must submit the tool again within 30 days of the survey. This submission addresses the choice of a conference call and any topics for discussion with Joint Commission staff.
- At the time of the organization's full survey, the surveyors will receive no information relating to the organization's Option 3 survey findings.

Joint Commission's Standards Interpretation Group (SIG) will review the accreditation report along with the health care organization's PPR. If an issue identified by the surveyor is identical to an issue in the PPR, the POA and MOS are appropriate, and the POA implementation date has not yet passed (or in the case of a PPR that has not yet received SIG approval and everything is acceptable), the RFI will remain in the report but will not count toward the accreditation decision.

Only those organizations submitting full PPR and PPR Option 2 are eligible for this consideration, as they are the only submission types that include the submission of actual compliance issues along with POA and MOS.

PPR Option 1 and PPR Option 3 do not submit identified compliance issues or POA and MOS and therefore are not eligible for this consideration.

Plans of Action

A Plan of Action (POA) is a detailed description of how a long term car organization plans to bring into compliance any standard identified as "not compliant" in the PPR (POAs are not required for standards where some EPs are marked "partial compliance" but where the standard does not meet the level of "not compliant"). The POA should include the planned action to be taken and target implementation dates. If the EP requires an MOS when lack of compliance exists, you must also describe the MOS or how you plan to measure your successful implementation of your plans of action.

The PPR will only affect an organization's accreditation decision if the organization fails to participate in the PPR process, whether the full or one of the three options, or through the PPR process an immediate threat to health or safety situation is identified and a special survey is conducted. If you need more information while completing your PPR, please contact your account representative at 630/792-3007.

Priority Focus Process

An important component of The Joint Commission's accreditation process is the Priority Focus Process (PFP), which guides the surveyor(s) in planning and conducting your on-site survey. This focuses survey activities on the organization-specific issues that are most relevant to safety and quality of care (referred to as *priority focus areas* [PFAs]). The PFP can be considered a process for standardizing the PFAs for review during survey. The PFP uses an automated tool, which takes available data from a variety of sources—including e-Apps for accreditation, previous survey findings, complaint data, and publicly available external data—and integrates them to identify CSGs and PFAs for your long term care organization. The PFP converts these data into information that focuses survey activities, increases consistency in the accreditation process, and customizes the accreditation process to make it specific to your organization, and guides tracer activities (*see* pages 53–57 for more information on the tracer methodology) and is a starting point for the survey.

Your long term care organization will receive PFP information for its top PFAs and CSGs on its secure extranet site. Complex organizations that are surveyed under more than one accreditation program will receive program-specific PFP information and organization-level PFP information that is a summary of all programs' data and information.

From these sources, the PFP identifies PFAs for each long term care organization on which surveyors initially will focus during the initial part of the on-site survey. Surveyors will use the PFP in the following ways:

- The surveyor(s) assigned to your long term care organization will have access to your organization's PFP information via the surveyor extranet
- The surveyor(s) will review the PFP information for organization–specific PFAs as well as for organization–specific CSGs
- As part of the planning process, the surveyor(s) will begin to assess and plan his or her tracer activities
- During the on-site survey, the surveyor(s) will use the long term care organization's active resident list to select tracer residents

As the survey progresses, the surveyor(s) may find other priority areas that need to be addressed and may begin to focus less on the PFP suggested list and more on what he or she is finding.

The PFP will also be used for a long term care organization undergoing its initial survey. The only difference with this type of organization (versus an organization that has already gone through a survey) is in the available data inputs that feed the PFP. Long term care organizations undergoing initial survey will not have previous requirements for improvement available to feed into the PFP. For initial surveys, The Joint Commission will only be able to feed e-App data, external data (as applicable), and Office of Quality Monitoring data into the PFP.

After these data are transformed to become the PFP information, the process for initial surveys is no different from the process for any other type of survey. The data will be aggregated in the same manner to determine the PFAs and CSGs for the long term care organization. PFP data are updated quarterly, as changes warrant. **Note:** *Organizations will receive an updated report only if there is a change to one or more PFAs and/or CSGs in their programs since the previous PFP Report. Due to the systems nature of the PFAs and CSGs, it is possible that there may not be a change from one quarter to the next.* The PFP Reports are shared with surveyors before the on-site survey to focus the survey and can also be used by organizations to support continuous performance improvement activities.

Priority Focus Areas

Priority focus areas (PFAs) are processes, systems, or structures in a health care organization that significantly impact safety and/or the quality of care provided. The list of PFAs was developed from information gathered through Joint Commission experience, published literature, and consensus. The Joint Commission categorized the different processes, systems, and structures leading to improved health care in 14 PFAs. The PFAs evolved from this process of identifying common patterns that are useful in building positive health care outcomes and safe, high-quality health care.

The PFAs provide a consistent yet customized approach to providing an initial focus for the on-site survey process, and they may assist the health care organization at the time of its PPR.

The PFAs are the following:

- Assessment and Care/Services
- Communication
- Credentialed Practitioners
- Equipment Use
- Infection Control
- Information Management
- Medication Management
- Organizational Structure
- Orientation & Training
- Patient Safety
- Physical Environment
- Quality Improvement Expertise/Activities
- Rights & Ethics
- Staffing

PFAs guide the surveyor with assessing standards compliance in relation to the individual tracer activities. Outside formal conferences/interviews, much of the survey will consist of reviewing issues in the form of tracer methodology (for more information, please *see* the "Tracer Methodology" section on page 53). The tracer methodology incorporates the use of the PFP information, follows the care experience for individuals initially identified by CSGs, and allows the surveyor to identify performance issues that may be related to PFAs for your organization.

Definitions for the PFAs follow.

Assessment and Care/Services Assessment and Care/Services for residents comprise the execution of a series of processes including, as relevant, screening; assessment; planning care, treatment, and/or services; provision of care; ongoing reassessment of care; and discharge planning, referral for continuing care, or discontinuation of services. Assessment and Care/Services are fluid in nature to accommodate a resident's needs. Although some elements of Assessment and Care/Services may occur only once, other aspects may be repeated or revisited as the resident's needs or care delivery priorities change. Successful implementation of improvements in Assessment and Care/Services rely on the full support of leadership.

Subprocesses of Assessment and Care/Services include the following:

- Screening
- Assessment
- Reassessment
- Planning care, treatment, or services
- Provision of care, treatment, or services
- Discharge planning or discontinuation of services

Communication Communication is the process by which information is exchanged between individuals, programs/services, or organizations. Effective communication successfully permeates every aspect of a health care organization, from the provision of care to performance improvement, resulting in a marked improvement in the quality of care delivery and functioning.

Subprocesses of Communication include the following:

- Provider and/or staff–resident communication
- Resident and family education
- Staff communication and collaboration
- Information dissemination
- Multidisciplinary teamwork

Credentialed Practitioners Credentialed Practitioners are health care professionals whose qualifications to provide resident care services have been verified and assessed, resulting in the assignment of clinical responsibilities. The category varies from organization to organization and from state to state. It includes licensed independent practitioners and others who are permitted to provide resident care services under the direction of a sponsoring physician. Licensed independent practitioners are permitted by law and the health care organization to provide care and services without clinical supervision or direction within the scope of their license and consistent with individually assigned clinical responsibilities.

Equipment Use Equipment Use incorporates the selection, delivery, setup, and maintenance of equipment and supplies to meet resident and staff needs. It generally includes movable equipment, as well as management of supplies that staff members use (for example, gloves, syringes). (Equipment Use does not include fixed equipment such as built-in oxygen and gas lines and central air conditioning systems; such items are included in the Physical Environment PFA.) Equipment Use includes planning and selecting; maintaining, testing, and inspecting; educating and providing instructions; delivery and setup; and risk prevention related to equipment and/or supplies.

Subprocesses of Equipment Use include the following:

- Selection
- Maintenance strategies
- Periodic evaluation
- Orientation and training

Infection Control Infection Control includes the surveillance/identification, prevention, and control of infections among residents, employees, physicians, and other licensed independent practitioners, contract service workers, volunteers, students, and visitors. This is a systemwide, integrated process that is applied to all programs, services, and settings.

Subprocesses of Infection Control include the following:

- Surveillance/identification
- Prevention and control
- Reporting
- Measurement

Information Management Information Management is the interdisciplinary field concerning the timely and accurate creation, collection, storage, retrieval, transmission, analysis, control, dissemination, and use of data or information, both within an organization and externally, as allowed by law and regulation. In addition to written and verbal information, supporting information technology and information services are also included in Information Management.

Subprocesses of Information Management include the following:

- Planning
- Procurement
- Implementation
- Collection
- Recording
- Protection
- Aggregation
- Interpretation
- Storage and retrieval
- Data integrity
- Information dissemination

Medication Management Medication Management encompasses the systems and processes an organization uses if an organization provides medication to individuals served by the organization. This is usually a multidisciplinary, coordinated effort of health care staff, implementing, evaluating, and constantly improving the processes of selecting, procuring, storing, ordering, transcribing, preparing, dispensing, administering (including self-administering), and monitoring the effects of medications throughout the residents' continuum of care. In addition, Medication Management involves educating residents and, as appropriate, their families, about each medication, its administration and use, and potential side effects.

Subprocesses of Medication Management include the following:

- Selection
- Procurement
- Storage
- Prescribing or ordering
- Preparing
- Dispensing
- Administration
- Monitoring

Organizational Structure The Organizational Structure is the framework for an organization to carry out its vision and mission. The implementation is accomplished through corporate bylaws and governing body policies, organization management, compliance, planning, integration and coordination, and performance improvement. Included are the organization's governance, as well as business ethics, contracted organizations, and management requirements.

Subprocesses of Organizational Structure include the following:

- Management requirements
- Corporate bylaws and governing body plans
- Organization management
- Compliance
- Planning

- Business ethics
- Contracted services

Orientation & Training Orientation is the process of educating newly hired staff in health care organizations to organizationwide, departmental, and job-specific competencies before they provide resident care, treatment, or services. *Newly hired staff* includes, but is not limited to, regular staff employees, contracted staff, agency (temporary) staff, float staff, volunteer staff, students, housekeeping, and maintenance staff.

Training refers to the development and implementation of programs that foster staff development and continued learning, address skill deficiencies, and thereby help ensure staff retention. More specifically, training entails providing opportunities for staff to develop enhanced skills related to revised processes that may have been addressed during orientation, new resident care techniques, or expanded job responsibilities. Whereas orientation is a one-time process, training is a continuous one.

Subprocesses of Orientation & Training include the following:
- Organizationwide orientation
- Program/service orientation
- Job-specific orientation
- Training and continuing or ongoing education

Patient Safety Effective Patient Safety entails proactively identifying the potential and actual risks to safety, identifying the underlying cause(s) of the potential, and making the necessary improvements to reduce risk. It also entails establishing processes to respond to sentinel events, identifying risks through root cause analysis, and making necessary improvements. This involves a systems-based approach that examines all activities within an organization that contribute to the maintenance and improvement of resident safety, such as performance improvement and risk management, to ensure that the activities work together, not independently, to improve care and safety. The systems-based approach is driven by organization leadership; anchored in the organization's mission, vision, and strategic plan; endorsed and actively supported by medical staff and nursing leadership; implemented by directors; integrated and coordinated throughout the organization's staff; and continuously re-engineered using proven, proactive performance improvement modalities. In addition, effective reduction of errors and other factors that contribute to unintended adverse outcomes in an organization requires an environment in which residents, their families, and organization staff and leaders can identify and manage actual and potential risks to safety.

Subprocesses of Patient Safety include the following:
- Planning and designing services
- Directing services
- Integrating and coordinating services
- Error reduction and prevention
- The use of *Sentinel Event Alerts*
- Joint Commission's National Patient Safety Goals
- Clinical practice guidelines
- Active resident involvement in their care

Physical Environment The Physical Environment refers to a safe, accessible, functional, supportive, and effective physical environment for residents, staff members, workers, and other individuals by managing physical design; construction and redesign; maintenance and testing; planning and improvement; and risk prevention, defined in terms of utilities, fire protection, security, privacy, storage, and hazardous materials and waste. The Physical Environment may include the home in the case of in-home programs and foster care.

Subprocesses of Physical Environment include the following:
- Physical design
- Construction and redesign
- Maintenance and testing
- Planning and improvement
- Risk prevention

Quality Improvement Expertise/Activities Quality Improvement identifies the collaborative and interdisciplinary approach to the continuous study and improvement of the processes of providing health care services to meet the needs of consumers and others. Quality improvement depends on understanding and revising processes on the basis of data and knowledge about the processes themselves. Quality improvement involves identifying, measuring, implementing, monitoring, analyzing, planning, and maintaining processes to ensure they function effectively. Examples of quality improvement activities include designing a new service, flowcharting a clinical process, collecting and analyzing data about performance measures or resident outcomes, comparing the organization's performance to that of other organizations, selecting areas for priority attention, and experimenting with new ways of carrying out a function.

Subprocesses of Quality Improvement Expertise/Activities include the following:
- Identifying issues and establishing priorities
- Developing measures
- Collecting data to evaluate status on outcomes, processes, or structures
- Analyzing and interpreting data
- Making and implementing recommendations
- Monitoring and sustaining performance improvement

Rights & Ethics Rights & Ethics includes resident rights and organizational ethics as they pertain to resident care. Rights & Ethics addresses issues such as resident privacy, confidentiality and protection of health information, advance directives (as appropriate), organ procurement, use of restraints, informed consent for various procedures, and the right to participate in care decisions.

Subprocesses of Rights & Ethics include the following:
- Resident rights
- Organizational ethics pertaining to resident care
- Organizational responsibility
- Consideration of resident
- Care sensitivity
- Informing residents and/or family

Staffing Effective Staffing entails providing the optimal number of competent personnel with the appropriate skill mix to meet the needs of a health care organization's residents based on that organization's mission, values, and vision. As such, it involves defining competencies and expectations for all staff (the competencies of licensed independent practitioners and medical staff are addressed in the Credentialed Practitioners PFA for all accreditation programs). Staffing includes assessing those defined competencies and allocating the human resources necessary for resident safety and improved resident outcomes.

Subprocesses of Staffing include the following:
- Competency
- Skill mix
- Number of staff

Clinical/Service Groups

Clinical/Service Groups (CSGs) categorize residents and/or services into distinct populations for which data can be collected. The Joint Commission created the list of CSGs based on data gathered from e-Apps from each accreditation program and on publicly available data from external sources. The list then underwent a thorough review to make sure that all categories were actually representative of populations served or services provided by the organizations surveyed by the individual accreditation programs. Joint Commission surveyors use a long term care organization's CSGs combined with other organization-specific data to get a better understanding of the organization's systems and the residents it serves. Tracer residents are selected according to CSGs.

The CSGs for long term care organizations follow.

Clinical/Service Groups for Long Term Care

- LTC—Hospital operated
- LTC—Freestanding
- Dementia care
- Geriatric psychiatric care
- Intermediate care
- Pediatric care
- Physical rehabilitation services
- Skilled nursing care/complex medical care
- Transitional care unit
- Traumatic brain injury services
- Ventilator services

Additional CSGs based on Centers for Medicare & Medicaid Services' Nursing Home Compare Data:

- Residents having delirium
- Residents having urinary tract infections
- Residents having loss of ability in activities of daily living
- Residents having mobility concerns
- Residents needing pain control

- Residents needing physical restraints
- Residents with declining physical activity
- Residents who lose too much weight
- Residents (short stay) with pressure sores
- Residents with high risk of pressure sores
- Residents with low risk of pressure sores
- Residents (short stay) given pneumonia vaccination
- Residents (short stay) given flu vaccination
- Residents given flu vaccination
- Residents given pneumonia vaccination
- Residents having depression
- Residents with low risk of bladder/bowel control problems
- Residents needing catheters

During the Survey

During an accreditation survey, The Joint Commission evaluates an organization's performance of functions and processes aimed at continuously improving resident outcomes. The survey process focuses on assessing performance of important resident-centered and organization functions that support the safety and quality of resident care. This assessment is accomplished through evaluating an organization's compliance with the applicable standards in this manual, based on the following:

- Tracing the care delivered to residents
- Verbal and written information provided to The Joint Commission
- On-site observations and interviews by Joint Commission surveyors
- Documents provided by the organization

The Joint Commission's accreditation process seeks to help organizations identify and correct problems and improve the safety and quality of care and services provided.

A survey is designed to be individualized to each organization, to be consistent, and to support the organization's efforts to improve performance. The Joint Commission determines the length of a survey based on information supplied in the e-App that describes the organization's size and scope of services. In addition, Joint Commission surveyors may conduct some survey activities on evenings, nights, and weekends, as necessary.

The On-Site Survey

This section includes information relevant to an organization that has applied for an accreditation survey and is ready for the survey process. It provides an overview of the survey process, including use of the PFP.

The Joint Commission's accreditation process focuses on systems critical to the safety and the quality of care, treatment, or services. It represents a shift from a focus on survey preparation to a focus on continuous operational improvement by encouraging long term care organizations to incorporate the standards as a guide for routine operations.

Under this accreditation process, the unannounced full survey is the on-site evaluation piece of a continuous process. (Organizations such as the Department of Defense, the

Bureau of Prisons, and organizations providing foster care will receive advance notice of their survey date.) The accreditation process encourages organizations to embed the standards into routine operations to achieve and maintain excellent operational systems on an ongoing basis. Initiatives such as the continuous PPR (discussed on page 35) and the sharing of PFP information (discussed on pages 39 and 40) facilitate this.

Unannounced Surveys

The Joint Commission conducts surveys in an unannounced fashion, with the following exceptions:

- Initial surveys (that is, for organizations that are undergoing their first Joint Commission survey), including both surveys conducted under the Early Survey Policy, unless deemed status requirements specify unannounced surveys
- Situations in which it would not be logical or feasible to conduct an unannounced survey, such as with the Bureau of Prisons or the Department of Defense facilities
- "Very small" organizations in certain situations
- PPR option 2 and option 3 surveys (*see* pages 37 and 38 for more information on these options)

See Table 3 on page 49 for exemptions to unannounced surveys.

An organization can have an unannounced survey between 18 and 39 months after its previous full unannounced survey. Pre-determined criteria based on Priority Focus Process (PFP) data across multiple quarters as well as trends in the performance of these data will determine the timing of an organization's full unannounced survey. For example, an organization that is due to have its next unannounced survey in January 2010 could have its survey as early as July 2008 or as late as April 1, 2010 (18 to 39 months).

With an *unannounced survey*, an accredited organization will receive *no notice* of its survey date prior to the start of the survey. In concert with the unannounced survey process, the following procedures will be implemented:

- Accredited organizations will be able to identify up to 10 days in their survey eligibility range (between 18 and 39 months after their last full unannounced survey) in which an unannounced survey should be avoided. These 10 days should not include federal holidays but may include regional events during which it may be difficult to conduct a survey. The Joint Commission will make every effort to accommodate the organization regarding avoiding these 10 days. However, The Joint Commission reserves the right to conduct a survey during an "avoid period" if the reason(s) given to avoid a survey at that time is such that a survey can be reasonably accomplished.
- Because an accredited organization will not be able to post its survey date and, therefore, individuals cannot request to have a Public Information Interview (PII), a new Accreditation Participation Requirement (APR) was established. This APR requires an organization to demonstrate how it communicates to its public that if members of the public have any quality of care or safety concerns, they should notify The Joint Commission.

Table 3. Exemptions to Unannounced Surveys

Subject	Exception
Initial surveys	Announced (except deemed status surveys for Medicare certification)
Early Survey Policy—1st and 2nd surveys	Announced
Department of Defense facilities	5 days within certain periods of time

- On the day of the unannounced survey, by 7:30 A.M. in the organization's local time zone (for organizations within the United States and its territories), The Joint Commission will post on the organization's secure *The Joint Commission Connect* extranet site the letter of introduction, the survey agendas, and the biographies and pictures of the surveyors assigned to conduct the survey. For organizations outside of these locations, notifications will continue to be posted by 7:00 A.M eastern standard time.
- If an organization knows of a surveyor who works or has worked at the organization or a competing organization or has had personal experience with the survey or that represents a potential conflict, the organization is asked to identify the individual(s) in its e-App.
- An organization will be invoiced approximately 7 to 10 days after its survey's completion to cover the direct costs of the survey (the indirect costs of the survey are covered in an organization's annual subscription payment).

Survey Agenda

The on-site survey process focuses on continuous operational improvement in support of safe, high-quality care, treatment, or services.

The survey agenda will include the following elements:*

Survey Planning Session. During this session, the surveyor(s) will review data and information about the long term care organizations MOS generated from the full PPR, Option 1, or Option 2, and plan the survey agenda. The surveyor(s) will also select initial tracer residents. As part of the survey process, surveyors will review the organization's MOS information.

Conducting a Public Information Interview. Because all surveys are now unannounced,† Public Information Interviews (PIIs) are conducted only if someone con-

---

* Please *see* the *Survey Activity Guide*, which is available on your extranet site or contact your account representative, if the guide is not available on the extranet site. For more detailed information on the survey process, call your account representative at 630/792-3007.

† Please *see* page 48 for exceptions to unannounced surveys.

tacts the surveyor(s) during an on-site survey to request a PII and the survey schedule can accommodate the PII. A PII is an opportunity for anyone who has information relevant to the accreditation of the surveyed organization to meet with the survey team and provide them with the information. The survey team will not make any conclusions based on a PII, but will use the information in their survey activities.

Leadership Session. During the leadership session, surveyors discuss the following with leaders:

- Information gathering and baseline assessment of leadership-level, system issues—system standards, management oversight and direction, and other leadership responsibilities
- Leadership's approach to the PPR and methods used to address areas needing improvement
- Ongoing initiatives to improve delivery of health care
- Safety program and National Patient Safety Goals
- Oversight by governance or the board
- PFP output related to CSGs and PFAs

Individual Tracers. During the individual tracer activity, the surveyor(s) will do the following:

- Follow the course of a type of care, treatment, or service provided to the resident by the long term care organization
- Assess the interrelationships among disciplines and services/programs and the important functions in the care, treatment, or services provided
- Evaluate the performance of processes relevant to the care, treatment, or service needs of the resident, with particular focus on the integration and coordination of distinct but related processes
- Identify vulnerabilities in the care processes

Individual-Based System Tracers. Individual-based system tracers are interactive sessions with the surveyor(s) and long term care organization staff that explore the performance of important resident-related functions that cross the organization. The surveyor(s) and organization staff will address critical risk points and provide education during the individual-based system tracer sessions. The following are the individual-based system tracers:

- Data use
- Infection control
- Medication management, if within the scope of the organization

As surveyors go through the individual tracers to determine standards compliance as it relates to care delivered to the selected resident, they also assess the organization's overall systems by conducting individual-based system tracers. Individual-based system tracers focus on high-risk processes across the organization.

Program-Specific Tracers. Program-specific tracers will be conducted if they apply to the organization being surveyed. *See* page 53 for more information.

Daily Briefings. During the daily briefing session, organization staff are briefed on the previous day's survey findings and any significant patterns or trends that are becoming evident in the survey. During the daily briefing, the surveyor(s) will do the following:

- Facilitate leadership's understanding of the survey process and the findings that contribute to the accreditation decision
- Report on findings from the previous day's survey activities
- Emphasize patterns or trends of significant concern that could lead to noncompliance determinations
- Highlight any positive findings or exemplary performance
- Allow the long term care organization to provide information that may have been missed during the previous survey day
- Review the agenda for the survey day ahead and make any necessary adjustments based on long term care organizations needs or the need for more intensive assessment of an issue

Special Issue Resolution. This session provides an opportunity for the surveyor(s) to follow up on potential findings that could not be resolved in other survey activities or address any requested Public Information Interviews.

Credentialing and Assigning of Clinical Responsibilities. This activity will help the organization and the surveyor(s) identify specific issues related to the following:

- Evaluation of the process the long term care organization uses to collect relevant data for decisions for credentialing
- Evaluation of consistent implementation of the credentialing and assigning of clinical responsibilities process
- Evaluation of processes for the privileges
- Determination that practitioners practice within the limited scope of assigned clinical responsibilities
- Linking of results of peer review and focused monitoring to the credentialing process
- Identification of vulnerabilities in the credentialing and assigning of clinical responsibilities

Environment of Care Session. This session will help the long term care organization and the surveyor(s) do the following:

- Identify vulnerabilities and strengths in the organization's processes
- Begin to identify or determine the action(s) necessary to address any identified vulnerabilities
- Begin the assessment or determine the organization's actual degree of compliance with relevant standards
- Identify environment of care processes requiring further evaluation of implementation
- Identify issues requiring further exploration

***Life Safety Code*®* Building Tour** (as applicable). This session will help the organization and the surveyor(s) do the following:

- Identify areas of concern in the organization's processes for designing buildings to *Life Safety Code* requirements

* *Life Safety Code*® is a registered trademark of the National Fire Protection Association, Quincy, MA.

- Identify areas of concern in the organization's processes for maintaining buildings to *Life Safety Code* requirements
- Identify areas of concern in the organization's processes for identifying and resolving *Life Safety Code* problems
- Determine the organization's degree of compliance with relevant *Life Safety Code* requirements
- Identify or determine the action(s) necessary to address any identified *Life Safety Code* problems

Clinical Leadership and Staff Discussion Session.* This group session focuses on the involvement of clinical leaders and staff in the provision of care. This activity is intended to do the following:

- Begin a dialogue with the surveyor(s) about the quality and safety of care provided by the organization
- Address the continuum of care provided to the residents by the organization in its various clinics and locations with particular focus on the integration and coordination of processes
- Assess the interrelationships and communication between and among disciplines, departments, programs, services, or settings (as applicable) in the organization
- Provide an opportunity to confirm the surveyor's observations and/or assessment of standards-based issues
- Identify potential opportunities for organizational improvement at the organization, system, or process level
- Provide consultation and education as time permits

Governance Discussion Session.* This session focuses on the organization's governance and is intended to address the following:

- The structure and composition of the governing body
- The functioning, participation, and involvement of the governing body in the oversight and operation of the organization
- The level of communication among the board members
- The governing body's perception of its role in the organization
- The knowledge of the governing body members with respect to federal law and regulation
- The governing body's understanding of performance improvement approaches and methods and involvement in the organization's approach to performance improvement
- Pertinent Leadership standards relevant to the governing body's role in the organization

Surveyor Team Meeting. On surveys being conducted by more than one surveyor, scheduled team meetings provide an opportunity for the surveyor(s) to share information and observations, plan for upcoming survey activities, and plan for communication and coordination with the organization.

---

* These on-site survey activities are only applicable to Bureau of Primary Health Care–supported organizations.

Surveyor Report Preparation. The surveyor(s) will use this time to compile, analyze, and organize the data he or she has collected throughout the survey into a report reflecting the organization's compliance with standards.

CEO Exit Briefing and Organization Exit Conference. During the CEO Exit Briefing the surveyor(s) will review the outcome of the survey, present the survey findings, discuss any concerns that the CEO has with the report, and determine the need for any special arrangements for the Organization Exit Conference.

During the Organization Exit Conference the surveyor(s) will report the outcome of the survey and present the survey findings if desired by the CEO, review the issues of standards compliance that have been identified during the survey, allow the organization a final on-site opportunity to question the survey findings or provide additional material regarding standards' compliance, and review required follow-up actions, as applicable.

Survey Team Composition

An accreditation survey may be conducted by a survey team rather than by an individual surveyor. The composition of an organization's survey team is based on the information provided in its e-App. Surveyors assess and provide education as part of the survey process.

The Survey Team Leader

If more than one surveyor is required, one of the surveyors on each organization survey team is designated as the "team leader." The team leader is responsible for integration, coordination, and communication of on-site survey activities. In addition to direct participation as an active member of the survey team, the team leader serves as the primary point of on-site contact between the organization and The Joint Commission. Among other responsibilities, the team leader leads the opening conference and the daily and exit briefings.

Tracer Methodology

The tracer methodology is the cornerstone of The Joint Commission on-site survey. The tracer methodology does the following:

- Incorporates the use of PFP information
- Follows the experience of care for a number of individuals (initially identified by CSGs) through the organization's entire health care process
- Allows the surveyor(s) to identify performance issues (that may be related to PFAs) in one or more steps of the process, or in the interfaces between processes

Program-Specific Tracers

The goal of the program-specific tracer activity is to identify safety concerns within different levels and types of care. Program-specific tracers bring a targeted focus on important issues relevant to the following information:

- Types of services offered by the organization
- Programs being surveyed
- The organization's PFAs

Table 4 on page 55 contains your organization-specific tracer activities, including applicability and objectives.

Topics for the program-specific tracers were identified through a review of expert literature, research, input from the field, and subject matter expertise. Program-specific tracers evaluate program-specific issues and compliance with relevant standards that impact resident safety.

Note: *Program-specific tracers will only be conducted if they apply to the specific organization being surveyed.*

Individual Tracer Activity

The individual tracer activity is an evaluation method that is conducted during an on-site survey and is designed to "trace" the care experiences that a resident had while at the long term care organization. The tracer methodology is a way to analyze an organization's system of providing care, treatment, or services using actual residents as the framework for assessing standards compliance. The surveyor(s) will use the following general criteria to select initial individual tracers:

- Residents in top CSGs for that organization
- Residents who cross programs (for example, long term care residents who present at a long term care organization or some care patients received from a long term care organization in complex organizations)
- Residents related to individual-based system tracer topics (*see* the "Individual-Based System Tracer Activity" section on page 56), such as infection control or medication management
- Residents receiving complex services, such as surgery or treatment in an intensive care unit*

Residents selected for initial individual tracer activity will most likely be those identified in the long term care organization's PFP information as listed in the CSGs. Based on identified CSGs, the surveyor(s) will identify individual tracers and follow specific residents through the organization's processes. A surveyor will not only examine the individual components of a system but will also evaluate how the components of a system interact with each other. In other words, a surveyor will look at the care, treatment, or services provided by each department/unit/program and service, as well as how departments/units/programs and services work together. The surveyor(s) may start where the resident is currently located. He or she can then move to where the resident first entered the organization's systems; an area of care provided to the resident that may be a priority for that organization; or to any areas in which the resident received care, treatment, or services. The order will vary. Along the way, the surveyor(s) will speak with the health care staff member(s) who actually provided the care to that individual tracer resident—or, if that staff member(s) is not available, will speak with another staff member(s) who provides the same type of care.

* Please *see* the *Survey Activity Guide*, which is available on the extranet or by calling your account representative, for more detailed information on other program-specific criteria for tracer selection.

Table 4. Program-Specific Tracer Applicability Objectives

Organization Type	Program-Specific Tracer	Applicability	Objectives
Long Term Care	Resident Centered	Long Term Care (not applicable to Medicare/Medicaid–Certification-Based Long Term Care)	• To learn how the organization supports the long term care resident's quality of life through direct and indirect observation and interviews • To evaluate the implementation of residents' rights by tracing and experiencing what the resident experiences • To identify long term care process- and possibly system-level issues contributing to a lack of resident-centered care
Long Term Care	Staffing	All Long Term Care	• To evaluate actions taken by the organization during turnover to ensure positive outcomes in resident care • To identify process- and possibly system-level issues contributing to negative resident outcomes in light of staff or administrative turnover

Based on the findings of the surveyor(s), he or she may select similar residents to trace. The tracer methodology permits surveyors to "pull the threads" if there is a reason to believe that an issue needs further exploration.

Individual-Based System Tracer Activity

Individual-based system tracers explore one specific system or process across the organization, focusing, when possible, on the experiences of specific residents or activities relevant to specific residents. This differs from individual tracers in that during individual tracers, the surveyor(s) follows an individual through his or her course of care, evaluating all aspects of care as opposed to a "system." During the individual-based system tracer sessions, the surveyor(s) evaluates the system/process, including the integration of related processes and the coordination and communication among disciplines and departments in those processes.

An individual-based system tracer includes an interactive session (involving a surveyor and relevant staff members) in tracing a "system" within the organization based on information from individual tracers. Points of discussion in the interactive session include the following:

- The flow of the process across your organization, including identification and management of risk points, integration of key activities, and communication among staff/units involved in the process
- Strengths in the process and possible actions to be taken in areas needing improvement
- Issues requiring further exploration in other survey activities
- A baseline assessment of standards compliance
- Education by the surveyor, as appropriate

The three topics evaluated with individual-based system tracers are data use, infection control, and medication management. Although the number of individual-based system tracers varies based on survey length, the data use individual-based system tracer is always performed. If survey length does not permit the conduct of an infection control or medication management system tracer, the area is assessed through other survey activities.

Data Use. The data use individual-based system tracer focuses on how your organization collects, analyzes, interprets, and uses data to improve resident safety and care.

Infection Control. The infection control individual-based system tracer explores your organization's infection control processes. The goals of this session are to assess your organization's compliance with the relevant infection control standards, identify infection control issues that require further exploration, and determine actions that may be necessary to address any identified risks and improve resident safety.

Medication Management. The medication management individual-based system tracer explores your organization's medication management processes while focusing on subprocesses and potential risk points (such as handoff points). This tracer activity helps the surveyor(s) evaluate the continuity of medication management from procurement of medications through the monitoring of their effects on residents.

The Role of Organization Staff in Tracer Methodology

To help the surveyor(s) in the tracer methodology process, staff will be asked to provide the surveyor(s) with a list of active residents, including the residents' names, current locations in the organization, and diagnoses, as appropriate. The surveyor(s) may request assistance from organization staff for selection of appropriate tracer residents. As the surveyor(s) moves around an organization, he or she will ask to speak with the staff members who have been involved in the tracer resident's care, treatment, or services. If those staff members are not available, the surveyor(s) will ask to speak to another staff member who would perform the same function(s) as the member who has cared for or is caring for the tracer resident. Although it is preferable to speak with the direct caregiver, it is not mandatory because the questions that will be asked are questions that any caregiver should be able to answer in providing care to the resident being traced.

Feedback Sessions

Surveyors will communicate their observations at daily briefings, if requested to do so by the organization. If the organization has additional information that would demonstrate compliance with a standard that a surveyor has indicated may be a requirement for improvement, the organization should supply that information to the surveyor(s) as soon as possible.

Final On-Site Survey Activities

At the organization exit conference, the survey team presents a written summary of the survey findings. A written report is not provided at the completion of a for-cause unannounced survey.

Threat to Health or Safety

The Joint Commission may consider for accreditation purposes a surveyor's finding that some aspect of an organization's operation is having or may potentially have a serious adverse effect on resident health or safety and that immediate action must be taken.

Surveyors notify the organization's CEO and Joint Commission headquarters staff immediately if they identify any condition they believe poses a serious threat to public or resident health or safety. The president of The Joint Commission, or if the president is unavailable, his or her designee, can then issue an expedited Preliminary Denial of Accreditation decision based on the threat. An organization notified of a Preliminary Denial of Accreditation decision* due to an immediate threat to health or safety situation does not have a right to "clarify" the survey findings relative to the situation. Since a Preliminary Denial of Accreditation is an official accreditation decision category, the decision is posted on Quality Check.

The organization's CEO and appropriate governmental authorities are informed of this decision and the findings that led to this action. The Accreditation Committee of The Joint Commission Board of Commissioners confirms or reverses the decision at its next meeting. The Accreditation Committee may take into consideration an organization's corrective actions or responses to a serious threat situation. The organization can provide information to demonstrate that the serious threat to health or safety situation has been corrected prior to the Accreditation Committee's consideration of the Preliminary Denial of Accreditation decision.

---

* After the Preliminary Denial of Accreditation (PDA) decision has been confirmed by The Joint Commission's Accreditation Committee, the organization has five days to notify The Joint Commission if it wishes to appeal the decision. If this is the case, The Joint Commission's published "Review and Appeal Procedures" on pages 88–100 apply.

In these situations, the corrective action is considered when a single issue leads to the adverse finding and the organization demonstrates that it did the following:

- Took immediate action to completely remedy the situation
- Prepared a thorough and credible root cause analysis
- Adopted systems changes to prevent a future recurrence of the problem

If the organization demonstrates that it has taken corrective action, The Joint Commission will conduct an on-site survey to validate the implementation of the corrective action and that the immediate threat situation is no longer present.

After notification of the Preliminary Denial of Accreditation decision, an organization has **up to 72 hours** to do the following:

- Eliminate the immediate threat to health or safety situation **entirely** (for example, removing adult medication doses from pediatric units)
  OR
- If the situation is such that it will take the organization more time to fully eliminate it, (such as situations involving building construction), then the organization must implement interim safety measures* to abate the risk to patients (for example, cease performing a certain procedure, implement additional safety measures) within 72 hours. If the situation is not fully eliminated within 72 hours, the organization will have, at a maximum, **up to 23 days** to do so.

Once The Joint Commission has been notified by the organization that it has abated the immediate threat to health or safety situation, it will conduct an "abatement" survey to validate the abatement. If the abatement survey confirms the absence of the immediate threat to health or safety situation, The Joint Commission will remove the Preliminary Denial of Accreditation decision (assuming there are no other reasons for the Preliminary Denial of Accreditation). Therefore, the sooner an organization eliminates the immediate threat to health or safety situation, the shorter the period of time the organization will be in Preliminary Denial of Accreditation.

Upon resolution of an immediate threat to health or safety situation, the organization's accreditation status will change from Preliminary Denial of Accreditation to Conditional Accreditation and remain as such until a Conditional Accreditation follow-up survey is conducted to assess the organization's sustained implementation of appropriate corrective actions.

See Figure 3 on page 59 for a visual representation of the Process Flow for Immediate Threat to Health and Safety Situations.

The Summary of Survey Findings Report

Following evaluation of an organization's performance of functions and processes, the surveyor (or survey team) reviews the results of integrated individual findings. Then, with the use of laptop-based decision support software, the surveyor (or survey team) produces the organization's Summary of Survey Findings Report. The surveyor (or sur-

* "Interim safety measure" refers to any safety measure implemented to preserve life, whether related to *Life Safety Code*® deficiencies or another immediate threat to health or safety situation. It has previously been defined as "a series of 11 administrative actions intended to temporarily compensate for significant hazards posed by existing National Fire Protection Association 101 2000 *Life Safety Code* deficiencies or construction activities."

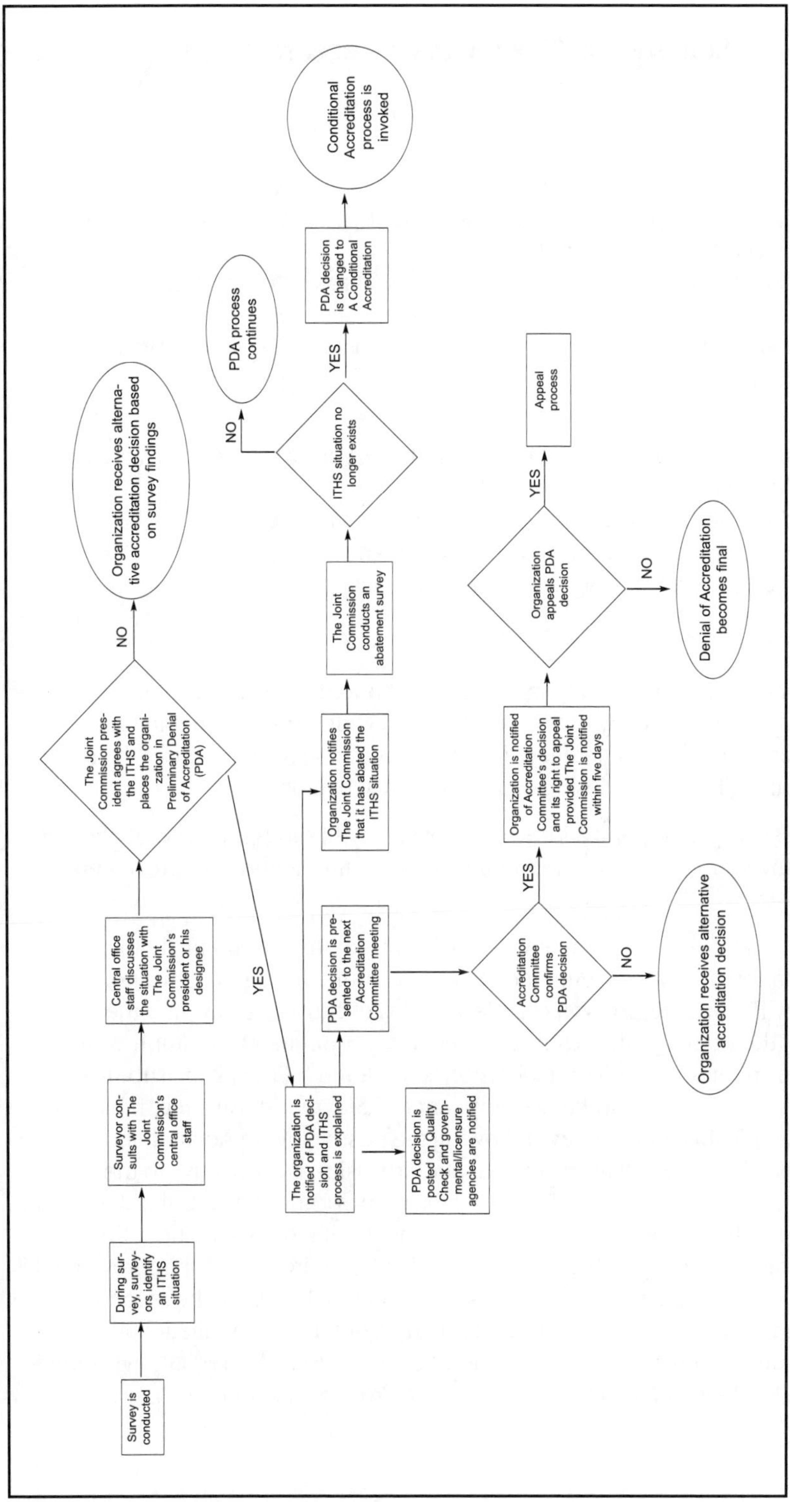

Figure 3. *Process flow for immediate threat to health and safety (ITHS) situations.*

Scoring of Elements of Performance

Beginning January 1, 2009, elements of performance (EPs) will be divided into the following two scoring categories:

1. "A" EPs
   - Usually relate to structural requirements (for example, policies or plans) that either exist or do not exist, and are scored either 0 or 2
   - May also address an issue that must be fully compliant even though it focuses on performance or outcome (for example, National Patient Safety Goals)
   - May also be related to a Medicare Condition of Participation that must always be fully compliant
2. "C" EPs
   - Frequency-based EPs that are scored based on the number of times a organization does not meet a particular EP.
   - Scored 2 if there are one or fewer occurrences of noncompliance
   - Scored 1 if there are two occurrences of noncompliance
   - Scored 0 if there are three or more occurrences of noncompliance

vey team leader) meets with the organization's CEO prior to the closing conference and provides him or her with a copy of the report. The CEO determines whether this report is distributed at the closing conference. The surveyor (or survey team) uses the report contents in making his or her closing conference presentations.

Shortly after a survey, an organization's report of survey findings is posted on the organization's secure extranet site. The report includes requirements for improvement, as appropriate.

If an organization does not receive any requirements for improvement, the organization's accreditation decision is rendered at the same time that the organization's Summary of Survey Findings Report is available, and it is effective the day after the completion of the survey. If an organization receives requirements for improvement, then the organization's accreditation decision is rendered following the submission of an acceptable Evidence of Standards Compliance (ESC) report. An acceptable ESC report is due within 45 calendar days following the posting of the Accreditation Survey Findings Report. The organization's accreditation decision is retroactive to the day after the last day of the survey, unless the organization is undergoing its first Joint Commission survey. In that case, the effective date for accreditation is set retroactively as the date on which an acceptable ESC that resolves all requirements for improvement is submitted. For an organization that receives a notification that it will be recommended for either Conditional Accreditation or Preliminary Denial of Accreditation, the accreditation decision is rendered by The Joint Commission's Accreditation Committee. (*See* "The Evidence of Standards Compliance Process" section beginning on page 65.)

After the Survey

This section includes information relevant to an organization that has recently participated in an accreditation survey. Material includes information on the ESC process, the MOS process, the types of accreditation decisions, how to request review of Preliminary Denial of Accreditation decisions, how to appeal Denial of Accreditation decisions, and how to use and display an accreditation award.

Scoring Categories and the Scale for Evaluating Compliance with Each Element of Performance

Elements of performance (EPs) are the performance expectations for determining if a standard is in compliance. EPs are scored on the following three point scale:

2 Satisfactory compliance
1 Partial compliance
0 Insufficient compliance
NA Not applicable

In addition to the requirements specifically stated in the EPs, EPs are also scored in accordance with the following track record achievements:

Score	Re-Survey
2	12 months
1	6 to 11 months
0	Fewer than 6 months

Overview of the Scoring and the Accreditation Decision Process

Beginning in 2009, accreditation decisions will be based on a "criticality" model. That is, the model is based on the premise that the immediacy of risk to quality of care and patient safety—based on noncompliance with Joint Commission standards and EPs—is variable, with certain situations constituting more immediate risks than others. Thus the more immediate the risk is to quality-of-care and patient safety, the shorter the period of time that the organization will have to address any relevant standards found to be noncompliant.

Criticality *is defined as the immediacy of risk to patient safety or quality of care as a result of non-compliance with a Joint Commission requirement (for example, an EP, National Patient Safety Goal, Universal Protocol).* The levels of criticality fall into the following four categories: 1) Immediate Threat to Health and Safety, 2) Situational Decision Rules, 3) Direct Impact Requirements, and 4) Indirect Impact Requirements.

Under the model, the immediacy of risk to the patient and to the organization's accreditation status increases as one moves from noncompliance with standards which have an "indirect" impact on patient care (the base or "blunt end" of the pyramid which is depicted in Figure 4 on page 62) to Immediate Threat to Health and Safety situations (the top or "sharp end" of the pyramid). Conversely, the timeframe within which organizations are expected to demonstrate resolution of instances of

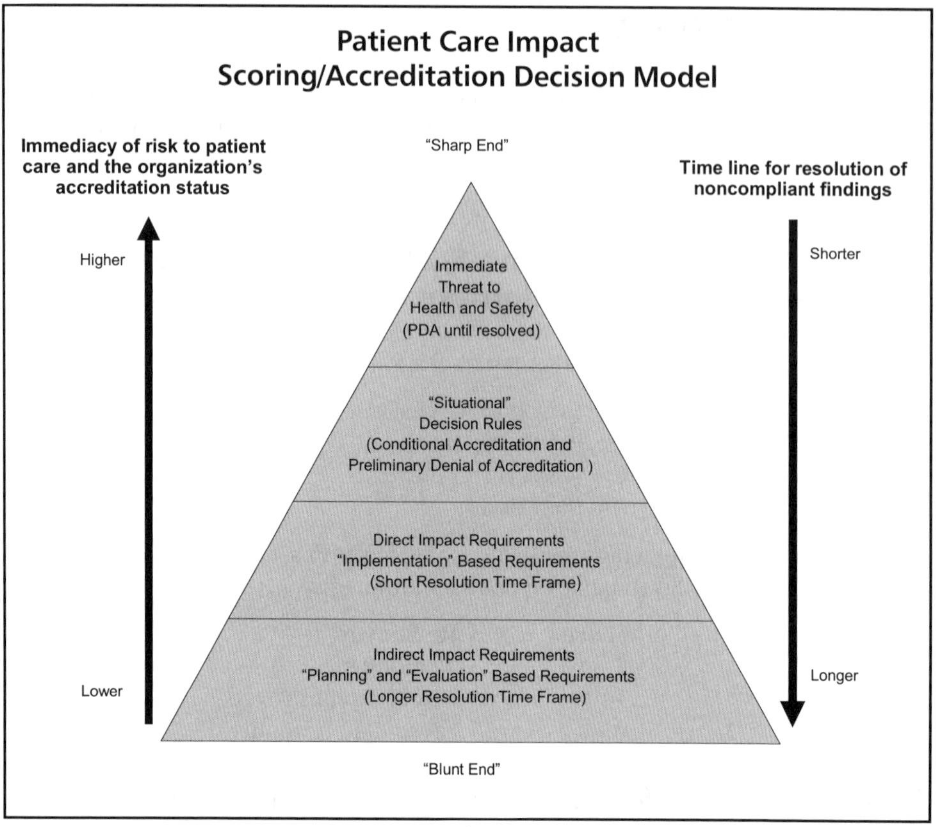

Figure 4. *Accreditation based on impact on patient care.*

noncompliance increases as one moves from the "sharp end" to the "blunt end" of the pyramid. The four "levels of risk" are defined as follows:

A. Immediate Threat to Health and Safety—Top (sharp end) of the pyramid representing the most immediate risk. This component of the model currently exists (*see* the "Threat to Health or Safety" section). While not linked to any specific standards or EPs, immediate threat to health or safety situations, which are identified on site, have or may potentially have serious adverse effects on patient health and safety. Upon resolution of an Immediate Threat to Health and Safety Situation, the organization's accreditation status will change from Preliminary Denial of Accreditation to Conditional Accreditation and remain as such until a Conditional Accreditation follow-up survey is conducted to assess the organization's sustained implementation of appropriate corrective actions.

B. Situational Decision Rules—Second level of the pyramid. These situations involve a recommendation for Preliminary Denial of Accreditation or Conditional Accreditation based on such issues as loss of facility licensure, provision of care by unlicensed individuals who require such a license, and failure to implement corrective action in response to identified *Life Safety Code* deficiencies. In follow-up to these situations, organizations must demonstrate resolution of the situation through the Evidence of Standards Compliance (ESC) process. An on-site survey is conducted to validate implementation of corrective action.

C. **Direct Impact Requirements**—Third level of the pyramid. A "Direct Impact" requirement (standard, elements of performance, National Patient Safety Goal, and Accreditation Participation Requirement) is a requirement that has a direct impact if noncompliance is likely to create an immediate risk to patient safety or quality of care. *The immediate risk usually results because there are no or few processes—or no or few protective defenses—intervening between the noncompliance and the impact on the safety or quality of a resident's care.*

   Evaluation of compliance with these requirements will be prioritized in the survey process. All instances of identified partial compliance or insufficient compliance with elements of performance which are associated with the Direct Impact requirements need to be resolved through the Evidence of Standards Compliance process **within 45 days**. The organization's accreditation decision would be held in abeyance pending demonstration of Evidence of Standards Compliance within the established time frame. Failure to resolve the instances of partial compliance or insufficient compliance with the associated elements of performance will lead to progressively more adverse accreditation decisions (Provisional Accreditation, Conditional Accreditation, and Preliminary Denial of Accreditation).

D. **Indirect Impact Requirements**—Bottom (blunt end) of the pyramid. These requirements pose less immediate risk to patient care and safety than Direct Impact requirements, but noncompliance increases risk to patient safety and quality of care over time. This risk may ultimately even exceed in scope or severity a direct impact.

   All instances of identified partial compliance and insufficient compliance with elements of performance under these requirements must be resolved through the Evidence of Standards Compliance process **within 60 days**. As above, the organization's accreditation decision will be held in abeyance pending demonstration of Evidence of Standards Compliance within the established time frames. As with the Direct Impact requirements, failure to resolve instances of partial compliance or insufficient compliance will lead to progressively more adverse accreditation decisions.

All partially compliant and insufficiently compliant EPs must be addressed via the ESC submission process. There will no longer be supplemental findings. The time line for completing the ESC submission will depend on the "criticality" of findings and immediacy of risk. EPs that are identified as having a direct impact on patient care as a result of partial or insufficient compliance will require the submission of an ESC within 45 days. EPs that are identified as having an "indirect impact" will require an ESC within 60 days.

In addition, if the number of noncompliant standards at the time of survey exceeds a predetermined threshold, a follow-up on-site survey will be required to validate implementation of the ESC.

The Accreditation Decision Process

The goal of the accreditation decision and reporting approach is to focus on the issues that pose the greatest risk to quality-of-care and patient safety. During the decision process, there are no numerical scores, and thus no scores are disclosed to the organizations or to the public. The lack of scores facilitates shifting the focus from passing the exam to continuous operational improvement. For more information on the accreditation decision rules for long term care organizations, *see* pages 80–88.

Key elements of the accreditation decision process include the following:

- Scoring of EPs is on the following scale: satisfactory compliance (2), partial compliance (1), insufficient compliance (0), or not applicable (NA).
- Standards are identified as compliant or not compliant based on the scoring pattern of their associated EPs.
- The surveyor(s) leaves a Summary of Survey Findings Report of findings on site (for special surveys, no report is left on site).
- The Accreditation Survey Findings Report will be posted on the organization's secure, password-protected extranet Web site space shortly after survey.
- If Requirements for Improvement (RFIs) are cited, the organization has a 45- or 60-day window to submit an ESC report to address correction of the RFIs. The accreditation decision is rendered following the submission of the ESC report. For organizations receiving a Preliminary Denial of Accreditation or Conditional Accreditation decision, the decision will be effective on the day the decision is rendered. For organizations that do not receive any RFIs, the accreditation decision will be effective the day after the last day of survey.

For more information on the scoring process, *see* pages 4–9 in the "How to Use This Book" (HB) chapter.

Accreditation Decision Categories

There are six categories of accreditation that an organization can achieve based on a Joint Commission full survey. The Joint Commission's accreditation decision categories are as follows:

- **Accredited.** The organization is in compliance with all standards at the time of the on-site survey or has successfully addressed all requirements for improvement in an Evidence of Standards Compliance (ESC) within 45 or 60 days following the posting of the Accreditation Survey Findings Report.
- **Provisional Accreditation.** The organization fails to successfully address all requirements for improvement in an ESC within 45 or 60 days following the posting of the Accreditation Survey Findings Report.
- **Conditional Accreditation.** The organization was previously in Preliminary Denial of Accreditation due to an Immediate Threat to Health or Safety situation, or failure to resolve the requirements of a Provisional Accreditation, or is not in substantial compliance with the applicable standards, as usually evidenced by a single issue or multiple issues that pose a risk to patient care or safety that was present at the time of survey. The organization must remedy identified problem areas through preparation and submission of Evidence of Standards Compliance and subsequently undergo an on-site, follow-up survey. In addition, an organization may

receive a Conditional Accreditation for failure to meet certain Joint Commission participation requirements, such as a Periodic Performance Review (PPR) or timely submission of data.

- **Preliminary Denial of Accreditation.** Justification to deny accreditation to the organization as evidenced by an Immediate Threat to Health or Safety situation, or failure to resolve the requirements of a Conditional Accreditation, or significant non-compliance with Joint Commission standards. The decision is subject to review and appeal prior to the determination to deny accreditation; the appeal process may also result in a decision other than Denial of Accreditation.
- **Denial of Accreditation.** The organization has been denied accreditation. All review and appeal opportunities have been exhausted.
- **Preliminary Accreditation.** The organization demonstrates compliance with selected standards in the surveys conducted under the Early Survey Policy.

See Table 5 (pages 66 and 67) for a description of each category and the conditions that lead to it.

The Evidence of Standards Compliance Process

After the survey, the surveyor(s) transmits their survey findings to The Joint Commission's Central Office. Your organization's official survey report will be posted on your organization's secure extranet site as soon as the Central Office's review is completed.

Every EP found not in compliance as the time of survey will generate a requirement for improvement. For every requirement for improvement cited in an organization's Accreditation Survey Findings Report, the organization must submit an Evidence of Standards Compliance (ESC). The ESC report is available for completion on the organization's secure extranet site at the same time that the organization's Accreditation Survey Findings Report is posted.

An acceptable ESC report must detail the action(s) that the organization took to bring itself into compliance with a standard or clarify why the organization believes that it is in compliance with the standard for which it received a requirement for improvement. An acceptable ESC must address compliance at the EP level and include an MOS, if applicable. An MOS is a numeric or quantifiable measure, usually related to an audit, that determines whether an action is effective and sustained.

An acceptable ESC report is due within 45 or 60 calendar days (depending on whether the EP relates to a "Direct" or "Indirect" Impact requirement) following the posting of the Accreditation Survey Findings Report. The required time frame will be specified in your report. Following a successful submission of the report, the organization receives an accreditation decision. However, the organization's accreditation decision is retroactive to the day after the last day of the survey, unless the organization is undergoing its first Joint Commission survey. In that case, the effective date for accreditation is the date on which the acceptable ESC is submitted.

If the organization implements actions to address its requirements for improvement, the organization's accreditation decision is Accredited. If an organization's ESC report does not acceptably address its requirements for improvement, then the organization's

Table 5. Joint Commission Accreditation Decisions

The Joint Commission has six accreditation decision categories. Each decision and the conditions that lead to it are described here.

Accreditation Decision Category	Conditions That Lead to This Type of Decision
Accredited	The organization is in compliance with all standards at the time of the on-site survey or has successfully addressed all requirements for improvement in an Evidence of Standards Compliance (ESC) response.
Provisional Accreditation	The organization fails to successfully address all requirements for improvement in an ESC.
Conditional Accreditation	The organization was previously in Preliminary Denial of Accreditation due to an Immediate Threat to Health and Safety situation, or failure to resolve the requirements of a Provisional Accreditation, or is not in substantial compliance with the applicable standards, as usually evidenced by a single issue or multiple issues that pose a risk to patient care or safety that was present at the time of survey. The organization must remedy identified problem areas through preparation and submission of Evidence of Standards Compliance and subsequently undergo an on-site, follow-up survey. In addition, an organization may receive a Conditional Accreditation for failure to meet certain Joint Commission participation requirements, such as a Periodic Performance Review (PPR) or timely submission of data.
Preliminary Denial of Accreditation	Justification to deny accreditation to the organization as evidenced by an Immediate Threat to Health and Safety situation, or failure to resolve the requirements of a Conditional Accreditation, or significant non-compliance with Joint Commission standards. The decision is subject to review and appeal prior to the determination to deny accreditation; the appeal process may also result in a decision other than Denial of Accreditation.

Table 5. Joint Commission Accreditation Decisions *(continued)*

Accreditation Decision Category	Conditions That Lead to This Type of Decision
Denial of Accreditation	The organization has been denied accreditation. All review and appeal opportunities have been exhausted.
Preliminary Accreditation	The organization demonstrates compliance with selected standards in the surveys conducted under the Early Survey Policy.

accreditation decision is Provisional Accreditation, which can eventually lead to a Conditional Accreditation or Preliminary Denial of Accreditation decision.

See Figures 5 and 6, page 68, for a time line of ESC and MOS submissions.

The organization's ESC submission(s) will be evaluated by Central Office staff using the same scoring guidelines used by the surveyors at the time of survey and by health care organizations when they conduct their PPR. The ESC(s) will be considered acceptable when the long term care organization has demonstrated resolution of all requirements for improvement. If the organization has not met a rule for Conditional Accreditation or Preliminary Denial of Accreditation and the ESC submission(s) are determined to be acceptable, its decision will be Accredited, and it will be required to submit the data for applicable MOS, if required, for each EP four months later.

If the long term care organization has not met a rule for Conditional Accreditation or Preliminary Denial of Accreditation and it is determined that a organization's ESC submission is unacceptable, its accreditation decision will be Provisional Accreditation, and it will be required to submit an acceptable ESC within 30 days. If the second ESC is determined to be acceptable, the organization's accreditation decision will remain Provisional Accreditation until it has submitted acceptable results of the corresponding MOS four months later. If the second ESC is determined to be unacceptable, a recommendation for Conditional Accreditation will be presented to the Accreditation Committee.

Central Office staff will evaluate the MOS results, when required. If it is determined that the MOS results are acceptable, no further action will be required of the organization, and if the organization had a Provisional Accreditation decision, its accreditation decision will be changed to Accredited. If it is determined that a organization's MOS submission is unacceptable and its accreditation decision is not currently Provisional Accreditation, its accreditation decision will be changed to Provisional Accreditation; the organization will be required to submit a second set of MOS results in another four months. If an organization whose accreditation decision is Provisional Accreditation

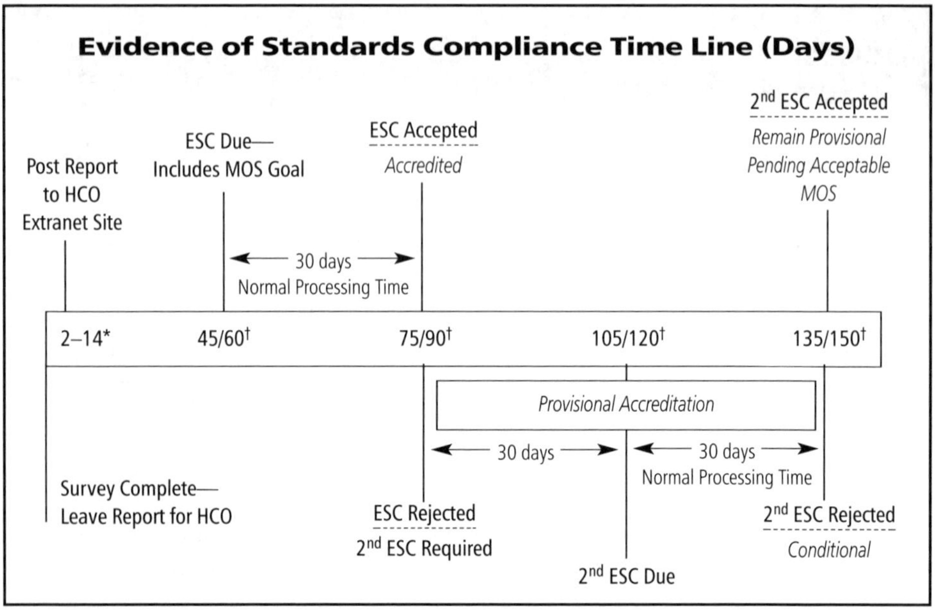

Figure 5. *This figure shows the Evidence of Standards Compliance (ESC) time line for 2009.*

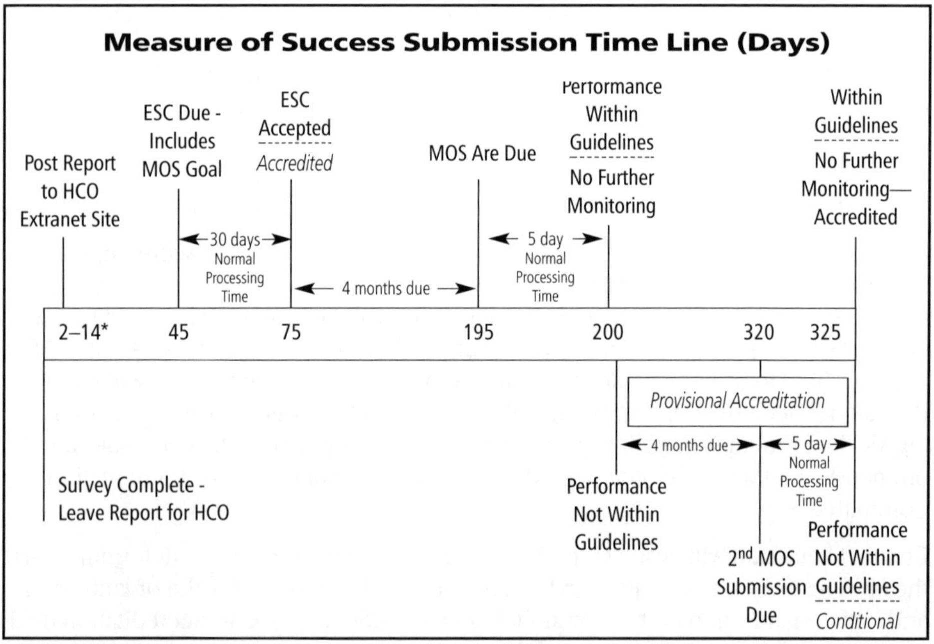

Figure 6. *This figure shows the measure of success (MOS) submission time line for 2009.*

* Those that go directly to the extranet are 2 days. If an account representative has to process it, it normally takes 14 days.

† The multiple time frames listed depend on whether the ESC is due in 45 days or 60 days.

because of an unacceptable first ESC submission submits an unacceptable first MOS submission, a recommendation for Conditional Accreditation will be presented to the Accreditation Committee.

If the organization's first ESC submission is determined to be acceptable and the second MOS submission is determined to be acceptable, its accreditation decision will be changed to Accredited, and no further action will be required of the organization. If the second MOS submission is determined to be unacceptable, a recommendation for Conditional Accreditation will be presented to the Accreditation Committee.

The organization's ESC submission and sustained implementation of it, including the MOS, are subject to review in random unannounced surveys.

A final decision letter will be posted to the organization's secure, password protected area of *The Joint Commission Connect* extranet site when its ESC has been reviewed and an accreditation decision has been rendered. A Quality Report will then be posted on Quality Check on The Joint Commission's Web site.

Clarification Process

After a survey event, organizations have the opportunity to submit clarifying Evidence of Standards Compliance (ESC) if they believe that their organization was in compliance with a particular standard at the time of survey.

The "clarification" is part of the ESC process, and must be submitted within the first ten days following the posting of your organization's report on the extranet site. The submission of "clarification" does not negate the requirement for submission of a "corrective" ESC within 45 or 60 days if the requirement for improvement continues, or provide an organization with additional time to submits its ESC. Therefore, if an organization submits "clarification" and still has to submit an ESC, the organization will have up to 45 or 60 days in total to submit both the "clarification" and the "corrective" ESC.

When submitting clarifying ESCs after a survey event, it is important to follow the directions in the submission tool. For "A" EPs, be sure to address each prompt, detailing why you believe that your organization was in compliance at the time of survey. Remember to address the EP as well as the actual surveyor observation.

For "C" EPs, an audit must be submitted that addresses the 30 days prior to the start of the survey. The sample sizes are defined in "How to Use This Book" (HB) chapter of this book and must be adhered to. Challenging specific surveyor observations will not result in the removal of a Requirement for Improvement (RFI). It is important to include all of the information regarding how the sample size was determined, how the sample was randomized, who conducted the audit, and the date range for the audit.

Conditional Accreditation, Preliminary Denial of Accreditation, and the ESC Report

If an organization is notified that a recommendation is to be made to The Joint Commission's Accreditation Committee for either Conditional Accreditation or Preliminary

Denial of Accreditation, the organization has 10 business days to provide information to clarify any of the requirements for improvement cited in its Accreditation Survey Findings Report through its ESC report.

After reviewing the organization's clarifying information and determining that the organization has no longer met the decision rule for Preliminary Denial of Accreditation or Conditional Accreditation, The Joint Commission will follow up with an on-site validation survey to do the following:

- Seek to validate the clarifying information submitted and determine if such information or data was available to the previous on-site survey team
- Determine whether the organization does or does *not* meet a decision rule for Preliminary Denial of Accreditation or Conditional Accreditation

If the organization does *not* meet a rule for Preliminary Denial of Accreditation or Conditional Accreditation, it will be awarded Accreditation (if it is compliant with all standards) or it will be required to submit an ESC (if it still has requirements for improvement). However, if the organization continues to meet a decision rule for Preliminary Denial of Accreditation or Conditional Accreditation, The Joint Commission staff will recommend to the Accreditation Committee that the organization remain in Preliminary Denial of Accreditation or Conditional Accreditation. If the results of the on-site validation survey suggest that the organization knowingly falsified its clarifying information, the staff will recommend to the Accreditation Committee that the Information Accuracy and Truthfulness Policy should apply.

A Clarification Validation Survey (CVS) will be conducted as part of the appeal process whenever an organization submits written or electronic information to demonstrate compliance with Joint Commission standards at the time of survey, and therefore no longer meets a rule for Preliminary Denial of Accreditation, even as part of the appeal process.

Under this process, whenever an organization submits written (or electronic) information after receiving a Preliminary Denial of Accreditation decision, the organization will undergo a CVS to validate the information and assure compliance with Joint Commission standards before The Joint Commission makes a final decision to remove the organization from the Preliminary Denial of Accreditation decision.

The CVS ensures that the organization was, in fact, in compliance with Joint Commission standards at the time of survey, instead of relying solely on written (or electronic) information submitted by the organization. Inclusion of the CVS to the appeal process helps maintain the integrity of the accreditation decision process and ensures that Joint Commission–accredited organizations are providing safe, high-quality care.

See Figures 7 and 8 on pages 71 and 72 for a visual representation of the process for the following situations:

1. Process Flow for a Preliminary Denial of Accreditation (PDA) Decision (Figure 7)
2. Process Flow for a Conditional Accreditation (CA) Decision (Figure 8)

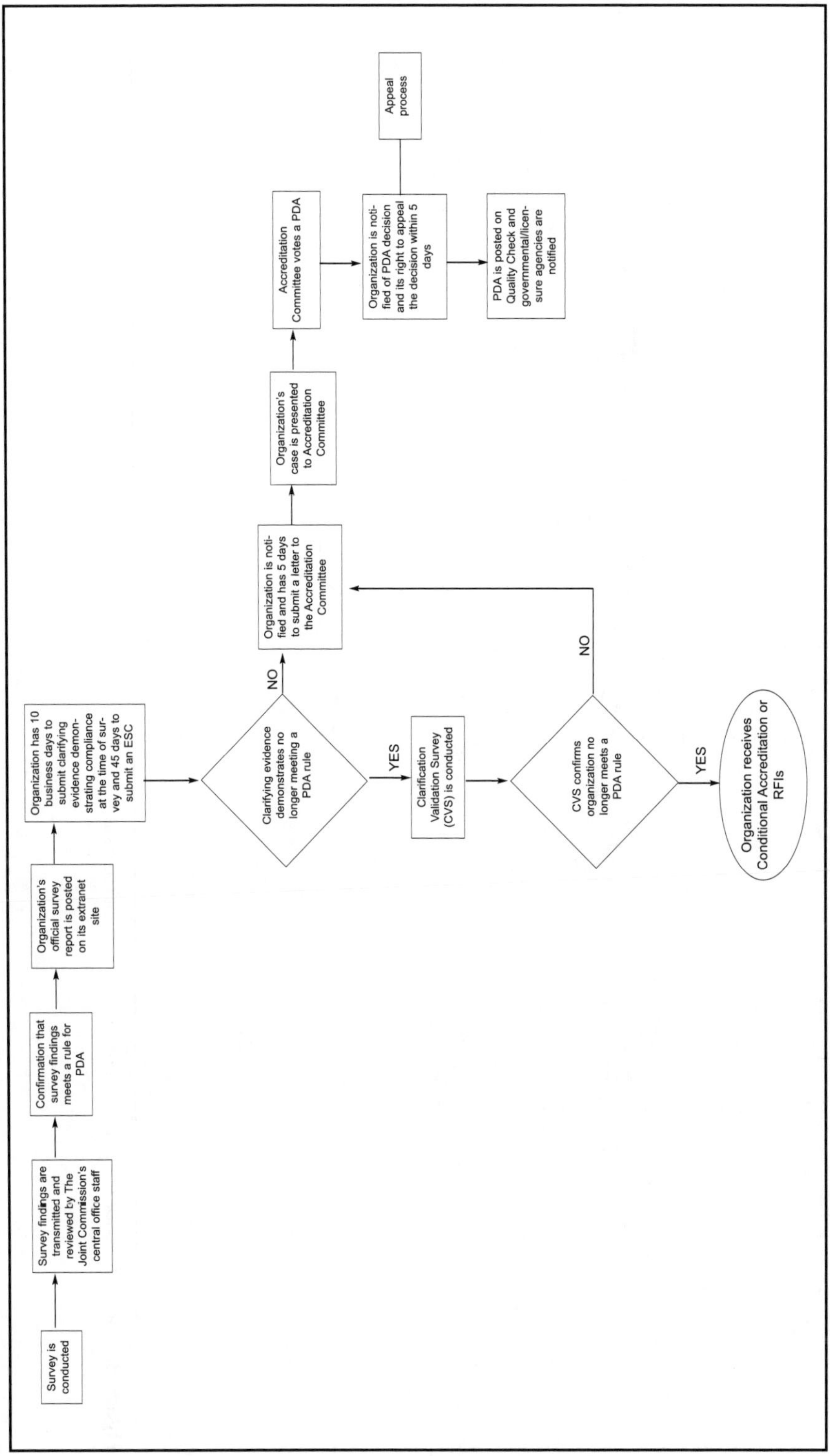

Figure 7. *Process flow for preliminary denial of accreditation (PDA) decision.*

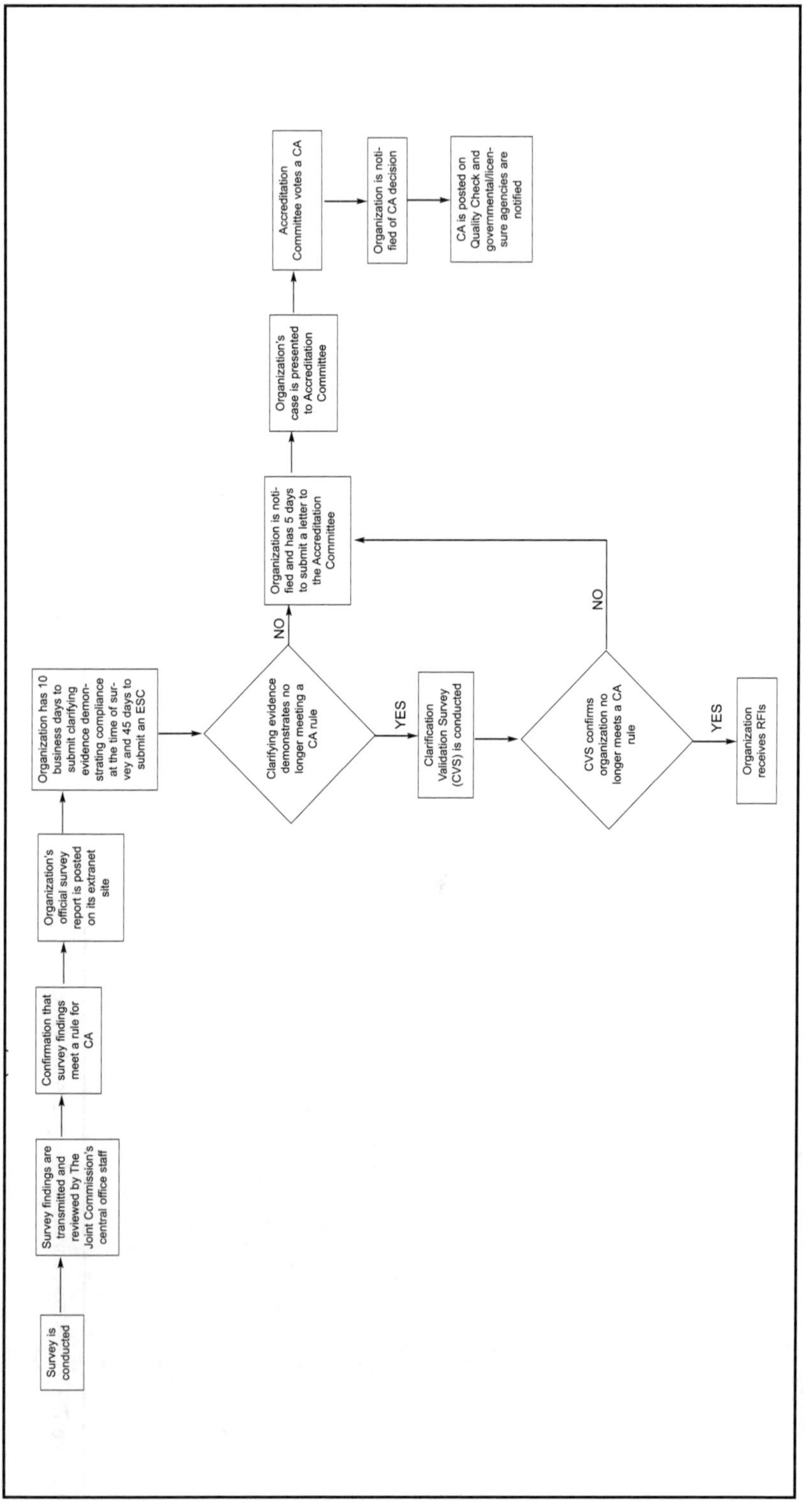

Figure 8. *Process flow for a conditional accreditation (CA) decision.*

Measure(s) of Success Report

If possible, an organization is required to submit a Measure of Success (MOS) report within four months of submitting an acceptable ESC report. The MOS report should demonstrate whether each MOS identified in the organization's ESC report was reached.

Accreditation Decisions

An organization's accreditation decision becomes official following submission of its acceptable ESC resolving all requirements for improvement, which is retroactive to the day after the last day of the full survey, or, in the case of Preliminary Denial of Accreditation, on the date the Accreditation Committee makes a decision. For organizations undergoing an initial survey, the accreditation decision becomes official the day of the Accreditation Committee meeting or an acceptable ESC resolving all requirements for improvement is submitted (if that occurs after the Accreditation Committee meeting). When an organization's accreditation decision becomes official, it is publicly disclosable. There are six possible accreditation decisions:

1. Accredited
2. Provisional Accreditation
3. Conditional Accreditation
4. Preliminary Denial of Accreditation
5. Denial of Accreditation
6. Preliminary Accreditation (Early Survey Policy)

See "The Accreditation Decision Process" section beginning on page 64 for more information.

Weighted Decision Rules

The weighted decision rules are applied to rendering accreditation decisions in complex organizations. When a secondary component of a complex organization meets rules of Conditional Accreditation or Preliminary Denial of Accreditation as a consequence of invoking the Threat to Health or Safety Policy or not complying with the Information Accuracy and Truthfulness Policy or an APR, that accreditation decision would apply equally to the component and the complex organization of which the component is a part.

See Table 6 on page 74 for more information on the weighted decision rules.

Withdrawing or Closing After Undergoing a Survey

An organization's request to withdraw from the accreditation process after undergoing survey (or that closes after undergoing survey) and before a final decision has been made does not terminate the decision-making process. The Joint Commission then issues a final accreditation decision.

Table 6. Weighted Decision Rules*

Primary Program	Secondary Programs
One program in a complex organization is to be identified as "primary" (this is not a change from the previous rule). If the primary program meets a rule for Provisional Accreditation, Conditional Accreditation, or Preliminary Denial of Accreditation, the overall decision for the organization is Provisional Accreditation, Conditional Accreditation, or Preliminary Denial of Accreditation, respectively. If the primary or any secondary program meets a rule for Provisional Accreditation, the overall decision for the organization is Provisional Accreditation.	If one of the secondary programs meets a rule for Preliminary Denial of Accreditation, the overall decision for the organization is Conditional Accreditation. If one of the secondary programs meets a rule for Conditional Accreditation, the overall decision for the organization is Provisional Accreditation. If two or more of the secondary programs meet rules for Preliminary Denial of Accreditation, the overall decision for the organization is Preliminary Denial of Accreditation. If two or more of the secondary programs meet rules for Conditional Accreditation, the overall decision for the organization is Conditional Accreditation. If the primary or any secondary program meets a rule for Provisional Accreditation, the overall decision for the organization is Provisional Accreditation.

* **Note:** *Weighted decision rules are not applicable when the laboratory is the secondary program.*

Review and Appeal of Preliminary Denial of Accreditation and Denial of Accreditation Decisions

The appeal procedures are set forth in the Review and Appeal Procedures section of this chapter, on pages 88–98. Two additional procedures specific to Preliminary Denial of Accreditation and Denial of Accreditation decisions are described here.

When an organization receives written notice from The Joint Commission that a recommendation of Preliminary Denial of Accreditation is proposed for submission to the Accreditation Committee, the organization has 10 business days from receipt of that notification to submit to The Joint Commission clarifying information that demonstrates that it was in fact in compliance with one or more standards in question at the time of survey.

If after Joint Commission review of any submitted materials, the Preliminary Denial of Accreditation recommendation will still be made, the organization will have five business days from receipt of this notification to submit a written response directly to the Accreditation Committee.

Award Display and Use

The Joint Commission provides each accredited organization with one certificate of accreditation per program. There is no charge for the initial certificate(s). Additional certificates may be purchased. Such requests should be sent to the certificate coordinator in the Division of Accreditation and Certification Operations at The Joint Commission.

The certificate and all copies remain The Joint Commission's property. They must be returned if either of the following situations occurs:

- The organization is issued a new certificate, reflecting a name change
  or
- The organization's accreditation decision is changed, withdrawn, or denied for any reason

An organization accredited by The Joint Commission must be accurate in describing to the public the nature and meaning of its accreditation and its award.* When an organization receives an accreditation award, The Joint Commission sends the organization guidelines for characterizing the accreditation award.

Accreditation award certificates include language about educating residents and their families on how to contact The Joint Commission.

An organization may not engage in any false or misleading advertising of an accreditation award. Any such advertising may be grounds for The Joint Commission to deny accreditation. For example, an organization may not represent its accreditation as being awarded by any of The Joint Commission's corporate members. These include the American College of Physicians, the American College of Surgeons, the American Dental Association, the American Hospital Association, and the American Medical Association. The Joint Commission has permission to reprint the seals of its corporate members on certificates of accreditation. However, these seals must not be reproduced or displayed separately from the certificate.

Any organization that materially misleads the public about any matter relating to its accreditation must undertake corrective advertising to a degree acceptable to The Joint Commission in the same medium in which the misrepresentation occurred. If an organization fails to undertake the required corrective advertising following the communication of false or misleading advertising about its accreditation decision, the organization may be subject to loss of accreditation.

The Joint Commission's logo is a registered trademark. An accredited organization may use the logo if it follows these guidelines:

- The logo must remain in the same proportional relationship as provided and should not be displayed any larger than an organization's own logo.
- The logo's format cannot be changed, the name may not be separated from the symbol, and the logo must be printed in the original color.
- Graphic devices such as seals, other words, or slogans cannot be added to the logo, except for the words "Accredited by."
- These guidelines apply to logo use on all print materials, Internet Web pages, and promotional items, such as coffee mugs, T-shirts, and notepads. Contact The Joint

* *See* APR.08.01.01 on page 139 in the "Accreditation Participation Requirements" (APR) chapter.

Commission Department of Communications at 630/792-5631 for questions about using The Joint Commission logo.

Additional Accreditation Activities

This section provides information that is relevant to organizations between Joint Commission surveys. Material includes the duration of an accreditation award; the process for continuing accreditation; how to notify The Joint Commission in the event of organization changes, including the opening or closing of a unit or services, addition or deletion of components, leadership changes, mergers, consolidations, and acquisitions; and unscheduled and unannounced for-cause surveys.

Reentering the Accreditation Process

For a previously accredited organization to be designated as "new," it must not have participated in the accreditation process during the previous six months. If an organization is reentering the accreditation process before six months have passed, it must demonstrate a continuing 12-month track record of compliance with the standards.

Duration of Accreditation Award

An accreditation award is continuous until the organization has its next full survey, which will be between 18 and 39 months after its previous full survey, unless accreditation is revoked for cause or as otherwise outlined in this chapter. An organization may request a full accreditation survey more frequently than when it is due to have a survey. The Joint Commission, at its discretion and in accordance with its mission, determines whether to honor the request. An organization should send such a request to its Joint Commission account representative.

Continuous Compliance

The Joint Commission expects an accredited organization to be in continuous compliance with all applicable standards and EPs. It may ask an organization to supply, in writing, information about compliance with standards. It may also survey an organization at any time with or without notice in response to complaints, media coverage, or other information that raises questions about the adequacy of resident health and safety protections (*see* the "For-Cause Surveys" section on page 79). The Joint Commission might also conduct a survey if an organization fails to respond to a request for more information.

The Joint Commission may view an organization's failure to permit a survey as the organization no longer wanting to participate in the accreditation process. In such a case, The Joint Commission begins proceedings to deny accreditation to the organization.*

Continuing Accreditation

An organization's accreditation cycle is continuous, as long as the organization:

- Has a full, unannounced survey within 39 months of its last survey; and
- Continues to meet all accreditation-related requirements as required, including, but not limited to, submission of an annual PPR, and an annual subscription payment.

---

* *See* APR.02.01.01 on page 136 in the "Accreditation Participation Requirements" (APR) chapter.

Duration of the Accreditation Decision

An organization's previous accreditation decision remains in effect until a decision is made either to accredit or to preliminarily deny accreditation to the organization.

Notifying The Joint Commission About Organizational Changes

Accreditation is neither automatically transferred nor continued if significant changes occur within an organization. When significant changes occur, the organization must notify The Joint Commission in writing or through its extranet site not more than 30 calendar days after such change is made. The organization must also notify The Joint Commission in writing if it opens or closes any units or services.

When an organization offers at least 25% of its services or programs at a new location or in a significantly altered physical plant, the organization must also fill out and submit to The Joint Commission Part 2: Basic Building Information of the Statement of Conditions™ (SOC) compliance document; Part 3E or 3F of the Statement of Fire Safety (SFS); and Part 4: Plan for Improvement, should *Life Safety Code* deficiencies be present. (For a copy of the SOC, visit The Joint Commission's Web site, at http://www.jointcommission.org, and select "Accredited Organizations," then your accreditation program, then "Standards," and then "Statement of Conditions.") Failure to provide timely notification to The Joint Commission of these changes may result in the organization's loss of accreditation. If completion dates for a PFI cannot be achieved, the organization is to contact The Joint Commission's engineering staff to request an extension.

Mergers, Consolidations, and Acquisitions

In the case of a merger, a consolidation, or an acquisition, The Joint Commission may decide that the organization responsible for services must have a survey. Barring exceptional circumstances, The Joint Commission continues the accreditation of the organization undergoing the kind of changes described here until it determines whether an extension survey is necessary.

Note: *If, after accreditation is rendered to an organization, the organization's structure changes whereby one or more of its services, programs, or related organizations are no longer part of the organization that was originally surveyed, the service, program, or related organization is no longer included in the organization's accreditation.*

When an accredited organization acquires another organization and an extension survey is conducted, the survey findings resulting from the extension survey are maintained separately from, and are not reflected in, the accreditation decision of the acquiring organization for 12 months following the acquisition. After the 12-month period, any outstanding standards compliance problems in the acquired component(s) are reflected in the accreditation decision of the acquiring organization.

Extension Surveys

An extension survey is conducted at an accredited organization or at a site that is owned and operated by the organization if the accredited organization's current accreditation is not due to expire for at least nine months and when at least one of the conditions below is met. The results of an extension survey may affect the organization's accreditation decision.

An extension survey of an organization may be necessary if the organization has done any of the following:

- Instituted a new service or program for which The Joint Commission has standards
- Changed ownership and has a significant number of changes in the management and clinical staff or operating policies and procedures
- Offered at least 25% of its services at a new location or in a significantly altered physical plant
- Expanded its capacity to provide services by 25% or more, as measured by resident volume, pieces of equipment, or other relevant measures
- Provided a more intensive level of service

  or
- Merged with, consolidated with, or acquired an unaccredited site, service, or program for which there are applicable Joint Commission standards and EPs

Accreditation Status of Organizations That Cease Services After a Disaster

The Joint Commission will discontinue the accreditation of organizations that have been closed or out of service for more than six months as a result of a disaster.

The Joint Commission's complete process for determining the accreditation status of organizations that cease services following a disaster is as follows.

For the first 30 days after a disaster and/or the organization's decision to cease operations, the organization's original Joint Commission accreditation status will stay in effect. When the organization resumes operation, the time frame for complying with any outstanding Joint Commission requirements (such as the PPR or ESC) will also resume. In most cases, The Joint Commission will not need to survey the affected organization to reassess its level of standards compliance. If The Joint Commission decides to conduct a survey, however, the organization's accreditation decision will be driven by the survey findings.

If the organization resumes services from 31 to 90 days after a disaster, The Joint Commission will conduct an extension survey to determine the organization's accreditation status. The circumstances surrounding the organization's closure will determine the survey's length and scope.

For organizations that resume services from 91 days up to six months after a disaster, The Joint Commission will require an environment of care on-site survey. This survey will preferably take place one to two weeks after services are resumed. It is assumed that these organizations have received clearance from the fire marshal and other local/state authorities before resuming services. In addition, The Joint Commission will conduct a second on-site survey approximately four months after services have been resumed to evaluate sustained compliance with Joint Commission standards and requirements. The track record requirement for demonstrating standards compliance will be four months.

If an organization does not resume services within six months after a disaster or the decision to cease operations, The Joint Commission will discontinue its accreditation. If the organization resumes services, it must reapply to become accredited. In such cases, the accreditation process will involve at least two surveys. The first survey will be conducted at the organization's request, and will assess the organization's ability to provide safe resident care. The organization may qualify for an accreditation award as a result of this survey. The second survey will be conducted approximately four months later to assess sustained compliance with Joint Commission requirements. The track record requirement for demonstrating standards compliance will be four months.

The Joint Commission will continue to list all affected organizations as Accredited up to six months after a disaster, unless survey findings dictate otherwise.

While working with affected health care organizations in the aftermath of a catastrophic event, The Joint Commission will be sensitive to these organizations' needs and will work with responsible state and federal agencies to help reestablish the organizations' operations as well as their qualification for accreditation.

For-Cause Surveys

The Joint Commission may perform a for-cause survey when it becomes aware of potentially serious standards compliance or resident care or safety issues, or when it has other valid reasons for surveying an accredited organization.*

Note: *For-cause unannounced surveys should not be confused with regular unannounced surveys, as described beginning on page 48.*

Reasons for for-cause surveys include occurrence of any event or series of events in an accredited organization that creates either of the following significant situations:

- Concern that a continuing threat may exist to the safety or care of residents at risk or
- Indication that the organization is not or has not been in compliance with The Joint Commission's Information Accuracy and Truthfulness Policy

Such a survey can either include all the organization's services or only those areas where a serious concern may exist.

A for-cause survey, which is usually unannounced, can take place at any point in an organization's accreditation cycle. No preliminary report is generated after a for-cause survey.

Note: *An organization is charged for a for-cause survey, regardless of the outcome. An organization can determine the cost of such a survey by calling The Joint Commission's Pricing Unit at 630/792-5115.*

The Joint Commission may deny an organization accreditation if the organization does not allow The Joint Commission to conduct an unscheduled or unannounced survey.

---

* *See* APR.02.01.01 on page 136 in the "Accreditation Participation Requirements" (APR) chapter.

Random Validation of Evidence of Standards Compliance

On an annual basis, a 5% random sample of all organizations that have been required to submit an Evidence of Standards Compliance (ESC), with or without an MOS will be selected for an unannounced on-site Validation Survey. The purpose of this survey is to maintain the credibility of the ESC process by validating statements made in the ESC submission. The surveyor will be surveying areas that were the subject of each RFI to determine whether the stated corrective actions were implemented as stated.

Depending on whether an organization is required to submit an ESC only or an ESC and an MOS will determine whether the organization will be included in the "pool" for organizations to have a validation survey in short proximity to the ESC submission or following the MOS submission. If an organization is required to submit an ESC and an MOS, the organization will not be included in the "pool" until after the MOS is submitted.

2009 Long Term Care and Long Term Care Deemed Status Decision Rules

The Joint Commission makes accreditation decisions by applying decision rules to the scored standards. Decision rules determine an accreditation decision that appropriately represents an organization's overall performance as measured by evidence of compliance with the applicable standards. Decision rules are approved by the Accreditation Committee. The Committee may exercise reasonable discretion in individual cases to determine whether to vary from applicable decision rules in furtherance of The Joint Commission's mission to help enhance the quality and safety of care.

"Weighted" decision rules have been in place to limit the impact that the performance of small or secondary components of a complex organization may have on the organization's overall accreditation decision. These rules were established based on the rationale that the poor performance of a small component of a large complex organization, as determined by standards noncompliance, should not determine the accreditation decision of the entire organization. As such, the performance factors contributing to the overall accreditation decision for a complex organization were "weighted" to account for a proportional impact on overall care. The current "weighted" decision rules can be found in Table 6 on page 74.

The decision rules long term care and long term care deemed status follow.

Denial of Accreditation

Denial of Accreditation will be recommended when one or more of the following conditions are met:

DA01 The organization does not permit the performance of any survey by The Joint Commission. (Accreditation Participation Requirement APR.02.01.01, EP 1)

DA02 The organization has failed to resolve a Conditional Accreditation status prior to withdrawing from the accreditation process.

DA03 The organization has failed to submit payment for survey fees or annual fees.

DA04 The organization, which was previously in Conditional Accreditation for failure to submit data and information to The Joint Commission within 61 days of the due date(s) has failed to meet all requirements for timely submission of data and information to The Joint Commission, within 91 days of the due date(s). (APR.01.01.01, EP 1)

DA05 The organization, which was previously in Conditional Accreditation for failure to submit the Periodic Performance Review 61 days after the due date, has failed to submit a Periodic Performance Review, and corrective action plan as appropriate, 91 days after the due date. The organization may also be required to participate in a scheduled consultative phone call with Central Office staff as specified in the description of the full Periodic Performance Review and the Periodic Performance Review options. (APR.03.01.01, EP 1)

Preliminary Denial of Accreditation

Preliminary Denial of Accreditation will be recommended when one or more of the following conditions are met:

PDA01 An immediate threat to patient/public health or safety exists within the organization.

PDA02 The organization's patients have been placed at risk for a serious adverse outcome because either (1) an individual who does not possess a license, registration, or certification is providing or has provided health care services in the organization that would, under applicable law or regulation, require such a license, registration, or certification; or (2) an individual is practicing outside the scope of his or her license, registration, or certification. (HR.1.20, EP 8; HR.4.10, EP 8; HR.4.20, EP 7)

PDA03 The Joint Commission is reasonably persuaded that the organization submitted falsified documents or misrepresented information in seeking to achieve or retain accreditation. Information provided by an organization and used by The Joint Commission for accreditation purposes must be accurate and truthful and may:

- be provided verbally, in writing, or electronically;
- be obtained through direct observation, interview or other communication by any Joint Commission employee;
- be derived from documents supplied by the organization to The Joint Commission including, but not limited to, an organization's root cause

analysis in response to a sentinel event, or an organization's application for accreditation;
- involve data or documents transmitted electronically to The Joint Commission, including but not limited to data or documents provided as part of the Periodic Performance Review process or the electronic application process.

If accreditation is denied following implementation of this rule, the organization shall be prohibited from participating in the accreditation process for a period of one year unless the president of The Joint Commission, for good cause, waives all or a portion of this waiting period. (APR.01.02.01, EP 1)

PDA04 The organization has been conditionally accredited on two consecutive full surveys in relation to the same issue or issues.

PDA05 New rule pending. Please refer to *The Joint Commission Perspectives®* for the text of this rule.

PDA06 The organization does not possess a license, certificate, and/or permit, as, or when, required by applicable law and regulation, to provide the health care services for which the organization is seeking accreditation. (LD.04.04.01, EP 1)

PDA07 The organization with a decision of Conditional Accreditation, as the result of a survey event, has failed to clear not compliant standards after two opportunities to do so as the result of:
- two failed Evidence of Standards Compliance (ESC) submissions,
- two failed Measure of Success (MOS) submissions,
- a combination of one failed ESC submission, one failed MOS submission and/or a failed Conditional Accreditation follow-up survey).

Note: *The opportunity is considered failed when the organization has not demonstrated resolution of all not compliant standards and continues to meet any of the decision rules requiring additional monitoring in the form of on-site follow-up, an Evidence of Standards Compliance submission, or a Measure of Success submission. In addition, a Conditional Accreditation follow-up survey is considered an opportunity to clear not compliant standards.*

PDA08 The result of a Conditional Accreditation follow-up survey is unacceptable.

Note: *The result of the Conditional Accreditation follow-up survey will be considered unacceptable if the organization continues to meet any of the rules or an exception to the rules that caused a recommendation of Conditional Accreditation or Preliminary Denial of Accreditation.*

PDA09 The organization has knowingly used Joint Commission employee to provide any accreditation-related consulting services. (APR.06.01.01, EP 1)

PDA10 The Joint Commission is notified that the Skilled Nursing Facility/Nursing Facility has been terminated for cause or voluntarily withdraws from the Medicare/Medicaid program. Applies to Medicare/Medicaid certification-based long term care only. (APR.10.01.01, EP 1)

Conditional Accreditation

Conditional Accreditation will be recommended when one or more of the following conditions are met:

CON01 New rule pending. Please refer to *The Joint Commission Perspectives®* for the text of this rule.

CON02 An individual who does not possess a license, registration, or certification is providing or has provided health care services in the organization that would, under applicable law or regulation, require such a license, registration, or certification; or an individual is practicing outside the scope of his or her license, registration, or certification. (HR.1.20, EP 8; HR.4.10, EP 8; HR.4.20, EP 7)

Note: *Except as provided under rule PDA02.*

CON03 The organization has failed to clear not compliant standards after two opportunities to do so (as the result of two failed Evidence of Standards Compliance [ESC] submissions, two failed Measure of Success [MOS] submissions, or a combination of one failed ESC submission and one failed MOS submission).

Note: *The opportunity is considered failed when the organization, which was not previously conditionally accredited, has not demonstrated resolution of all not compliant standards and continues to meet any of the decision rules requiring additional monitoring in the form of on-site follow-up, an Evidence of Standards Compliance submission, or a Measure of Success submission.*

CON04 The organization has failed to implement or make sufficient progress toward the corrective actions described in a Statement of Conditions™, Part 4, Plan for Improvement, which was previously accepted by The Joint Commission, or has failed to implement or enforce applicable interim life safety measures. (LS.01.01.01, EP 3; LS.01.02.01, EP 3)

CON05 The organization, which was previously in Provisional Accreditation for failure to submit data and information to The Joint Commission within 31 days of the due date(s), has failed to meet all requirements for timely submission of data and information to the Joint Commission, within 61 days of the due date(s). (APR.01.01.01, EP 1)

CON06 The organization, which was previously in Provisional Accreditation for failure to submit the Periodic Performance Review 31 days after the due date, has failed to submit a Periodic Performance Review, and corrective action plan as appropriate, 61 days after the due date. The organization may also be required to participate in a scheduled consultative phone call with Central Office staff as specified in the description of the full Periodic Performance Review and the Periodic Performance Review options. (APR.03.01.01, EP 1)

Conditional Accreditation Follow-up

A Conditional Accreditation Follow-up survey will be recommended when one or more of the following conditions are met:

CONF01 A Conditional Accreditation follow-up survey will be scheduled for organizations with a Conditional Accreditation decision.

Note: *The date of the survey will be established at the time the final Conditional Accreditation decision is awarded. (Conditional Accreditation follow-up surveys typically occur at approximately six months from the date when the organization is notified of its official Conditional Accreditation decision.)*

CONF02 A second Conditional Accreditation follow-up survey will be scheduled when as the result of a conditional follow-up survey, one or more of the original Requirements for Improvement remain unresolved.

Note: *This accreditation decision results when the organization which was awarded Conditional Accreditation as the result of an on-site survey has passed its first ESC submission, but the Conditional Accreditation follow-up survey finds that one or more of the original Requirements for Improvement remain unmet, and none of the other rules for Preliminary Denial of Accreditation or Conditional Accreditation have been met.*

Provisional Accreditation

Provisional Accreditation will be recommended when one or more of the following conditions are met:

PROV01 The organization has failed to demonstrate resolution of all requirements for improvement at the time of its first ESC or first MOS submission. This accreditation decision results when at least one standard is scored not compliant and none of the rules for Preliminary Denial of Accreditation or Conditional Accreditation have been met.

Note 1: *Not compliant standards must be resolved within stipulated time frames (through an on-site MOS as provided in rule MOS03, submission of an ESC, or submission of an MOS by the organization) to maintain accreditation.*

Note 2: *When an organization is placed in Provisional Accreditation as the result of a failed first ESC or failed first MOS submission, it will remain in Provisional Accreditation until an MOS submission has been determined to be acceptable.*

PROV02 The organization has failed to meet all requirements for timely submission of data and information to The Joint Commission, within 31 days of the due date(s). (APR.01.01.01, EP 1)

PROV03 The organization has failed to submit a Periodic Performance Review, and corrective action plan as appropriate, 31 days after the due date. The organization may also be required to participate in a scheduled consultative phone call with Central Office staff as specified in the description of the full Periodic Performance Review and the Periodic Performance Review options. (APR.03.01.01, EP 1)

Evidence of Standards Compliance (ESC)

An Evidence of Standards Compliance (ESC) is a report submitted by a surveyed organization within 45 days of its survey, which details the action(s) that it took to bring itself into compliance with a standard or clarifies why the organization believes that it was in compliance with the standard for which it received a Requirement for Improvement. An ESC must address compliance at the EP level and include a Measure of Success (MOS) for all applicable EP corrections.

An ESC will be required when one or more of the following conditions are met:

ESC01 An organization has one or more standards scored not compliant at the time of a survey event.

ESC02 Failure to demonstrate continued compliance with all not compliant standards in the first ESC submission will result in Provisional Accreditation. The organization will be required to submit a second ESC within 30 days of the official notification that the first ESC was unacceptable.

On-site ESC survey

An on-site ESC survey, due in 45 days, will be scheduled when the following condition is met:

ESC03 If a determination is made that on-site evaluation is required to assess compliance with the relevant standards, the assigned follow-up activity may be in the form of an on-site ESC survey rather than an ESC submission.

Note: *A written ESC submission may still be required.*

Measure of Success (MOS)

A Measure of Success (MOS) is a numerical or quantifiable measure, usually related to an audit that determines if an action was effective and sustained, due four months after Evidence of Standards Compliance approval.

An MOS for all applicable EP corrections will be required when one or more of the following conditions are met:

MOS01 An organization has submitted a successful ESC.

MOS02 Failure to demonstrate continued compliance with all not compliant standards in the first MOS submission will require the submission of a second MOS four months after official notification of the failure of the first MOS.

Note: *If the organization determines that the corrective action documented in its first ESC submission was not effective, the organization may elect to submit a second ESC that identifies new corrective action, rather than submitting a second MOS. In this case, the first MOS submission will be considered failed. If this second ESC or the second MOS fails, the organization's decision will be changed to Conditional or Preliminary Denial of Accreditation as appropriate.*

On-site MOS Survey

A four-month on-site MOS survey will be scheduled when the following condition is met:

MOS03 If a determination is made that on-site evaluation is required to assess compliance with the relevant standards, the assigned follow-up activity may be in the form of an on-site MOS survey rather than an MOS submission.

Note: *A written ESC submission may still be required.*

Preliminary Accreditation

Preliminary Accreditation will be recommended when the following condition is met:

PA01 Preliminary Accreditation will be recommended when an organization has demonstrated compliance with the selected standards used in the first of two surveys conducted under the Early Survey Policy.

Note: *The first survey is conducted using a defined subset of applicable standards. The second survey is a full survey conducted approximately six months later to allow the organization sufficient time to demonstrate a track record of performance. Preliminary Accreditation remains until the organization completes the second —that is, initial—survey.*

Accredited

Accreditation will be recommended when one or more of the following conditions are met:

A01 An organization's accreditation decision will be changed to Accredited when it is in compliance with all standards at the time of the on-site survey or has successfully addressed all Requirements for Improvement, in its first ESC submission.

Note: *Organizations that are in Provisional Accreditation as a result of a failed ESC will have their accreditation decision changed to Accredited when a second ESC submission and MOS as required has been determined to be acceptable.*

A02 An organization's accreditation decision will be changed to accredited when as a result of a Conditional Accreditation follow-up survey, all of the original Requirements for Improvement have been met.

Note: *The organization must provide evidence of standards compliance for standards, that were not the subject of the Conditional Accreditation follow-up survey, that are identified as not compliant at the time of the follow-up survey. An organization which is in Conditional Accreditation as a result of two failed ESC submissions, will have their accreditation status changed to Accredited when their MOS submission has been determined to be acceptable.*

Administrative Rules

Administrative rules will be used when one or more of the following conditions are met:

ADM01 The follow-up time frames and nature of follow-up activity for demonstrating compliance with all not compliant standards may be changed from that stated in these decision rules when the severity of the issue requires an earlier response.

ADM02 If the primary program meets a rule for Provisional Accreditation, Conditional Accreditation, or Preliminary Denial of Accreditation, the overall decision for the organization is Provisional Accreditation, Conditional Accreditation, or Preliminary Denial of Accreditation, respectively.

ADM03 If the primary or any secondary program meets a rule for Provisional Accreditation, the overall decision for the organization is Provisional Accreditation.

ADM04 If one of the secondary programs meets a rule for Preliminary Denial of Accreditation, the overall decision for the organization is Conditional Accreditation.

Note: *This rule is not applicable when the laboratory is the secondary program and the hospital is the primary program.*

ADM05 If one of the secondary programs meets a rule for Conditional Accreditation, the overall decision for the organization is Provisional Accreditation.

Note: *This rule is not applicable when the laboratory is the secondary program and the hospital is the primary program.*

ADM06 If two or more of the secondary programs meet rules for Preliminary Denial of Accreditation, the overall decision for the organization is Preliminary Denial of Accreditation.

ADM07 If two or more of the secondary programs meet rules for Conditional Accreditation, the overall decision for the organization is Conditional Accreditation.

Sentinel Event Policy Follow-up

SE01 An organization that has experienced a sentinel event subject to review under the Sentinel Event Policy is required to complete a thorough and credible root cause analysis and action plan and submit them to The Joint Commission, or otherwise provide evidence of an acceptable response to the sentinel event, in a manner and time frame acceptable to The Joint Commission as specified in the Sentinel Event Policy.

SE02 Follow-up will be scheduled, per the Sentinel Event Policy, when a sentinel event, subject to review under the Sentinel Event Policy, has occurred and The Joint Commission has determined that the organization has completed a thorough and credible root cause analysis and action plan. The purpose of the follow-up activity is to assess the implementation and effectiveness of the organization's action plan.

Review and Appeal Procedures

After any Preliminary Denial of Accreditation decision, the organization has the right to make a detailed presentation before a Review Hearing Panel. The Accreditation Committee then reviews the findings of the Review Hearing Panel and either denies accreditation to the organization or selects an appropriate alternative accreditation decision. The organization may appeal any decision of the Accreditation Committee to deny accreditation before the decision becomes the final decision of The Joint Commission.

See Figure 9 on page 89 for a visual representation of the Process Flow for Appeal of a Preliminary Denial of Accreditation Decision.

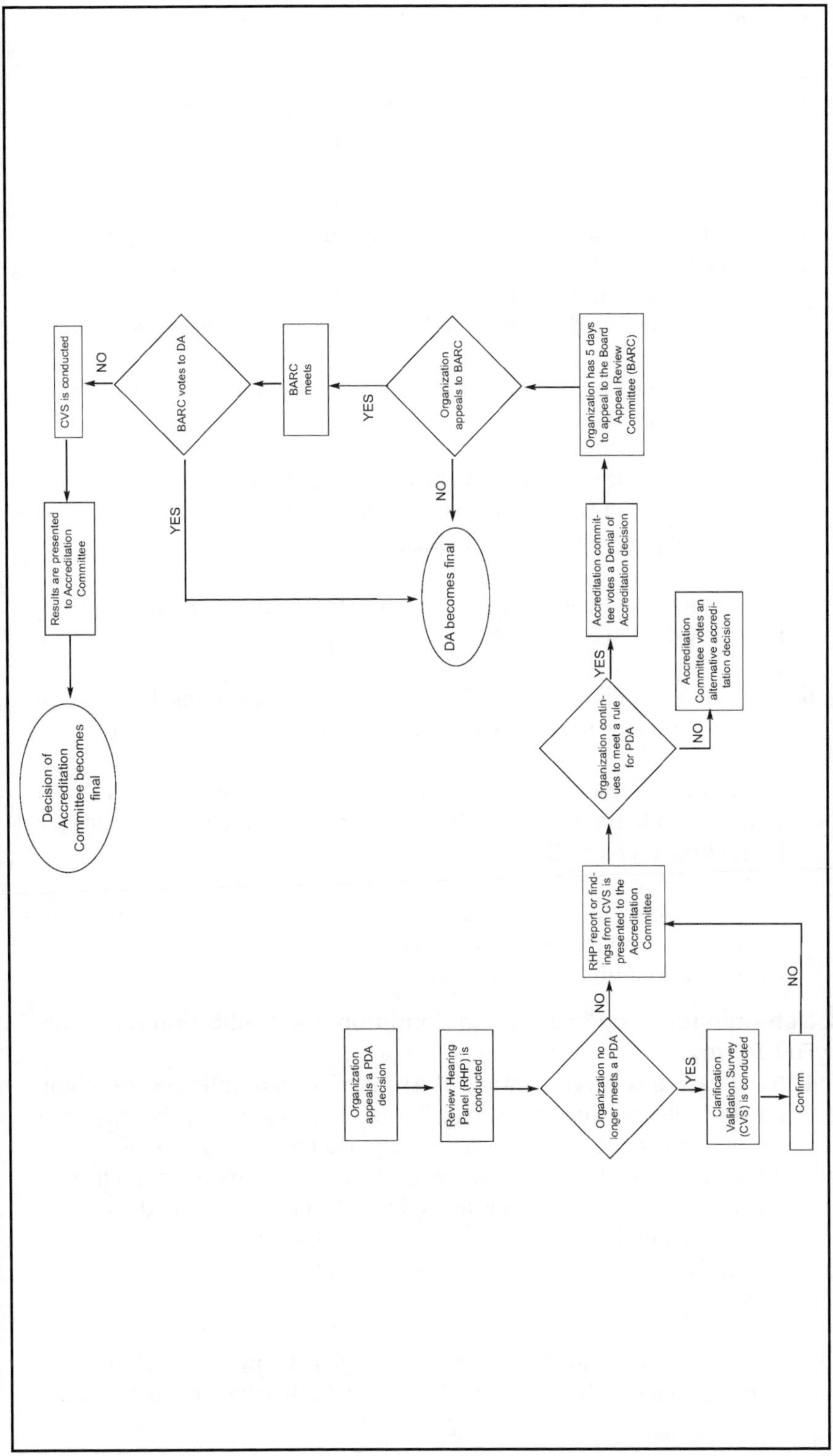

Figure 9. *Process flow for appeal of a preliminary denial of accreditation decision.*

The following outline details the review and appeal procedures:

I. Evaluation by Joint Commission Staff

A. Review and Determination by Joint Commission Staff.

Following any survey activity, The Joint Commission staff shall review survey findings, survey documents, and any other relevant materials or information received from any source. Except as provided in paragraphs I.B, I.C, and I.D, Joint Commission staff shall, in accordance with decision rules approved by the Accreditation Committee of the Board of Commissioners, do the following:

1. Determine or recommend to the Accreditation Committee that the organization be accredited, as described in paragraph VII of these procedures
   or
2. Recommend to the Accreditation Committee that the organization be conditionally accredited
   or
3. Determine that the organization be conditionally accredited, if the organization does not submit Evidence of Standards Compliance (ESC) in accordance with paragraph I.B.I.a or I.B.I.b
   or
4. Recommend to the Accreditation Committee that the organization be preliminarily denied accreditation
   or
5. Defer consideration while additional information regarding the organization's compliance status is reviewed by The Joint Commission staff
   or
6. Determine or recommend to the Accreditation Committee that the organization be preliminarily accredited in accordance with the Early Survey Policy set forth on pages 29–32
   or
7. Recommend to the Accreditation Committee that the organization be initially denied Preliminary Accreditation in accordance with the Early Survey Policy set forth on pages 29–32

B. Determination to Recommend Conditional Accreditation Based on Full Surveys.

1. **Notification to Organization of Areas of Noncompliance with Standards.** In the case of a full survey, if Joint Commission staff, based on survey findings, survey documents and any other relevant materials or information received from any source, determine to recommend that the organization be conditionally accredited, it will outline its findings and determination. The organization may do the following:
   a. Accept the findings and determination of the staff through submission of the ESC
   or
   b. Submit to The Joint Commission, through ESC any clarification of its compliance with Joint Commission standards at the time of the survey

that is not reflected in the Accreditation Survey Findings Report, along with an explanation of why such documentation was not available for review at the time of the survey

2. **Consideration of the Organization's Response.** Joint Commission staff shall review the organization's submission of any additional information and shall, in accordance with decision rules approved by the Accreditation Committee, do the following:
   a. Recommend to the Accreditation Committee that the organization be conditionally accredited
   or
   b. Recommend to the Accreditation Committee that the organization be preliminarily denied accreditation
   or
   c. Recommend to the Accreditation Committee that the organization be accredited, as described in paragraph VII of these procedures

C. Determination to Recommend that Accreditation Be Preliminarily Denied Based on Full or Other Survey Activity.

1. **Notification to Organization of Areas of Noncompliance with Standards.** In the case of a full survey, if Joint Commission staff, based on survey findings, survey documents, and any other relevant materials or information received from any source, determine, in accordance with decision rules approved by the Accreditation Committee, to recommend to the Accreditation Committee that the organization be preliminarily denied accreditation, it will outline its findings and determination. The organization may do the following:
   a. Accept the findings and determination of the staff through submission of the ESC
   or
   b. Submit to The Joint Commission, through the ESC, any clarification of its compliance with Joint Commission standards at the time of the survey that is not reflected in the Accreditation Survey Findings Report, along with an explanation of why such information was not available for review at the time of the survey
2. **Consideration of the Organization's Response.** Joint Commission staff members shall review the organization's submission of any additional information and shall, in accordance with decision rules approved by the Accreditation Committee, do the following:
   a. Recommend to the Accreditation Committee that the organization be conditionally accredited
   or
   b. Recommend to the Accreditation Committee that the organization be preliminarily denied accreditation
   or
   c. Recommend to the Accreditation Committee that the organization be accredited, as described in paragraph VII of these procedures.

D. Decisions by the President of The Joint Commission. Notwithstanding anything outlined in paragraphs I.A–I.C.1 of these procedures to the contrary, if the findings of any survey identify any condition that poses a threat to public or resident safety, the president of The Joint Commission, or, if the president is not available, a vice president of The Joint Commission designated by the president to do so, may promptly decide that the organization be immediately placed in Preliminary Denial of Accreditation. This action and the findings that led to this action shall be reported by telephone and in writing to the organization's chief executive officer and in writing to the authorities having jurisdiction. The president's or his or her designee's decision shall be promptly reviewed by the Accreditation Committee in accordance with paragraph II of these procedures.

II. Review by the Accreditation Committee

A. Scope of Review. The Accreditation Committee shall consider The Joint Commission president's, or the president's designee's, decision and Joint Commission staff's report and recommendation and may review the survey findings, survey documents, and any other relevant materials or information received from any source, including any additional information supplied by the organization in response to this information or, in the case of a Preliminary Denial of Accreditation decision by the president or his or her designee, information supplied by the organization regarding corrective actions taken in response to the identification of a serious threat to resident or public health or safety.

B. Decision. Following such consideration, the Accreditation Committee shall do the following:

1. Accredit the organization, as described in paragraph VII of these procedures
   or
2. Conditionally accredit the organization
   or
3. Preliminarily deny accreditation to the organization or confirm a decision by the president or his or her designee to preliminarily deny accreditation
   or
4. Defer consideration while additional information regarding the organization's compliance status is gathered and reviewed by Joint Commission staff
   or
5. Order a resurvey or partial resurvey of the organization and an evaluation of the results, to the extent appropriate, by The Joint Commission staff. Thereafter, Joint Commission staff shall transmit its report and recommendation to the Accreditation Committee for action, as provided in paragraph II.C of these procedures.
   or
6. Preliminarily accredit the organization
   or

7. Initially deny Preliminary Accreditation to those organizations that apply for the Early Survey Policy

C. Deferred Consideration. When the Accreditation Committee defers consideration pursuant to paragraph II.B.4 or II.B.5 of these procedures, Joint Commission staff shall review and report to the Accreditation Committee concerning the organization's compliance decision. The Accreditation Committee may order any resurvey or partial resurvey necessary to determine such decision.

Following such consideration and review, the Accreditation Committee shall do the following:

1. Accredit the organization, as described in paragraph VII of these procedures
   or
2. Conditionally accredit the organization
   or
3. Preliminarily deny accreditation or confirm a decision of the president or his or her designee to preliminarily deny accreditation to the organization
   or
4. Defer consideration while additional information regarding the organization's compliance status is gathered and reviewed by The Joint Commission staff
   or
5. Order an additional resurvey or partial resurvey of the organization and an evaluation of the results, to the extent appropriate, by The Joint Commission staff. Thereafter, Joint Commission staff shall transmit its report and recommendations to the Accreditation Committee for action, as provided in paragraph II.C of these procedures.
   or
6. Preliminarily accredit the organization
   or
7. Preliminarily deny Preliminary Accreditation to those organizations applying under the Early Survey Policy

III. Conditional Accreditation

A. Survey to Determine Implementation of the Evidence of Standards Compliance (ESC). Within approximately six months from the date the organization is notified of its Conditional Accreditation decision, The Joint Commission shall conduct a survey of the organization to determine the degree to which deficiencies have been corrected or improvements implemented, although The Joint Commission upon occasion may shorten that time period, as appropriate.

B. Review and Determination by Joint Commission Staff. Joint Commission staff shall review the survey findings, survey documents, and any other relevant materials or information received from any source. In accordance with decision rules approved by the Accreditation Committee, The Joint Commission staff shall do the following:

1. Determine or recommend to the Accreditation Committee that the organization be accredited, as described in paragraph VII of these procedures
   or
2. Recommend to the Accreditation Committee that the organization be preliminarily denied accreditation
   or
3. Defer consideration while additional information regarding the organization's compliance status is gathered and reviewed by The Joint Commission staff. At the conclusion of this review, one of the recommendations outlined in paragraph III.C of these procedures shall be made to the Accreditation Committee.

C. **Action by the Accreditation Committee.** Following review of the recommendations of The Joint Commission staff, the Accreditation Committee shall do the following:
1. Accredit the organization, as described in paragraph VII of these procedures
   or
2. Preliminarily deny accreditation to the organization
   or
3. Defer consideration while additional information regarding the organization's compliance status is gathered and reviewed by The Joint Commission staff
   or
4. Order a resurvey or partial resurvey of the organization and an evaluation of the results, to the extent appropriate, by The Joint Commission staff. Thereafter, Joint Commission staff shall transmit its report and recommendation to the Accreditation Committee for action, as provided in paragraph III.C of these procedures.

D. **Charges to the Organization.** The full costs of the Conditional Accreditation process shall be paid by the organization that receives Conditional Accreditation.

IV. Review Hearing Panels

A. **Right to a Hearing Before a Review Hearing Panel.** An organization that has been preliminarily denied accreditation* or initially denied Preliminary Accreditation pursuant to paragraph II.B.3, II.B.7, II.C.3, II.C.7, or III.C.2 of these procedures is entitled to a hearing in which to make a detailed presentation before a Review Hearing Panel if The Joint Commission receives the organization's written request for the hearing within five business days after the organization receives the written notice of the Accreditation Committee's decision, including confirmation of a decision by the president, or his or her designee, to preliminarily deny accreditation, as provided in paragraph I.D of these procedures. A Review Hearing Panel shall be composed of two health

* The Preliminary Denial of Accreditation decision, if subsequently changed to other than Denial of Accreditation, following review and action by the Accreditation Committee, is no longer disclosable as part of the organization's accreditation decision history.

care professionals not on the Accreditation Committee and one member of the Accreditation Committee who is familiar with the organization's decision.

B. Notice of the Time and Place of the Presentation Before a Review Hearing Panel. The presentation before the Review Hearing Panel shall be held at The Joint Commission's headquarters except when the president of The Joint Commission, or his or her designee, determines otherwise for good cause shown. At least 30 calendar days before the presentation, The Joint Commission shall send the organization written notice of the time and place of the hearing and copies of any supplemental materials or information received from any source that the organization does not already have and that may affect any accreditation decision. The notice shall advise the organization of the agenda to be followed and, if feasible, of the identity and professional qualifications of the panel members. At least 10 calendar days before the scheduled hearing date, the organization must submit to The Joint Commission any materials it wishes to be considered by the Review Hearing Panel.

C. Procedure for the Conduct of a Hearing. A Review Hearing Panel may proceed with only two of the three panel members present, provided one of them is the member of the Accreditation Committee. Representatives of the organization may make oral and written presentations and may be accompanied by legal counsel. The organization's representatives may present information relevant to the facts at the time of survey to the panel members. Presentations or information concerning actions taken by the organization subsequent to the survey upon which the Preliminary Denial of Accreditation decision was based are not considered relevant to the validity of the decision. A Joint Commission surveyor who participated in the survey will ordinarily appear at the hearing.

D. Report of Review Hearing Panel. After a hearing has been completed, the Review Hearing Panel shall review the facts regarding the original Preliminary Denial of Accreditation decision. The panel will submit a written report of its findings on factual matters for consideration by the Accreditation Committee. The Joint Commission shall send the organization a copy of the report of the Review Hearing Panel at least 15 calendar days before the meeting of the Accreditation Committee at which the report will be considered. The notice shall inform the organization of the meeting date and of the organization's right to submit written responses or comments for consideration by the Accreditation Committee. Any such written responses or comments must be received by The Joint Commission at least 10 calendar days before the meeting of the Accreditation Committee.

E. Charges to the Organization. The organization will be charged a nominal fee for the conduct of a Review Hearing Panel.

V. Second Consideration by the Accreditation Committee

A. Scope of Review. The report of the Review Hearing Panel shall be considered by the Accreditation Committee.

B. Decision. Following such consideration, the Accreditation Committee shall do the following:

1. Accredit or preliminarily accredit the organization, as described in paragraph VII of these procedures
   or
2. Conditionally accredit the organization
   or
3. Deny accreditation to the organization
   or
4. Defer consideration while additional information regarding the organization's compliance status is gathered and reviewed by Joint Commission staff
   or
5. Order a resurvey or partial resurvey of the organization and an evaluation of the results, to the extent appropriate, by The Joint Commission staff

VI. Review by the Board Appeal Review Committee

A. Review Request. An organization that has been denied accreditation or Preliminary Accreditation pursuant to paragraph V.B.3 of these procedures is entitled to request a review of the decision by the Board Appeal Review Committee if The Joint Commission receives the organization's request for review within five business days after the organization receives the written notice of the Accreditation Committee's decision. The Board Appeal Review Committee is composed of four members of the Board of Commissioners who are not members of the Accreditation Committee.

B. Notice of Time and Procedure for Review. The Joint Commission shall send the organization a copy of the report of the Review Hearing Panel at least 20 business days before the meeting of the Board Appeal Review Committee at which the organization's request for review will be considered. Two members of the Board Appeal Review Committee will constitute a quorum. This meeting will generally be held by telephone conference, except when it is held in conjunction with meetings of the Board of Commissioners or other committee(s) of the Board of Commissioners. The organization must submit any materials that it wishes the Board Appeal Review Committee to consider at least 10 calendar days before the scheduled meeting date. The Board Appeal Review Committee shall review the decision of the Accreditation Committee, which considered the report of the Review Hearing Panel, and any written materials submitted by the organization, and shall do one of the following:

1. Deny accreditation or Preliminary Accreditation to the organization, after finding that there is substantial evidence to support the Accreditation Committee's decision

or

2. Make an independent evaluation of the Accreditation Committee's decision and then decide to conditionally accredit, preliminarily accredit, or accredit the organization, as described in paragraph VII of these procedures

The action taken by the Board Appeal Review Committee shall constitute the final accreditation decision of The Joint Commission.

C. Participation. No member of the Accreditation Committee or of the Review Hearing Panel who participated in an accreditation decision or review of findings on factual matters concerning an organization shall participate in any deliberations or vote of the Board Appeal Review Committee in its review of that accreditation decision or report of findings on factual matters. This provision shall not preclude any commissioner who participated in a review hearing as a member of the Review Hearing Panel from presenting and responding to questions about the report of that Review Hearing Panel to the Board Appeal Review Committee.

VII. Procedure Relating to Not Compliant Standards and Determination of Corrected Not Compliant Standards

A. A decision of The Joint Commission staff pursuant to paragraph I.A.1, I.B.2.c, or I.C.2.c of these procedures, of the Accreditation Committee pursuant to paragraph II.B.1, II.C.1, or III.C.1 of these procedures, or of a Board Appeal Review Committee, as provided in paragraph VI.B of these procedures, to accredit an organization may be made contingent upon satisfactory correction of not compliant standards or, when appropriate, upon compliance with interim life safety measures. The organization may be conditionally accredited or its accreditation may be withdrawn if it does not correct or document the correction of the specified not compliant standards within the time specified in the notice of the decision to the organization, or, when applicable, fails to demonstrate compliance with the interim life safety measures. Joint Commission staff, through the use of surveys or partial surveys or through other means, such as ESC and MOS, shall determine whether the organization has corrected the not compliant standards within the time provided or, when applicable, has demonstrated compliance with interim life safety measures, and shall report its findings to the organization. If The Joint Commission staff determines that the organization has not corrected the not compliant standards within the time provided or, when applicable, has not demonstrated compliance with interim life safety measures, the organization's status will change to Provisional Accreditation. The Joint Commission shall report its findings to the organization, and, after reviewing any comments of the organization, as appropriate and in accordance with decision rules approved by the Accreditation Committee, do the following:

1. Provide another opportunity to the organization to correct or document the correction of not compliant standards, as provided in any applicable decision rules approved by the Accreditation Committee

or

2. Determine or recommend that the organization be placed in Conditional Accreditation status with a conditional follow-up survey in approximately four months or other time, as appropriate
   or
3. Recommend to the Accreditation Committee that the organization be preliminarily denied accreditation, if certain not compliant standards, specified in decision rules approved by the Accreditation Committee, have not been corrected or the correction of which has not been documented after the specified number of opportunities given to the organization to do so, and, when applicable and as specified in decision rules approved by the Accreditation Committee, the organization has failed to demonstrate compliance with interim life safety measures

B. If The Joint Commission staff determines to recommend to the Accreditation Committee that the organization be preliminarily denied accreditation in accordance with paragraph VII.A.3, or be conditionally accredited in accordance with VII.A.2, the staff shall submit its recommendation and any comments of the organization to the Accreditation Committee for action, as provided in paragraph II.B.1 through II.B.7.

VIII. Final Accreditation Decision

A. The action taken by The Joint Commission staff shall constitute the final decision of The Joint Commission to do the following:

1. Accredit the organization, when taken pursuant to paragraph I.A.1, I.B.2.c, or I.C.2.c of these procedures
   or
2. Conditionally accredit the organization, when taken pursuant to paragraph I.A.3 or VII.A.2 of these procedures
   or
3. Preliminarily accredit the organization, when taken pursuant to paragraph I.A.6 of these procedures

B. The action taken by the Accreditation Committee shall constitute the final decision of The Joint Commission to do the following:

1. Accredit the organization, when taken pursuant to paragraph II.B.1, II.C.1, or III.C.1 of these procedures
   or
2. Conditionally accredit the organization, when taken pursuant to paragraph II.B.2 or II.C.2 of these procedures
   or
3. Deny accreditation to the organization, when taken pursuant to paragraph II.B.3, II.C.3, III.C.2, or VII.B of these procedures, and the organization does not request the opportunity to make a presentation before a Review Hearing Panel pursuant to paragraph IV.A of these procedures
   or
4. Preliminarily accredit the organization, when taken pursuant to paragraph II.B.6 of these procedures

or

5. Deny Preliminary Accreditation to the organization, when taken pursuant to paragraph II.B.7 of these procedures, and the organization applying for the Early Survey Policy does not request the opportunity to make a presentation before a Review Hearing Panel pursuant to paragraph IV.A of these procedures

C. The action taken by the Board Appeal Review Committee shall constitute the final decision of The Joint Commission to do the following:

1. Accredit the organization, conditionally accredit the organization, or deny accreditation, when taken pursuant to paragraph VI.B of these procedures

IX. Status of the Organization Pending a Final Decision and Effective Date of a Final Decision

A. The accreditation status of an accredited organization shall continue in effect pending any final accreditation decision.

B. A final decision to accredit, preliminarily accredit, or conditionally accredit an organization that follows an initial Accreditation Committee decision of Preliminary Denial of Accreditation pursuant to paragraph II.B shall be considered effective as of the first day after completion of the organization's survey from which the decision results.

C. A final decision to deny accreditation or Provisional Accreditation to an organization shall become effective as follows:

1. As of the date of the decision made by the Board Appeal Review Committee pursuant to paragraph VI.B of these procedures

   or

2. At the expiration of the time during which an organization may, but does not, request a review by the Board Appeal Review Committee, pursuant to paragraph VI.A of these procedures

   or

3. At the expiration of the time during which an organization may, but does not, request the opportunity to make a presentation before a Review Hearing Panel pursuant to paragraph IV.A of these procedures

   or

4. On receipt by The Joint Commission, before a final decision, of notification from the organization that it withdraws its request for review of a Preliminary Denial of Accreditation decision before a Review Hearing Panel or its request for appeal of a Denial of Accreditation decision before the Board Appeal Review Committee

X. Notice

Any notice required by these accreditation procedures to be given to an organization shall be addressed to the organization at its post office address as shown in Joint Commission records and shall be sent to the organization by certified letter as forwarded by a recognized package delivery service. Any notice required to be given to The Joint Commission by the organization shall be sent by the organization in the same manner and shall be addressed to the Office of the Executive Vice President for Accreditation Operations, Joint Commission on Accreditation of Healthcare Organizations, One Renaissance Boulevard, Oakbrook Terrace, IL 60181.

2009

SLTC

Sentinel Events (SE)

SE

SE

Sentinel Events

I. Sentinel Events

In support of its mission to continuously improve the safety and quality of health care provided to the public, The Joint Commission reviews organizations' activities in response to sentinel events in its accreditation process, including all full accreditation surveys and random unannounced surveys, and, as appropriate, for-cause surveys.

- A sentinel event is an unexpected occurrence involving death or serious physical or psychological injury, or the risk thereof. Serious injury specifically includes loss of limb or function. The phrase *or the risk thereof* includes any process variation for which a recurrence would carry a significant chance of a serious adverse outcome.
- Such events are called *sentinel* because they signal the need for immediate investigation and response.
- The terms *sentinel event* and *medical error* are not synonymous; not all sentinel events occur because of an error, and not all errors result in sentinel events.

II. Goals of the Sentinel Event Policy

The policy has four goals:

1. To have a positive impact in improving resident care, treatment, and services and preventing sentinel events
2. To focus the attention of an organization that has experienced a sentinel event on understanding the causes that underlie the event and on changing the organization's systems and processes to reduce the probability of such an event in the future
3. To increase the general knowledge about sentinel events, their causes, and strategies for prevention
4. To maintain the confidence of the public and accredited organizations in the accreditation process

III. Standards Relating to Sentinel Events

Standards

Each Joint Commission accreditation manual contains standards in the "Improving Organization Performance" (PI) and "Leadership" (LD) chapters that relate specifically to the management of sentinel events.

Organization-Specific Definition of *Sentinel Event*

LD.04.04.05, EPs 7 and 8, requires each accredited organization to define *sentinel event* for its own purposes in establishing mechanisms to identify, report, and manage these events. While this definition must be consistent with the general definition of sentinel event as published by the Joint Commission, accredited organizations have some latitude in setting more specific parameters to define *unexpected, serious,* and *the risk thereof.* At a minimum, an organization's definition must include those events that are subject to review under the Sentinel Event Policy, as defined in Section IV of this chapter.

Expectations Under the Standards for an Organization's Response to a Sentinel Event

Accredited organizations are expected to identify and respond appropriately to all sentinel events (as defined by the organization in accordance with the preceding paragraph) occurring in the organization or associated with services that the organization provides or provides for. Appropriate response includes conducting a timely, thorough, and credible root cause analysis; developing an action plan designed to implement improvements to reduce risk; implementing the improvements; and monitoring the effectiveness of those improvements.

Root Cause Analysis

Root cause analysis is a process for identifying the basic or causal factors that underlie variation in performance, including the occurrence or possible occurrence of a sentinel event. A root cause analysis focuses primarily on systems and processes, not on individual performance. It progresses from special causes* in clinical processes to common causes† in organizational processes and systems and identifies potential improvements in processes or systems that tend to decrease the likelihood of such events in the future or determines, after analysis, that no such improvement opportunities exist.

Action Plan

The product of a root cause analysis is an action plan that identifies the strategies that the organization intends to implement to reduce the risk of similar events occurring in the future. The plan should address responsibility for implementation, oversight, pilot testing as appropriate, time lines, and strategies for measuring the effectiveness of the actions.

Survey Process

When conducting an accreditation survey, The Joint Commission seeks to evaluate the organization's compliance with the applicable standards and to score those standards based on performance throughout the organization over time (for example, the preceding 12 months for a full accreditation survey or the preceding 4 months for an initial survey). Surveyors are instructed not to seek out specific sentinel events beyond those already known to The Joint Commission.

If, in the course of conducting the usual survey activities, a sentinel event is identified, the surveyor will take the following steps:

- Inform the CEO that the event has been identified
- Inform the CEO the event will be reported to The Joint Commission for further review and follow-up under the provisions of the Sentinel Event Policy

---

* **Special cause** is a factor that intermittently and unpredictably induces variation over and above what is inherent in the system. It often appears as an extreme point (such as a point beyond the control limits on a control chart) or some specific, identifiable pattern in data.

† **Common cause** is a factor that results from variation inherent in the process or system. The risk of a common cause can be reduced by redesigning the process or system.

During the on-site survey, the surveyor(s) will assess the organization's compliance with sentinel event–related standards in the following ways:

- Review the organization's process for responding to a sentinel event
- Interview the organization's leaders and staff about their expectations and responsibilities for identifying, reporting, and responding to sentinel events
- Ask for an example of a root cause analysis that has been conducted in the past year to assess the adequacy of the organization's process for responding to a sentinel event. Additional examples may be reviewed, if needed, to more fully assess the organization's understanding of, and ability to conduct, root cause analyses. In selecting an example, the organization may choose a "closed case" or a "near miss"* to demonstrate its process for responding to a sentinel event.

IV. Reviewable Sentinel Events

Definition of Occurrences That Are Subject to Review by the Joint Commission Under the Sentinel Event Policy

The definition of a reviewable sentinel event takes into account a wide array of occurrences applicable to a wide variety of health care organizations. Any or all occurrences might apply to a particular type of health care organization. Thus, not all of the following occurrences might apply to your particular organization. The subset of sentinel events that is subject to review by the Joint Commission includes any occurrence that meets any of the following criteria:

- The event has resulted in an unanticipated death or major permanent loss of function, not related to the natural course of the resident's illness or underlying condition†‡

  or
- The event is one of the following (even if the outcome was not death or major permanent loss of function unrelated to the natural course of the resident's illness or underlying condition):
  - Suicide of any resident receiving care, treatment, or services in a staffed around-the-clock care setting or within 72 hours of discharge
  - Unanticipated death of a full-term infant

---

* **Near miss** Used to describe any process variation that did not affect an outcome but for which a recurrence carries a significant chance of a serious adverse outcome. Such a near miss falls within the scope of the definition of a sentinel event but outside the scope of those sentinel events that are subject to review by The Joint Commission under its Sentinel Event Policy.

† A distinction is made between an adverse outcome that is primarily related to the natural course of the resident's illness or underlying condition (not reviewed under the Sentinel Event Policy) and a death or major permanent loss of function that is associated with the treatment (including "recognized complications") or lack of treatment of that condition, or otherwise not clearly and primarily related to the natural course of the resident's illness or underlying condition (reviewable). In indeterminate cases, the event will be presumed reviewable and the organization's response will be reviewed under the Sentinel Event Policy according to the prescribed procedures and time frames without delay for additional information such as autopsy results.

‡ *Major permanent loss of function* means sensory, motor, physiologic, or intellectual impairment not present on admission requiring continued treatment or life-style change. When major permanent loss of function cannot be immediately determined, applicability of the policy is not established until either the resident is discharged with continued major loss of function, or two weeks have elapsed with persistent major loss of function, whichever occurs first.

- Abduction of any resident receiving care, treatment, or services
- Discharge of an infant to the wrong family
- Rape*
- Hemolytic transfusion reaction involving administration of blood or blood products having major blood group incompatibilities
- Surgery on the wrong resident or wrong body part†
- Unintended retention of a foreign object in a resident after surgery or other procedure
- Severe neonatal hyperbilirubinemia (bilirubin >30 milligrams/deciliter)
- Prolonged fluoroscopy with cumulative dose >1500 rads to a single field or any delivery of radiotherapy to the wrong body region or >25% above the planned radiotherapy dose

Examples of reviewable sentinel events and nonreviewable events are provided in Table 1 (*see* page 105).

How the Joint Commission Becomes Aware of a Sentinel Event

Each organization is encouraged, but not required, to report to the Joint Commission any sentinel event meeting the preceding criteria for reviewable sentinel events. Alternatively, the Joint Commission might become aware of a sentinel event by some other means such as communication from a resident, a family member, an employee of the organization, a surveyor, or through the media.

Reasons for Reporting a Sentinel Event to the Joint Commission

Although self-reporting a sentinel event is not required and there is no difference in the expected response, time frames, or review procedures, whether the organization voluntarily reports the event or the Joint Commission becomes aware of the event by some other means, there are several advantages to an organization that self-reports a sentinel event:

- Reporting the event enables the addition of the "lessons learned" section to the Joint Commission's Sentinel Event Database, thereby contributing to the general knowledge about sentinel events and to the reduction of risk for such events in many other organizations.
- Early reporting provides an opportunity for consultation with Joint Commission staff during the development of the root cause analysis and action plan.

---

* *Rape*, as a reviewable sentinel event, is defined as unconsented sexual contact involving a resident and another resident, staff member, or other perpetrator while being treated or on the premises of the health care organization, including oral, vaginal, or anal penetration or fondling of the resident's sex organ(s) by another individual's hand, sex organ, or object. One or more of the following must be present to determine reviewability:

- Any staff-witnessed sexual contact as described above
- Sufficient clinical evidence obtained by the organization to support allegations of unconsented sexual contact
- Admission by the perpetrator that sexual contact, as described above, occurred on the premises

† All events of surgery on the wrong resident or wrong body part are reviewable under the policy, regardless of the magnitude of the procedure or the outcome.

Table 1. Examples of Sentinel Events That Are Reviewable and Events That Are Not Reviewable Under The Joint Commission's Sentinel Events Policy*

Examples of Sentinel Events That Are Reviewable Under the Joint Commission's Sentinel Event Policy

Any resident death, paralysis, coma, or other major permanent loss of function associated with a medication error.

A resident commits suicide within 72 hours of being discharged from an organization setting that provides staffed around-the-clock care.

Any elopement, that is, unauthorized departure, of a resident from an around-the-clock care setting resulting in a temporally related death (suicide, accidental death, or homicide) or major permanent loss of function.

An organization operates on the wrong side of the resident's body.

Any intrapartum (related to the birth process) maternal death.

Any perinatal death unrelated to a congenital condition in an infant having a birth weight greater than 2500 grams.

A resident is abducted from the organization where he or she receives care, treatment, or services.

Assault, homicide, or other crime resulting in resident death or major permanent loss of function.

A resident fall that results in death or major permanent loss of function as a direct result of the injuries sustained in the fall.

Hemolytic transfusion reaction involving major blood group incompatibilities.

A foreign body, such as a sponge or forceps, that was left in a resident after surgery.

> **Note:** An adverse outcome that is *directly related* to the natural course of the resident's illness or underlying condition, for example, terminal illness present at the time of presentation, is *not* reportable *except* for suicide in, or following elopement from, a 24-hour care setting (see above).

Examples of Events That Are Not Reviewable Under the Joint Commission's Sentinel Event Policy

Any "near miss."

Full or expected return of limb or bodily function to the same level as prior to the adverse event by discharge or within two weeks of the initial loss of said function.

Any sentinel event that has not affected a recipient of care (patient, client, resident).

Medication errors that do not result in death or major permanent loss of function.

(continued on next page)

Table 1. Examples of Sentinel Events That Are Reviewable and Events That Are Not Reviewable Under The Joint Commission's Sentinel Events Policy *(continued)*

Suicide other than in an around-the-clock care setting or following elopement from such a setting.

A death or loss of function following a discharge against medical advice (AMA).

Unsuccessful suicide attempts unless resulting in major permanent loss of function.

Minor degrees of hemolysis not caused by a major blood group incompatibility and with no clinical sequelae.

> **Note:** In the context of its performance improvement activities, an organization may choose to conduct intensive assessment, for example, root cause analysis, for some nonreviewable events. Please refer to the "Improving Organization Performance" chapter.

* **Note:** *This list might not apply to all settings.*

- The organization's message to the public that it is doing everything possible to ensure that such an event does not happen again is strengthened by its acknowledged collaboration with the Joint Commission to understand how the event happened and what can be done to reduce the risk of such an event in the future.

Required Response to a Reviewable Sentinel Event

If the Joint Commission becomes aware (either through voluntary self-reporting or otherwise) of a sentinel event that meets the preceding criteria (*see* page 103) and the event has occurred in an accredited organization, the organization is expected to do the following:

- Prepare a thorough and credible root cause analysis and action plan within 45 calendar days of the event or of becoming aware of the event
- Submit to the Joint Commission its root cause analysis and action plan, or otherwise provide for Joint Commission evaluation of its response to the sentinel event under an approved protocol (*see* Section VI), within 45 calendar days of the known occurrence of the event

The Joint Commission will then determine whether the root cause analysis and action plan are acceptable. If the determination that an event is reviewable under the Sentinel Event Policy occurs more than 45 calendar days following the known occurrence of the event, the organization will be allowed 15 calendar days for its response. If the organization fails to submit an acceptable root cause analysis within the 45 calendar days (or within 15 calendar days, if the 45 calendar days have already elapsed), the following consequences will result (depending on the length of time the organization fails to submit a root cause analysis):

- If the organization has failed to submit a root cause analysis within an additional 30 days following its due date, its accreditation decision will automatically be changed to Provisional Accreditation, and both the organization and the Accreditation Committee will be notified.
- If the organization has failed to submit a root cause analysis within 60 days following its due date, its accreditation decision will automatically be changed to Conditional Accreditation, and both the organization and the Accreditation Committee will be notified.
- If the organization then continues to fail to submit a root cause analysis for 90 days following its due date, a recommendation for Denial of Accreditation will be presented to the Accreditation Committee. The organization would then be given the opportunity to submit a response to the Accreditation Committee. However, if the committee were to reach a Denial of Accreditation decision because the organization has failed to submit any root cause analysis, the organization would not have access to the appeals process.

Please note that an organization that experiences a sentinel event as defined by the organization but that does not meet the criteria for review under the Sentinel Event Policy is still expected to complete a root cause analysis (as required by standard LD.04.04.05) but does not need to submit it to The Joint Commission.

Review of Root Cause Analyses and Action Plans

A root cause analysis will be considered *acceptable* if it has the following characteristics:

- The analysis focuses primarily on systems and processes, not on individual performance.
- The analysis progresses from special causes in clinical processes to common causes in organizational processes.
- The analysis repeatedly digs deeper by asking "Why?"; then, when answered, "Why?" again, and so on.
- The analysis identifies changes that could be made in systems and processes (either through redesign or development of new systems or processes), which would reduce the risk of such events occurring in the future.
- The analysis is thorough and credible.

To be *thorough,* the root cause analysis must include the following:

- A determination of the human and other factors most directly associated with the sentinel event and the process(es) and systems related to its occurrence
- An analysis of the underlying systems and processes through a series of "Why?" questions to determine where redesign might reduce risk
- An inquiry into all areas appropriate to the specific type of event, as described in Table 2 (*see* page 108)
- An identification of risk points and their potential contributions to this type of event
- A determination of potential improvement in processes or systems that would tend to decrease the likelihood of such events in the future, or a determination, after analysis, that no such improvement opportunities exist

Table 2. Minimum Scope of Root Cause Analysis for Specific Types of Sentinel Events

Detailed inquiry into these areas is expected when conducting a root cause analysis for the specified type of sentinel event. Inquiry into areas not checked (or listed) should be conducted as appropriate to the specific event under review.

	Suicide (24-Hour Care)	Medication Error	Procedural Complication	Wrong-Site Surgery	Treatment Delay	Restraint Death	Elopement Death	Assault/Rape/Homicide	Transfusion Death	Patient Abduction	Unanticipated Death of Full-Term Infant	Unintended Retention of Foreign Body	Fall Related
Behavioral assessment process*	X					X	X	X					
Physical assessment process†	X	X	X	X	X	X	X				X		X
Individual identification process		X		X					X				
Individual observation procedures	X				X	X	X	X	X		X		X
Care planning process	X		X			X	X				X		X
Continuum of care	X	X			X	X							X
Staffing levels	X	X	X	X	X	X	X	X	X	X		X	X
Orientation and training of staff	X	X	X	X	X	X	X	X	X	X	X	X	X
Competency assessment/ credentialing	X	X	X	X	X	X	X	X	X	X	X	X	X
Supervision of staff‡	X	X	X		X	X			X			X	
Communication with individual/ family	X	X		X	X	X	X			X			X
Communication among staff members	X	X	X	X	X	X	X	X	X	X	X	X	X
Availability of information	X	X	X	X	X	X			X		X		X
Adequacy of technological support		X	X										
Equipment maintenance/ management		X	X		X	X					X		X
Physical environment§	X	X	X	X		X	X	X	X	X			X
Security systems and processes	X						X	X		X			
Medication management‖		X	X		X				X		X		X

* Includes the process for assessing individual's risk to self (and to others, in cases of assault, rape, or homicide where an individual is the assailant).

† Includes search for contraband.

‡ Includes supervision of physicians-in-training.

§ Includes furnishings; hardware (for example, bars, hooks, rods); lighting; distractions.

‖ Includes selection and procurement; storage; ordering and transcribing; preparing and dispensing; administration; and monitoring.

To be *credible,* the root cause analysis must do the following:

- Include participation by the leadership of the organization and by individuals most closely involved in the processes and systems under review
- Be internally consistent (that is, not contradict itself or leave obvious questions unanswered)
- Provide an explanation for all findings of "not applicable" or "no problem"
- Include consideration of any relevant literature

An action plan will be considered *acceptable* if it does the following:

- Identifies changes that can be implemented to reduce risk or formulates a rationale for not undertaking such changes
- Identifies, in situations where improvement actions are planned, who is responsible for implementation, when the action will be implemented (including any pilot testing), and how the effectiveness of the actions will be evaluated

All root cause analyses and action plans will be considered and treated as confidential by the Joint Commission. A detailed listing of the minimum scope of root cause analysis for specific types of sentinel events is included in Table 2.

Follow-up Activities

After The Joint Commission has determined that an organization has conducted an acceptable root cause analysis and developed an acceptable action plan, The Joint Commission will notify it that the root cause analysis and action plan are acceptable and will assign an appropriate follow-up activity, typically one or more sentinel event Measures of Success (SE MOS) due in four months. (*See* page 112 for more details.)

V. The Sentinel Event Database

To achieve the third goal of the Sentinel Event Policy, "to increase the general knowledge about sentinel events, their causes, and strategies for prevention," The Joint Commission collects and analyzes data from the review of sentinel events, root cause analyses, action plans, and follow-up activities. These data and information form the content of The Joint Commission's Sentinel Event Database.

The Joint Commission is committed to developing, maintaining, and using this Sentinel Event Database in a fashion that protects the confidentiality of the organization, the caregiver, and the resident. Included in this database are three major categories of data elements:

1. Sentinel event data
2. Root cause data
3. Risk reduction data

Deidentified aggregate data relating to root causes and risk reduction strategies for sentinel events that occur with significant frequency will form the basis for future error-prevention advice to organizations through *Sentinel Event Alert* and other media. The Sentinel Event Database is also a major component of the evidence base for the National Patient Safety Goals.

VI. Procedures for Implementing the Sentinel Event Policy

Voluntary Self-Reporting of Reviewable Sentinel Events to the Joint Commission

If an organization wishes to report an occurrence in the subset of sentinel events that are subject to review by The Joint Commission, the organization will be asked to complete a form accessible through its extranet home page. From the home page, select "Self Report Sentinel Event" from the "Continuous Compliance Tools" section.

Each organization is encouraged, but not required, to report to The Joint Commission any sentinel event meeting the preceding criteria for reviewable sentinel events. Alternatively, The Joint Commission may become aware of a sentinel event by some other means, such as communication from a patient, a family member, an employee of the organization, a surveyor, or the media.

Reviewable Sentinel Events That Are Not Reported by the Organization

If The Joint Commission becomes aware of a sentinel event subject to review under the Sentinel Event Policy that was not reported to The Joint Commission by the organization, the CEO of the organization is contacted, and a preliminary assessment of the sentinel event is made. An event that occurred more than one year before the date The Joint Commission became aware of the event will not, in most cases, be reviewed under the Sentinel Event Policy. In such a case, a written response will be requested from the organization, including a summary of processes in place to prevent similar occurrences.

Determination That a Sentinel Event Is Reviewable Under the Sentinel Event Policy

Based on available factual information received about the event, Joint Commission staff will apply the preceding definition (page 101) to determine whether an event is reviewable under the Sentinel Event Policy. Challenges to a determination that an event is reviewable will be resolved through consultation with senior Joint Commission staff.

Initial On-Site Review of a Sentinel Event

An initial on-site review of a sentinel event will usually not be conducted unless it is determined that there is a potential ongoing immediate threat to resident health or safety or potentially significant noncompliance with Joint Commission standards. Immediate Threat to Health and Safety incidents include situations in which the organization's noncompliance with one or more standards has caused, or is likely to cause, serious injury, harm, impairment, or death to a resident and is likely to continue. Complaints are assigned this priority if the information indicates immediate corrective action is necessary. All are immediately referred to Joint Commission Executive Leadership for authorization to conduct an unannounced for-cause survey. If an on-site (for-cause) review is conducted, the organization will be billed an appropriate amount based on the established fee schedule to cover the costs of conducting such a survey.

Disclosable Information

If The Joint Commission receives an inquiry about the accreditation decision of an organization that has experienced a reviewable sentinel event, the organization's accreditation decision will be reported in the usual manner, without making reference to the sentinel event. If the inquirer specifically references the specific sentinel event, The Joint Commission will acknowledge that it is aware of the event and currently is working or has worked with the organization through the sentinel event review process.

Submission of Root Cause Analysis and Action Plan

An organization that experiences a sentinel event subject to the Sentinel Event Policy is asked to submit two documents: (1) the complete root cause analysis, including its findings, and (2) the resulting action plan that describes the organization's risk reduction strategies and measures for evaluating their effectiveness. This information will be submitted to The Joint Commission Central Office, using an online root cause analysis collection tool, also accessible from the "Continuous Compliance Tools" section of the extranet home page, under the "Sentinel Event Activities" link.

The root cause analysis and action plan are not to include the name(s) of caregivers and residents involved in the sentinel event.

Alternatively, if the organization has concerns about waivers of confidentiality protections as a result of sending the root cause analysis documents to The Joint Commission, the following alternative approaches to a review of the organization's response to the sentinel event are acceptable:

1. A review of the root cause analysis and action plan documents brought to Joint Commission headquarters by organization staff and taken back to the organization on the same day. (This meeting is arranged by appointment only.)
2. An on-site visit by a specially trained surveyor to review the root cause analysis and action plan.
3. An on-site visit by a specially trained surveyor to review the root cause analysis and findings without directly viewing the root cause analysis documents through a series of interviews and a review of relevant documentation. For purposes of this review activity, *relevant documentation* includes, at a minimum, any documentation relevant to the organization's process for responding to sentinel events, the resident's medical record, and the action plan resulting from the analysis of the subject sentinel event. The latter serves as the basis for appropriate follow-up activity.
4. When the organization affirms that it meets specified criteria respecting the risk of waiving confidentiality protections for root cause analysis information shared with The Joint Commission, an on-site visit by a specially trained surveyor is conducted to do the following:
   a. Interview and review relevant documentation, including the resident's medical record, to obtain information about the following:
      - The process the organization uses in responding to sentinel events
      - The relevant policies and procedures preceding and following the organization's review of the specific event and the implementation thereof, sufficient to permit inferences about the adequacy of the organization's response to the sentinel event
   b. A standards-based survey that traces a resident's care, treatment, and services and the organization management functions relevant to the sentinel event under review*

Any one of the four alternatives will result in a charge to the organization sufficient to cover the average direct costs of the visit. Inquiries about the fee should be directed to The Joint Commission's Pricing Unit at 630/792-5115.

* For more information about the tracer methodology, *see* "The Accreditation Process," chapter, pages 53–56.

The Joint Commission must receive a request for review of an organization's response to a sentinel event using any of these alternative approaches within at least five business days of the self-report of a reviewable event or of the initial communication by The Joint Commission to the organization that it has become aware of a reviewable sentinel event.

The Joint Commission's Response

Joint Commission staff assess the acceptability of the organization's response to the reviewable sentinel event, including the thoroughness and credibility of any root cause analysis information reviewed and the organization's action plan. If the root cause analysis and action plan are found to be thorough and credible, the response will be accepted, and one or more SE MOS will be assigned (*see* below for more details).

If the response is unacceptable, staff will provide consultation to the organization on the criteria that have not yet been met and will allow an additional 15 calendar days beyond the original submission period for the organization to resubmit its response.

If the response does not meet established criteria, the organization's accreditation decision automatically will be changed to Provisional Accreditation, and both the organization and the Accreditation Committee will be notified. Joint Commission staff will provide additional consultative support to the organization and allow an additional 10 business days to submit an acceptable root cause analysis and action plan. The organization's accreditation decision reverts to Accredited when the root cause analysis and action plan are determined to be acceptable.

If the third submission continues to not meet established criteria, The Joint Commission staff will recommend that the organization's accreditation decision be changed to Conditional Accreditation, and both the organization and the Accreditation Committee will be notified. The organization will have one final 45-day period in which to submit an acceptable root cause analysis and action plan. If the submitted root cause analysis and action plan still do not meet established criteria, the Accreditation Committee of The Joint Commission will be requested to change the organization's accreditation decision to Preliminary Denial of Accreditation.

When the organization's response (initial or revised) is found to be acceptable, The Joint Commission issues a letter that does the following:

- Reflects The Joint Commission's determination to continue or modify the organization's current accreditation decision
- Assigns an appropriate follow-up activity, typically one or more SE MOS due in four months

Sentinel Event Measure of Success

The organization's follow-up activity will be conducted through the Measure of Success (MOS) process. An MOS is a numerical or quantifiable measure usually related to an audit that determines if a planned action was effective and sustained. The SE MOS are due four months after the root cause analysis and action plan are determined acceptable. If the planned action can be associated with a standard or National

Patient Safety Goal requirement, it will have a level of compliance expectation based on the type of element of performance (EP) for the associated standard or National Patient Safety Goal requirement. That is, if the action is equivalent to an EP that is identified as an "A" EP, the level of compliance expectation for the SE MOS for that action will be 100%. If the action is equivalent to an EP that is identified as a "C" EP, the minimum required level of compliance for the SE MOS for that action will be 90%. If the action cannot be associated with an existing standard or National Patient Safety Goal requirement, the organization will identify the level of compliance expectation, which must be at least 85%, subject to approval by The Joint Commission. The following information further outlines the SE MOS requirement:

- If an SE MOS is 30 or more days late, the organization's accreditation status will automatically be changed to Provisional Accreditation, and both the organization and the Accreditation Committee will be notified.
- If an SE MOS is 60 or more days late, the Joint Commission staff will recommend that the organization's accreditation decision be changed to Conditional Accreditation, and both the organization and the Accreditation Committee will be notified.
- If an SE MOS is 90 or more days late, the Joint Commission staff will recommend to the Accreditation Committee that the organization decision be changed to Denial of Accreditation. In accordance with the Accreditation Committee policy, such an organization will not be afforded any appeal.
- If an SE MOS is submitted on time but does not meet established levels of compliance, the Joint Commission staff will request an additional four months of data. The organization's accreditation decision will be changed to Provisional Accreditation, and both the organization and the Accreditation Committee will be notified.
- If the second set of data meet established levels of compliance, the organization will be restored to Accredited.
- If the second set of data does not meet established levels of compliance, the Joint Commission staff will recommend that the organization's accreditation decision will be changed to Conditional Accreditation, and both the organization and the Accreditation Committee will be notified. Any further actions will be based on the standards-based MOS decision rules.

A decision to maintain or change the organization's accreditation decision as a result of the follow-up activity or to assign additional follow-up requirements will be based on existing decision rules unless otherwise determined by the Accreditation Committee.

Handling Sentinel Event–Related Documents

The handling of any submitted root cause analyses and action plans is restricted to specially trained staff in accordance with procedures designed to protect the confidentiality of the documents.

Upon completion of the Joint Commission review of any submitted root cause analyses and action plans, and the abstraction of the required data elements for the Joint Commission's Sentinel Event Database, the original root cause analysis documents and any copies will be destroyed. Upon request, the original documents will be returned to the organization. With the new electronic process, the information contained in the electronically submitted root cause analysis tool will be de-identified when the review is completed.

The action plan resulting from the analysis of the sentinel event will initially be retained to serve as the basis for the SE MOS. Once the action plan has been implemented and meets the established levels of compliance as determined through the SE MOS, the Joint Commission will destroy the action plan. If the SE MOS was submitted electronically, the information will likewise be de-identified upon completion of the review.

Oversight of the Sentinel Event Policy

The Accreditation Committee of the Joint Commission's Board of Commissioners is responsible for overseeing the implementation of this policy and procedure. In addition to reviewing and deciding individual cases involving changes in an organization's accreditation decision, the senior staff in Accreditation and Certification Operations will periodically audit the root cause analyses and SE MOS and report these findings to the Accreditation Committee. For the purposes of these audits, the Joint Commission temporarily retains random samples of these documents. Upon completion of the audit, these documents are also destroyed.

For more information about the Joint Commission's Sentinel Event Policy and procedures, visit the Joint Commission's Web site at http://www.jointcommission.org or call the Sentinel Event Hotline at 630/792-3700.

2009 SLTC National Patient Safety Goals (NPSG)

NPSG

NPSG

National Patient Safety Goals (NPSG)

Overview

This chapter addresses the requirements of the 2009 National Patient Safety Goals (NPSGs). The purpose of The Joint Commission's NPSGs is to promote specific improvements in patient safety. The goals highlight problematic areas in health care and describe evidence- and expert-based consensus as solutions to these problems. Because sound system design is intrinsic to the delivery of safe, high-quality health care, the goals generally focus on system-wide solutions, whenever possible.

Note: *The term* implementation expectations *has been changed to* elements of performance (EPs) *and the numbering system has been modified to be consistent with the method used for the accreditation standards.*

The broadly representative Sentinel Event Advisory Group (SEAG) works with Joint Commission staff on a continuing basis to prioritize and develop goals, requirements, and EPs. As part of this development process, candidate goals, requirements, and EPs are sent to the field for review and comment. The Advisory Group annually recommends selected existing and new goals, requirements, and EPs to The Joint Commission's Board of Commissioners for review and approval.

Long term care organizations providing services relevant to these goals are responsible for implementing the applicable requirements or effective alternatives. If a long term care organization thinks that an alternative approach to meeting an EP fulfills the intent of the requirement and wishes to implement such an alternative, the organization must obtain Joint Commission approval of the alternative. The SEAG also assists The Joint Commission in evaluating potential alternatives to goal requirements that have been suggested by individual organizations. Compliance with these requirements is assessed throughout the accreditation cycle, through on-site surveys, and through the Periodic Performance Review (PPR), when required by The Joint Commission. When an organization does not fully comply with a requirement, the organization will be assigned a Requirement for Improvement (RFI) in the same way that noncompliance with an accreditation EP generates an RFI. All RFIs must be addressed during the Evidence of Standards Compliance (ESC) process. Failure to resolve an RFI affects an organization's accreditation status, which could ultimately lead to a loss of accreditation.

The Joint Commission provides guidance on how to comply with each goal's requirements. This guidance includes detailed answers to Frequently Asked Questions (FAQs), which are posted on The Joint Commission Web site (http://www.jointcommission.org).

Rationale for NPSG.14.01.01

Pressure ulcers (decubiti) continue to be problematic in all heath care settings. Most pressure ulcers can be prevented, and deterioration at Stage I can be halted. The use of clinical practice guidelines can effectively identify residents and define early intervention for prevention of pressure ulcers.

Elements of Performance for NPSG.14.01.01

A 1. The organization has a written plan for the prediction, prevention, and early treatment of pressure ulcers, which addresses the following:
- Identifying individuals at risk for pressure ulcers and the specific factors that place them at risk
- Maintaining and improving tissue tolerance to pressure in order to prevent injury
- Protecting against the adverse effects of external mechanical forces
- Reducing the incidence of pressure ulcers through staff educational programs

C Ⓜ 2. An initial assessment for the risk of pressure ulcers is performed for each resident at admission. ⚠3

C Ⓜ 3. A systematic risk assessment for pressure ulcers is conducted using a validated risk assessment tool such as the Braden Scale or Norton Scale. ⚠3

C Ⓜ 4. Pressure ulcer risk is reassessed at periodic intervals. ⚠3

C Ⓜ 5. The organization takes action to address any identified risks to the resident for pressure ulcers. ⚠3

2009 SLTC

Accreditation Participation Requirements (APR)

2009

SLTC

Ethics, Rights, and Responsibilities (RI)

RI

RI

RI.2.100
RI.2.110
RI.2.120
RI.2.130
RI.2.140
RI.2.150
RI.2.160
RI.2.170
RI.2.180
RI.2.190
RI.2.195
RI.2.200
RI.2.210
RI.2.220
RI.2.230
RI.2.240
RI.2.250

Ethics, Rights, and Responsibilities (RI)

Overview

The **goal** of the ethics, rights, and responsibilities function is to improve care, treatment, services, and outcomes by recognizing and respecting the rights of each resident and by conducting business in an ethical manner. Care, treatment, and services are provided in a way that respects and fosters dignity, autonomy, positive self regard, civil rights, and involvement of residents. Care, treatment, and services consider the resident's abilities and resources, the relevant demands of his or her environment, and the requirements and expectations of the providers and those they serve. The family is involved in care, treatment, and services decisions with the resident's approval.

An organization's adherence to ethical care and business practices significantly affects the resident's experience of and response to care, treatment, and services. The standards in this chapter address the following processes and activities related to ethical care and business practices:

- Managing the organization's relationships with residents and the public in an ethical manner
- Considering the values and preferences of residents, including the decision to discontinue care, treatment, and services
- Helping residents understand and exercise their rights
- Informing residents of their responsibilities in care, treatment, and services
- Recognizing the organization's responsibilities under law

Residents deserve care, treatment, and services that safeguard their personal dignity and respect their cultural, psychosocial, and spiritual values. These values often influence the resident's perceptions and needs. By understanding and respecting these values, providers can meet care, treatment, and services needs and preferences.

Key: 0 = Insufficient compliance; 1 = Partial compliance; 2 = Satisfactory compliance; NA = Not applicable; **A** indicates scoring category A; **C** indicates scoring category C; ▲(2) indicates situational decision rules apply; △(3) indicates direct impact requirements apply; (M) indicates Measure of success is needed

and interests. Residents can have items such as pictures, clothing, photos, radios, furniture, afghans, and the like to help them personalize their living space. Staff recognizes that the need and choice for such items may change over time and supports the unique needs and choices of each resident. The long term care organization controls any risks and problems these items could cause to other residents.

Elements of Performance for RI.2.140

A 1. The environment of care supports the positive self-image of residents and preserves their human dignity.

A 2. The organization provides sufficient storage space to meet the personal needs of the residents.

A 3. The organization allows residents to keep and use personal clothing and possessions, unless this infringes on others' rights or is medically or therapeutically contraindicated (as appropriate to the setting or service).

A 4. The environment's essential components include the following:
- Homelike surroundings
- Sufficient space with access to personal living space
- Appropriate communication about room and roommate assignments or changes
- Environmental adaptations to help those with dementia, cognitive impairment, or temporary confusion
- Appropriate accommodations for married couples and clients with significant others regardless of sexual orientation, unless any limitations consistent with the organization's mission and philosophy have been disclosed to the resident at the time of or before admission

Standard RI.2.150

Residents have the right to be free from mental, physical, sexual, and verbal abuse, neglect, and exploitation.*

Elements of Performance for RI.2.150

A 1. The organization addresses how it will, to the best of its ability, protect residents from real or perceived abuse; neglect, including involuntary seclusion; or exploitation from anyone, including staff, students, volunteers, other residents, visitors, or family members. △3

Note: *See Standard PC.3.10, which addresses assessing and reporting of abuse, neglect, and exploitation.*

C Ⓜ 2. All allegations, observations, or suspected cases of abuse, neglect, or exploitation that occur in the organization are explored by the organization and, based on the type of event, are referred to the appropriate authorities for investigation. △3

* **Exploitation** Taking advantage of another for one's own advantage or benefit.

Standard RI.2.160

Residents have the right to pain management.

Rationale for RI.2.160

Residents may experience pain. Unrelieved pain has adverse physical and psychological effects. The organization respects and supports the right of residents to pain management. In accordance with the organization's mission, this may occur through referral.

Element of Performance for RI.2.160

A 1. The organization plans, supports, and coordinates activities and resources to ensure that pain is recognized and addressed appropriately and in accordance with the care, treatment, and services provided, including the following:
- Assessing for pain
- Educating all relevant providers about assessing and managing pain
- Educating residents and families, when appropriate, about their roles in managing pain and the potential limitations and side effects of pain treatments ⚠3

Standard RI.2.170

Residents have a right to access protective and advocacy services.

Elements of Performance for RI.2.170

C Ⓜ 1. When the organization serves a population of residents who often need protective services (that is, guardianship and advocacy services, conservatorship, and child or adult protective services), it provides resources to help the family and the courts determine the resident's needs for such services.

A 2. When appropriate, the organization maintains a list of names, addresses, and telephone numbers of pertinent state client advocacy groups such as the state authority and the protection and advocacy network.

C Ⓜ 3. The list is given to residents when requested.

A 4. The organization develops and implements policies and procedures for the above requirements.

Applicable to Long Term Care Programs Participating in Research

Standard RI.2.180

The organization protects research subjects and respects their rights during research, investigation, and clinical trials involving human subjects.

Rationale for RI.2.180

An organization that conducts research, investigations, or clinical trials involving human subjects knows that its first responsibility is to the health and well-being of the

2009 SLTC

Provision of Care, Treatment, and Services (PC)

PC

PC

Provision of Care, Treatment, and Services* (PC)

Overview

Care, treatment, and services are provided through the successful coordination and completion of a series of processes that include appropriate initial assessment of needs; development of a plan for care, treatment, and services; the provision of care, treatment, and services; ongoing assessment of whether the care, treatment, and services provided are meeting the resident's needs; and either the successful discharge of the resident or referral or transfer of the resident for continuing care, treatment, and services.

The provision of care, treatment, and services to residents consists of four core processes or elements:

1. Assessing resident needs
2. Planning care, treatment, and services
3. Providing the care, treatment, and services the resident needs
4. Coordinating care, treatment, and services

These core elements may also include the following activities:

- Providing access to the appropriate levels of care and/or disciplines for residents
- Providing interventions based on the plan for care, treatment, and services
- Teaching residents what they need to know about their care, treatment, and services
- Coordinating care, treatment, and services, if needed, when the resident is referred, transferred, or discharged

The elements that make up the provision of care, treatment, and services are related to each other through an integrated and cyclical process that may occur over minutes, hours, days, weeks, months, or years, depending on the setting and the needs of the resident. This cyclical process may occur among multiple organizations or within a single organization. The standards in this chapter address the processes in this cycle, including those provided for resident populations with unique needs or residents who are receiving interventions or services that are problem prone.

The core processes or elements of the provision of care, treatment, and services should not be seen as separate steps, rather as interrelated activities in an integrated and ongoing care process. The activities related to the provision of care, treatment, and services should be capable of moving easily between elements as required to meet residents' needs and maintain the continuity of care, treatment, and services.

* This chapter is a compilation of the former "Assessment," "Care," "Education," and "Continuum of Care" chapters.

Key: 0 = Insufficient compliance; 1 = Partial compliance; 2 = Satisfactory compliance; NA = Not applicable; **A** indicates scoring category A; **C** indicates scoring category C; ▲(2) indicates situational decision rules apply; △(3) indicates direct impact requirements apply; (M) indicates Measure of success is needed

Standards

The following is a list of all standards for this function. They are presented here for your convenience without footnotes or other explanatory text. If you have a question about a term used here, please check the Glossary.

Note: *A revised standard numbering system is being used with the reformatted standards. The revised numbering system will allow for more flexibility to add standards while maintaining the current label for each standard.*

Entry to Care, Treatment, and Services

PC.1.10 The organization accepts for care, treatment, and services only those residents whose identified, care, treatment, and service needs it can meet.

Assessment

PC.2.10 Not applicable

PC.2.20 The organization defines in writing the data and information gathered during assessment and reassessment.

PC.2.30 Through PC.2.110 Not applicable

PC.2.120 The organization defines in writing the time frame(s) for conducting the initial assessment(s).

PC.2.130 Initial assessments are performed as defined by the organization.

PC.2.140 Not applicable

PC.2.150 Residents are reassessed as needed.

Additional Standard for Victims of Abuse

PC.3.10 Residents who may be victims of abuse, neglect, or exploitation are assessed. (*See* standard RI.2.150.)

PC.3.20 Through PC.3.220 Not applicable

Diagnostic Services

PC.3.230 Diagnostic testing necessary for determining the resident's health care needs is performed.

Planning Care, Treatment, and Services

PC.4.10 Development of a plan for care, treatment, and services is individualized and appropriate to the resident's needs, strengths, limitations, and goals.

PC.4.20 Through PC.4.120 Not applicable

Providing Care, Treatment, and Services

PC.5.10 The organization provides care, treatment, and services for each resident according to the plan for care, treatment, and services.

PC.5.20 Not applicable

PC.5.30 The attending physician prescribes the medical requirements of care for the residents he or she admits.

PC.5.40 The attending physician visits the resident in accordance with the resident's needs and at least once during the 30 days after admission.

PC.5.50 Care, treatment, and services are provided in an interdisciplinary, collaborative manner.

PC.5.60 The organization coordinates the care, treatment, and services provided to a resident as part of the plan for care, treatment, and services and consistent with the organization's scope of care, treatment, and services.

PC.5.70 Not applicable

Education

PC.6.10 The resident receives education and training specific to the resident's needs and as appropriate to the care, treatment, and services provided.

PC.6.20 Not applicable

PC.6.30 The resident receives education and training specific to the resident's abilities as appropriate to the care, treatment, and services provided by the organization.

PC.6.40 Not applicable

PC.6.50 The organization provides academic education to children and youth as needed.

PC.6.60 Through PC.6.180 Not applicable

Nutritional Care

PC.7.10 The organization has a process for preparing and/or distributing food and nutrition products.

Pain

PC.8.10 Pain is assessed in all residents.

Restorative Services

PC.8.20 When necessary, residents receive appropriate restorative services, including assistance with activities of daily living, such as eating, dressing, grooming, bathing, oral hygiene, ambulation, and toilet activities.

Preventive Care

PC.8.30 Residents at risk for health-related complications receive appropriate preventive care.

Social and Diversional Activities

PC.8.40 Residents are helped so they can participate in social and diversional activities according to their functional levels.

Access to the Outdoors

PC.8.50 Not applicable

PC.8.60 Not applicable

End-of-Life Care

PC.8.70 Comfort and dignity are optimized during end-of-life care.

Specific Procedures

Administering Blood and Blood Components

PC.9.10 Blood and blood components are administered safely, as appropriate to the settings.

Responding to Life-Threatening Emergencies

PC.9.20 The organization responds to life-threatening emergencies according to organization policy and procedure.

PC.9.30 Through PC.11.70 Not applicable

Restraint and Seclusion

PC.11.80 The organization designs a system to achieve a restraint-free environment.

PC.11.90 When alternatives to restraint are ineffective, restraint is safely and appropriately used.

PC.11.100 Through PC.12.190 Not applicable

Standards for Additional Special Procedures

Sedation and Anesthesia Care for Subacute Services

PC.13.10 Licensed independent practitioners define the scope of assessment for operative or other procedures and/or the administration of moderate or deep sedation or anesthesia.

PC.13.20 Operative or other procedures and/or the administration of moderate or deep sedation or anesthesia are planned.

PC.13.30 Residents are monitored during the procedure and/or administration of moderate or deep sedation or anesthesia.

PC.13.40 Residents are monitored immediately after the procedure and/or administration of moderate or deep sedation or anesthesia.

Additional Special Procedures

PC.13.50 Through PC.14.30 Not applicable

Discharge or Transfer from the Organization

PC.15.10 A process addresses the needs for continuing care, treatment, and services after discharge or transfer.

PC.15.20 The transfer or discharge of a resident to another level of care, treatment, and services, different professionals, or different settings is based on the resident's assessed needs and the organization's capabilities.

PC.15.30 When residents are transferred or discharged, appropriate information related to the care, treatment, and services provided is exchanged with other service providers.

PC.15.40 Not applicable

PC.15.50 The organization tells residents and their families of its bed-hold policy.

Waived Testing

PC.16.10 The director named on the CLIA certificate establishes policies and procedures that define the context in which waived test results are used in resident care, treatment, and services.

PC.16.20 The director named on the CLIA certificate identifies the staff responsible for performing and supervising waived testing.

PC.16.30 Staff receive specific training and orientation for the tests they perform and demonstrate satisfactory levels of competence.

PC.16.40 Policies and procedures governing specific testing-related processes are current, approved, and readily available.

PC.16.50 Quality control checks are conducted on each procedure.

PC.16.60 Quality control and test result records are maintained.

PC.17.10 Not applicable

PC.17.20 Not applicable

PC.17.30 Not applicable

Standards, Rationales, Elements of Performance, and Scoring

Entry to Care, Treatment, and Services

Agreeing to provide care, treatment, and services for a resident should be based both on the resident's needs and the scope of the services provided by the organization. To do this, the organization does the following:

- Establishes criteria to determine entry eligibility
- Defines the minimum information necessary to determine the resident's eligibility for entry to a program or service
- Defines the appropriate professionals and settings needed to provide the services offered consistent with the organization's mission
- Makes entry decisions for appropriate care, treatment, and services offered by the organization based on these criteria

Standard PC.1.10

The organization accepts for care, treatment, and services only those residents whose identified care, treatment, and service needs it can meet.

Elements of Performance for PC.1.10

A 1. The organization has a defined written process that includes the following:
- The information to be gathered to determine eligibility for entrance into the organization
- The populations of residents accepted or not accepted by the organization, for example, programs designed to treat adults that do not treat young children
- The criteria to determine eligibility for entry into the system
- The procedures for accepting referrals

C Ⓜ 2. Residents are screened for appropriateness at the point of first contact (including contact by phone) with the organization.

A 3. The interdisciplinary team is consulted when necessary to determine whether a prospective resident meets admission criteria.

C Ⓜ 4. If a resident is not accepted after referral and preadmission screening, the reasons for denying admission are stated.

A 5. The staff refers the resident to another appropriate organization, making reasonable referral efforts.

A 6. The staff explains to the referring organization its reasons for not accepting the resident and, when possible, suggests a more appropriate organization.

A 7. When warranted by need, separate specialized screening, assessment, and reassessment processes are identified for the various populations served.

8. Not applicable

C Ⓜ 9. The organization accepts residents for care, treatment, and services according to established processes.

Assessment

The goal of assessment is to determine the appropriate care, treatment, and services to meet a resident's initial needs as well as his or her changing needs while in the setting.

Identifying and delivering appropriate care, treatment, and services depends on three processes:

1. *Collecting data* about each resident's health history; physical, functional, and psychosocial status; and needs as appropriate to the setting and circumstances
2. *Analyzing data* to produce information about residents' needs for care, treatment, and services and to identify the need for additional data
3. *Making care, treatment, and services decisions* based on information developed about each resident's needs and his or her response to care, treatment, and services

Qualified staff assesses each resident's care needs throughout the resident's contact with the organization through assessments or screenings. These activities may also identify the need for additional assessments or planning. These assessments are as follows:

- Defined by the organization
- Individualized to meet each resident's needs
- Address the needs of special populations

The process defined by the organization identifies the resident's physical, cognitive, behavioral, emotional, and psychosocial status. This assessment identifies facilitating factors and possible barriers to the resident reaching his or her goals, including the presenting problems and needs, such as the following:

- Symptoms that might be associated with a disease, condition, or treatment (such as pain, nausea, or dyspnea)
- Social barriers, including cultural and language barriers
- Social and environmental factors
- Physical disabilities
- Vision and hearing impairments and disabilities
- Developmental disabilities
- Communicative disorders
- Cognitive disorders
- Emotional, behavioral, and mental disorders
- Substance abuse, dependence, and other addictive behaviors

The depth and frequency of the assessment or screening depend on a number of factors, including the resident's needs; program goals; and the care, treatment, and services provided. Assessment or screening activities may vary between settings, as defined by the clinical and other leaders of the organization. Resident screenings, assessments, and reassessments need to be done and documented within a reasonable time frame to identify the resident's needs and determine whether these needs are being met.

Information gathered at the first contact can indicate the need for more data or a more intensive assessment of the resident's physical, psychological, cognitive, and communicative skills or development or social functioning. At a minimum, the need for further assessment is determined by the care, treatment, and services sought; the client's presenting condition(s); and whether the client agrees to care, treatment, and services.

Standard PC.2.10

Not applicable

Standard PC.2.20

The organization defines in writing the data and information gathered during assessment and reassessment.

Rationale for PC.2.20

A full assessment involves obtaining relevant information from multiple sources. This may include obtaining information from the resident, a family member, or other sources including other providers. Sources might also include mediums that the resident has sought out to convey information to those who may provide care, treatment, or services. These include databases, medical jewelry, and paper or electronic documents. Whatever the source, information to complete a comprehensive assessment should be sought out from all available sources.

Elements of Performance for PC.2.20

A 1. The organization's written definition of the data and information gathered during assessment and reassessment includes the following:
- The scope of assessment and reassessment activities by each discipline
- The content of the assessment and reassessment
- The criteria for when an additional or more in-depth assessment is done by each discipline*

A 2. The screening, assessment, and reassessment activities described are within the scope of practice, state licensure laws, applicable regulations, or certification of the discipline doing the assessment.

A 3. If applicable, separate specialized assessment and reassessment information is identified for the various populations served.

---

* For example, nutritional or functional risk assessments may be defined for at-risk residents. In such cases, nutritional risk criteria should be developed by dieticians or other qualified individuals, and functional risk criteria should be developed by rehabilitation specialists or other qualified individuals.

4. Through 11. Not applicable

A 12. The information defined by the organization to be gathered during the initial assessment(s) includes the following, as relevant to the care, treatment, and services:
- Current diagnosis(es)
- Pertinent history
- Medication history, including drug allergies and sensitivities
- Current medications, including prescribed and over-the-counter medications
- Current treatments

The information defined by the organization to be gathered during the initial assessment(s) also includes the following (EPs 13–20):

A 13. The resident's physical and neuropsychiatric status, including the following:
- Musculoskeletal status
- Cardiorespiratory status
- Gastrointestinal status
- Integumentary status
- Foot care needs
- Mental, affective, and cognitive status and needs

A 14. The resident's communication status, including the following:
- Ability to hear
- Ability to speak
- Predominant language(s)
- Modes of expression

A 15. The resident's functional status, including the following:
- Ability to perform activities of daily living
- Mobility, balance, and strength
- Ability to swallow
- Physical limitations and precautions
- Rehabilitation status, needs, and potential
- Orientation

A 16. The resident's activity status, needs, and potential, including the following:
- Personal preferences regarding schedules and grooming
- The resident's activity and recreational skills, based on his or her cognitive abilities and the limitations of his or her illness or treatment
- Hobbies, recreational interests, associated needs, and potential
- Ability to participate in structured and group activities

A 17. The resident's nutritional* and hydration status and needs, including the following:
- Potential nutritional risk, deficiencies, and needs
- Cultural, religious, or ethnic food preferences
- Nutrient-intake patterns and special dietary requirements
- Dietary/food allergies
- Food and fluid consumption
- Bowel and urinary output
- Skin integrity
- Swallowing problems
- Appropriate laboratory tests
- Weight (at least monthly)
- Criteria used to evaluate weight gain and loss to determine the need for further assessment

A 18. The resident's dental status and oral health, including the following:
- Dental status and oral health, including the condition of the oral cavity, teeth, and tooth-supporting structures
- The presence or absence of natural teeth or dentures and the ability to function with or without natural teeth or dentures

A 19. The resident's pain, including the following:
- Pain status, including its origin, location, severity, and alleviating and exacerbating factors
- Current treatment for pain and response to treatment

A 20. The resident's psychosocial and spiritual status, including the following:
- Cultural and ethnic factors that influence care, treatment, and services
- Current emotional status
- Social skills
- Current living situation
- Family relationships and circumstances
- Relevant past history of roles
- Response to stress caused by the illness and required treatment
- Spiritual orientation, status, and needs
- The dying resident's concerns related to hope, despair, guilt, or forgiveness

A 21. In addition, when the bereavement process is a significant factor, the psychosocial assessment includes the social, spiritual, and cultural variables that influence the perceptions and expressions of grief by the resident or family.

---

* The content of the nutritional screening criteria that the organization develops (which may include the minimum data set [MDS]), is at the discretion of the organization but should be contained in an approved policy. The standards also reflect that, based on the results of the nutrition screen, further nutrition assessment is completed when indicated and the resident is reassessed at determined intervals.

Standards PC.2.30 Through PC.2.110

Not applicable

Standard PC.2.120

The organization defines in writing the time frame(s) for conducting the initial assessment(s).

Elements of Performance for PC.2.120

A 1. The organization defines the time frame(s) for conducting the initial assessment(s).

2. Through 7. Not applicable

A Ⓜ 8. At a minimum, the organization specifies the following time frames for assessments: Each resident's initial Minimum Data Set/interdisciplinary assessment is to be completed within 14 days of admission or as required by law and regulation.

Note: *Consideration should be given to residents with complex needs or short lengths of stay when establishing time frames for completion.*

9. Not applicable.

A 10. At a minimum, the organization specifies the following time frames for assessments: The attending physician or licensed independent practitioner performs a *medical assessment.* These time frames apply for all admissions and re-admissions. Any previous medical history does not have to be completely redone. It can be updated with information about the most recent illness and hospitalization since the date the last history was taken within a time frame appropriate to the resident's condition. This time frame must not exceed 24 hours before admission or within 72 hours after admission.

Durable, legible originals or reproductions of a medical history and physical examination, obtained from the attending physician or licensed independent practitioner and completed within 30 days before admission or readmission, are acceptable, provided that there is a summary of the resident's condition and course of care during the interim period, and the summary also includes the resident's current physical/psychosocial status.

A 11. If the attending physician or licensed independent practitioner other than the attending physician performed the medical assessment that is being transferred, and that assessment was performed within 30 days before admission, then within 24 hours before admission or within 72 hours after admission, the attending physician or attending licensed independent practitioner must do the following:

- Review the physical examination
- Conduct a second medical assessment to confirm the information and findings

- Update any information and findings as necessary, including a summary of the resident's condition and course of care during the interim period and the current physical/psychosocial status
- Sign and date the additional information to attest to its currency

A 12. At a minimum, the organization specifies the following time frames for assessments: The assessment findings are recorded in the medical record on admission within time frames noted in EP 11.

A 13. At a minimum, the organization specifies the following time frames for assessments: Each resident's oral health assessment is to be performed and documented within 90 days before admission or within 14 days after admission.

14. Not applicable

15. Not applicable

16. Not applicable

C Ⓜ 17. For residents with complex needs or who require short lengths of stay, the organization completes assessments within five calendar days after admission for all disciplines pertinent to the reason for admission or as required by law and regulation.

Standard PC.2.130

Initial assessments are performed as defined by the organization.

Elements of Performance for PC.2.130

C Ⓜ 1. Each resident is assessed per organization policy. ⚠3

C Ⓜ 2. Each resident's initial assessment is conducted within the time frame specified by the needs of the resident, organization policy, and law and regulation. ⚠3

A 3. A registered nurse assesses the resident's need for nursing care in all settings, as required by law, regulation, or organization policy. ⚠3

C Ⓜ 4. Residents who exhibit symptoms of dementia are evaluated, and a differential diagnosis is established. ⚠3

C Ⓜ 5. The evaluation* of residents who exhibit symptoms of dementia is performed by a neurologist, a psychiatrist, or a geriatrician, if available, or another qualified physician. ⚠3

Standard PC.2.140

Not applicable

* Guidelines for conducting such an evaluation are available from the "Guidelines for Dignity" from the Alzheimer's Association. The guidelines include a history and physical examination; a mental status evaluation; a neurologic examination; a blood workup; a psychiatric evaluation; a neuropsychiatric assessment; a psychological assessment; CT/MRI, as indicated; and any reversible causes for the presenting symptoms.

Standard PC.2.150

Residents are reassessed* as needed.

Rationale for PC.2.150

Each resident may be reassessed for many reasons, including the following:

- To evaluate his or her response to care, treatment, and services
- To respond to a significant change in status and/or diagnosis or condition
- To satisfy legal or regulatory requirements
- To meet time intervals specified by the organization
- To meet time intervals determined by the course of the care, treatment, and services for the resident

Elements of Performance for PC.2.150

C Ⓜ 1. Each resident is reassessed as needed. ⚠3

C Ⓜ 2. Reassessment occurs in conjunction with the interdisciplinary care plan schedule or in response to change(s) in the resident's condition or as required by law and regulation. ⚠3

Additional Standard for Victims of Abuse

Standard PC.3.10

Residents who may be victims of abuse, neglect, or exploitation are assessed. (*See* standard RI.2.150.)

Rationale for PC.3.10

Victims of abuse, neglect, or exploitation may come to an organization in a variety of ways. The resident may be unable or may be reluctant to speak of the abuse, and it may not be obvious to the casual observer. Staff needs to be able to identify abuse, neglect, and exploitation as well as the extent and circumstances of the abuse, neglect, or exploitation, to give the resident appropriate care.

Criteria for identifying and assessing victims of abuse, neglect, or exploitation should be used throughout the organization. The assessment of the resident must be conducted within the context of the requirements of the law to preserve evidentiary materials and support future legal actions.

Elements of Performance for PC.3.10

A 1. The organization develops or adopts criteria† for identifying victims in each of the following situations:
- Physical assault
- Rape
- Sexual molestation

---

* The scope and intensity of any further assessments are based on the resident's diagnosis; the setting; the resident's desire for care, treatment, and services; and the resident's response to any previous care, treatment, and services.

† The Family Violence Prevention Fund is one resource that can be contacted for further information at http://www.fvpf.org.

- Domestic abuse
- Elder neglect or abuse
- Child neglect or abuse
- Exploitation

A 2. Appropriate staff* is educated about abuse, neglect, or exploitation and how to refer as appropriate.

A 3. A list of private and public community agencies that provide or arrange for assessment and care of abuse victims is maintained to facilitate appropriate referrals.

A 4. Victims of abuse, neglect, or exploitation are identified using the criteria developed or adopted by the organization at entry into the system and on an ongoing basis. ⚠3

A 5. The organization's staff refers appropriately or conducts the assessment of victims of abuse, neglect, or exploitation. ⚠3

A 6. All cases of possible abuse, neglect, or exploitation are reported to appropriate agencies according to organization policy and law and regulation. ⚠3

A 7. All cases of possible abuse, neglect, or exploitation are immediately reported in the organization. ⚠3

Standards PC.3.20 Through PC.3.220

Not applicable

Diagnostic Services

Standard PC.3.230

Diagnostic testing† necessary for determining the resident's health care needs is performed.

Elements of Performance for PC.3.230

C Ⓜ 1. Diagnostic testing and procedures are performed as ordered. ⚠3

C Ⓜ 2. Diagnostic testing and procedures are performed in a timely manner as defined by the organization. ⚠3

---

* Staff should be able to screen for abuse and neglect as indicated by the resident's needs or conditions. The organization may define who conducts the full assessment for alleged or suspected abuse or neglect or refer to another organization.

† Diagnostic testing includes laboratory, radiologic, electrodiagnostic, and other functional tests and imaging technologies.

C Ⓜ 3. When a test report requires clinical interpretation, relevant information is provided with the request. ⚠3

4. Not applicable

A 5. Radiologic and other diagnostic services, including pathology and clinical laboratory services, are available 24 hours a day, seven days a week. ⚠3

Planning Care, Treatment, and Services

Planning includes creating an initial plan for care, treatment, and services appropriate to the resident's specific assessed needs and then revising or maintaining the plan based on the resident's response. Planning for care, treatment, and services is individualized to meet the resident's unique needs and circumstances. Performed by qualified individuals, planning for care, treatment, and services involves using an interdisciplinary approach and involving the resident to the extent possible.

The plan may be modified or terminated based on reassessment; the resident's need for further care, treatment, and services; or the achievement of plan of care goals. This modification may result in planning for the resident's transfer to another setting or service or discharge from the organization.

An interdisciplinary approach is used to plan and manage care, treatment, and services and ultimately guide the outcomes of care, treatment, and services. This approach may draw from internal staff and external consultants from the areas of activities, dietetic, medical, nursing, pharmacy, rehabilitation, social services, and other disciplines whose roles and responsibilities are determined by the following:

- Professional skills, competence, and credentials
- The component of care, treatment, and services being provided
- Licensure, certification, regulation, scope of practice, and job description

Standard PC.4.10

Development of a plan for care, treatment, and services is individualized and appropriate to the resident's needs, strengths, limitations, and goals.

Rationale for PC.4.10

Planning care, treatment, and services is not limited to developing a written plan. Rather, planning is a dynamic process that addresses the execution of care, treatment, and services. The plan for care, treatment, and services must be consistently re-evaluated to ensure that the resident's needs are met. Planning for care, treatment, and services includes the following:

- Integrating assessment findings in the care-planning process
- Developing a plan for care, treatment, and services that includes resident care goals that are reasonable and measurable
- Regularly reviewing and revising the plan for care, treatment, and services
- Determining how the planned care, treatment, and services will be provided

- Documenting the plan for care, treatment, and services
- Monitoring the effectiveness of care planning and the provision of care, treatment, and services
- Involving residents and/or families in care planning

Elements of Performance for PC.4.10

A 1. Care, treatment, and services are planned to ensure that they are individualized to the resident's needs.

2. Not applicable

A 3. The interdisciplinary team identifies and prioritizes each resident's care needs based on the analysis of assessment data.

C Ⓜ 4. An individualized, interdisciplinary plan for care, treatment, and services is developed by an interdisciplinary team representing all appropriate health care professionals as soon as possible after admission, but no later than 7 calendar days after comprehensive assessments are completed. △3

5. Not applicable

6. Not applicable

A 7. The plan identifies the following:
- The care, treatment, and settings
- The frequency at which care, treatment, and services and interventions will occur
- The team members responsible for providing care, treatment, and services
- The financial implications of care, treatment, and services
- Interventions to facilitate the resident's return to the community or discharge to an appropriate level of care

C Ⓜ 8. An interim plan for care, treatment, and services is developed for each resident immediately after the resident is admitted. △3

A 9. A process is in place for gathering input, collaborating on care plan development, and reporting the final plan to team members not available to participate in care planning.

A 10. Policies and procedures define how care plans can be modified between team meetings.

A 11. The organization implements a process for evaluating the plan for care, treatment, and services and its effectiveness, which includes the following:
- 90-day evaluation intervals or more frequent intervals in response to a significant change in the resident's physical, communicative, psychosocial, functional, or emotional status
- Care plan revisions that reflect the resident's current needs, problems, goals, care, treatment, and services
- Review and revision by the interdisciplinary team of all components of care, treatment, and services needed by the resident

C Ⓜ 12. Evaluation of the resident is based on the resident care goals and the resident's plan for care, treatment, and services. ⚠3

C Ⓜ 13. The goals of care, treatment, and services are revised when necessary.

A 14. Plans for care, treatment, and services are revised when necessary.

A 15. The interdisciplinary team revises care plans in collaboration with residents, family, and the individual responsible for financial resource monitoring.

C Ⓜ 16. The care plan review occurs quarterly, or more frequently when indicated by change in the resident's condition, or as required by law and regulation.

Standard PC 4.20 Through PC 4.120

Not applicable

Providing Care, Treatment, and Services

Caring for residents involves providing individualized, planned, and appropriate interventions in settings responsive to specific individual needs. "Care" includes care, treatment, services, rehabilitation, habilitation, or another intervention provided to the resident by the organization.

The goal of providing effective care, treatment, and services is met when the following are performed well:

- Intervening in a collaborative manner (in light of assessed resident needs)
- Educating the resident
- Promoting health and providing appropriate preventive care
- Providing supportive care, treating a disease or condition, and/or treating symptoms (such as pain, nausea, or dyspnea) using accepted professional standards of practice
- Meeting the resident's nourishment needs, if appropriate to the setting
- Helping residents with appropriate restorative services, including assistance with activities of daily living, such as eating, dressing, grooming, bathing, oral hygiene, ambulation, and toilet activities
- Rehabilitating physical, communicative, or psychosocial impairment or maintaining the resident's level of functioning
- Coordinating the care, treatment, and services provided to a resident
- Optimizing comfort and dignity during end-of-life care
- Involving families as indicated and acceptable to the resident

All interventions should respect and encourage the resident's ability to make choices, to develop and maintain a sense of achievement about attaining their personal health goals, and to choose to continue or modify participation in the care process.

The activities comprising care, treatment, and services may be performed by a variety of staff whose roles and responsibilities are determined by the component of care, treatment, and services being provided; relevant licensure; law and regulation; registration; certification; scope of practice; job description; or privileges. The actions or interventions may also be carried out by the resident, family, volunteers, or other caregivers.

Standard PC.5.10

The organization provides care, treatment, and services for each resident according to the plan for care, treatment, and services.

Elements of Performance for PC.5.10

C Ⓜ 1. The organization provides care, treatment, and services for each resident according to the plan for care, treatment, and services. ⚠3

2. Not applicable

3. Not applicable

4. Use at least two resident identifiers (neither to be the resident's room number) whenever administering medications or blood products; taking blood samples and other specimens for clinical testing, or providing any other treatments or procedures.

   Note: *The preceding requirement is not scored here. It is scored at NPSG.01.01.01.*

Standard PC.5.20

Not applicable

Standard PC.5.30

The attending physician prescribes the medical requirements of care for the residents he or she admits.

Elements of Performance for PC.5.30

C Ⓜ 1. Orders* are obtained from the physician or other authorized individuals according to law and regulation and professional practice acts before providing care, treatment, and services. ⚠3

C Ⓜ 2. The order is tailored to each resident's needs and includes all elements required by law and regulation. ⚠3

C Ⓜ 3. All orders are renewed or updated to reflect the following:
- Changes in the care, treatment, and services being provided
- Changes in the resident's physical or psychosocial condition
- The resident's response to care, treatment, and services
- The resident's outcome related to care, treatment, and services
- Changes in diagnosis, treatment (including procedures and medications), and equipment

* These orders may be verbal or written and include prescriptions.

- The minimum review time frame defined by the organization
- Applicable law and regulation ⚠3

C Ⓜ 4. The organization provides care, treatment, and services according to the most recent order. ⚠3

C Ⓜ 5. Each attending physician designates an alternate physician whom the organization can contact to obtain regular or emergency care when the attending physician is not available.

Standard PC.5.40

The attending physician visits the resident in accordance with the resident's needs and at least once during the 30 days after admission.

Elements of Performance for PC.5.40

A 1. The attending physician visits the resident in accordance with the resident's needs. ⚠3

C Ⓜ 2. The attending physician visits the resident at least once during the 30 days after admission.

C Ⓜ 3. For planned stays of less than 30 days, the resident's attending physician visits the resident at least once before discharge.

C Ⓜ 4. The resident is seen within 72 hours of admission when the long term care physician is different from the resident's primary physician.

C 5. Physicians' visiting schedules comply with law, regulation, and organization policy regarding the following:
- Frequency and timing of visits
- Visits by physician assistants or advanced practice registered nurses instead of attending physicians

Standard PC.5.50

Care, treatment, and services are provided in an interdisciplinary, collaborative manner.

Rationale for PC.5.50

A collaborative, interdisciplinary approach to meeting the resident's needs and goals helps coordinate care, treatment, and services and achieve optimal outcomes. The mix of disciplines involved and the intensity of the collaboration will vary as appropriate to each resident and the scope of services provided by the organization. An interdisciplinary approach should not be interpreted as a requirement for the signing of other individual's notes.

Elements of Performance for PC.5.50

A 1. Care, treatment, and services are provided in an interdisciplinary, collaborative manner* as appropriate to the needs of the resident and the organization's scope of services.

2. Not applicable

A 3. Changes in the resident's condition are communicated to the physician or other authorized health care professionals, the resident, and his or her family.

C Ⓜ 4. Information from consultation and evaluation reports is communicated to the physician.

C Ⓜ 5. The organization provides this information on a timely basis as defined by the organization and required by law and regulation.

Standard PC.5.60

The organization coordinates the care, treatment, and services provided to a resident as part of the plan for care, treatment, and services and consistent with the organization's scope of care, treatment, and services.

Rationale for PC.5.60

Throughout the provision of care, treatment, and services, residents should be matched with appropriate internal and external resources to meet their ongoing needs in a timely manner. Care, treatment, and services should be coordinated between providers and between settings, independent of whether they are provided directly or through written agreement.

Elements of Performance for PC.5.60

A 1. The organization coordinates the care, treatment, and services provided through internal resources to a resident.

A 2. When external resources are needed, the organization participates in coordinating care, treatment, and services with these resources.

A 3. The organization has a process to receive or share relevant resident information to facilitate appropriate coordination and continuity when residents are referred to other care, treatment, and service providers.

A 4. There is a process to resolve duplication or conflict with either internal or external resources.

A 5. The activities detailed in the plan of care, treatment, and services is designed to occur in a time frame that meets the resident's health needs.

---

* The process is designed to ensure coordinated participation of all appropriate health care professionals from the appropriate settings and includes identifying interdisciplinary team members' responsibilities, holding interdisciplinary team meetings, providing for resolution of differences among interdisciplinary team members, documenting interdisciplinary team members' participation in the medical record, and discussing and modifying the resident's interdisciplinary care plan.

6. Not applicable

A 7. Services are made available directly or through arrangement to meet the following resident needs:
- 24-hour emergency dental services
- Spiritual services
- Behavioral health services,* including counseling on a continuing basis in individual, family, and group services, as appropriate
- Activity services for ambulatory and nonambulatory residents at various functional levels as well as those who are unable to attend group activities
- Assistance with guardianship and conservatorship, when indicated
- Services to facilitate family support, social work, nursing care, dental care, rehabilitation, primary physician care, or discharge

Standard PC.5.70

Not applicable

Education

Standard PC.6.10

The resident receives education and training specific to the resident's needs and as appropriate to the care, treatment, and services provided.

Rationale for PC.6.10

Residents must be given sufficient information to make decisions and to take responsibility for self-management activities related to their needs. Residents and, as appropriate, their families are educated to improve individual outcomes by promoting healthy behavior and appropriately involving residents in their care, treatment, and services decisions.

Elements of Performance for PC.6.10

A 1. Education provided is appropriate to the resident's needs.

C Ⓜ 2. The assessment of learning needs addresses cultural and religious beliefs, emotional barriers, desire and motivation to learn, physical or cognitive limitations, and barriers to communication as appropriate.

A 3. As appropriate to the resident's condition and assessed needs and the organization's scope of services, the resident is educated about the following:
- The plan for care, treatment, and services
- His or her condition or illness and preventive interventions

* These services may be provided by various disciplines (for instance, social workers, psychologists, clinical nurse specialists, or other appropriately educated consultants).

- Basic health practices and safety
- The safe and effective use of medications
- Nutrition interventions, modified diets, or oral health
- Safe and effective use of medical equipment or supplies when provided by the organization
- Understanding pain, the risk for pain, the importance of effective pain management, the pain assessment process, and methods for pain management
- Habilitation or rehabilitation techniques to help them reach the maximum independence possible
- Environmental and physical plant safety issues, such as fire safety, evacuation, storage of chemical agents, and so on
- Use of nonmedical equipment, including, but not limited to, operating call lights, beds, and personal appliances
- How to carry out self-care
- Transfer techniques
- Personal safety and mobility
- Bathroom safety
- Available resources to meet identified needs and how to access such resources
- When to seek and how to obtain follow-up or continuing care, treatment, and services

Standard PC.6.20

Not applicable

Standard PC.6.30

The resident receives education and training specific to the resident's abilities as appropriate to the care, treatment, and services provided by the organization.

Rationale for PC.6.30

Learning styles vary, and the ability to learn can be affected by many factors, including individual learning preferences and readiness to learn. Educational activities must be tailored to meet the resident's needs and abilities.

Elements of Performance for PC.6.30

A 1. Education provided is appropriate to the resident's abilities.

A 2. Education is coordinated among the disciplines providing care, treatment, and services.

A 3. The content is presented in an understandable manner.

A 4. Teaching methods accommodate various learning styles.

C Ⓜ 5. Comprehension is evaluated.

2009

SLTC

Medication Management (MM)

MM

MM

Medication* Management (MM)

Overview

Medication management is often an important component in the palliative, symptomatic, and curative treatment of many diseases and conditions. A safe medication management system addresses an organization's medication processes, including the following (as applicable):

- Selection and procurement
- Storage
- Ordering and transcribing
- Preparing and dispensing
- Administration
- Monitoring

Effective and safe medication management involves multiple services and disciplines working closely together. These standards address activities involving various individuals within an organization's medication management system, such as licensed independent practitioners and other health care staff involved in medication management processes.

A well-planned and implemented medication management system supports resident safety and improves the quality of care by doing the following:

- Reducing practice variation, errors, and misuse
- Monitoring medication management processes with regard to efficiency, quality, and safety
- Standardizing equipment and processes across the organization to improve the medication management system
- Using evidence-based good practices to develop medication management processes
- Managing critical processes associated with medication management to promote safe medication management throughout the organization
- Handling all medications in the same manner, including sample medications

---

* For the purpose of these standards, *medication* includes prescription medications, sample medications, herbal remedies, vitamins, nutraceuticals, over-the-counter drugs, vaccines, diagnostic and contrast agents used on or administered to persons to diagnose, treat, or prevent disease or other abnormal conditions; radioactive medications; respiratory therapy treatments; parenteral nutrition; blood derivatives; intravenous solutions (plain, with electrolytes and/or drugs); and any product designated by the Food and Drug Administration (FDA) as a drug. The definition of *medication* does not include enteral nutrition solutions (which are considered food products), oxygen, and other medical gases.

Key: 0 = Insufficient compliance; 1 = Partial compliance; 2 = Satisfactory compliance; NA = Not applicable; **A** indicates scoring category A; **C** indicates scoring category C; ▲2 indicates situational decision rules apply; △3 indicates direct impact requirements apply; Ⓜ indicates Measure of success is needed

An effective medication management system includes mechanisms for reporting potential and actual medication-related errors and a process to improve medication management processes and resident safety based on this information. The most effective feedback and improvement systems usually operate in organizations that have a nonpunitive culture.

The "Medication Management" chapter (MM.1.10 through MM.8.10) addresses critical medication management processes, including those undertaken by the organization and those provided through contracted pharmacy services. When pharmacy services are provided on a contracted basis, the contract addresses responsibility for these standards and performance expectations. An organization that contracts with a pharmacy for services must monitor the performance of contracted services. When an on-site pharmacy exists, the pharmacy is responsible for the control and distribution of all medications used in the organization. When medications are dispensed by outside pharmacies, the long term care facility, in conjunction with the consultant pharmacist, designs, monitors, and determines if the medication management system meets applicable law or regulation, accepted standards of practice, and organization policies and procedures.

Standards

The following is a list of all standards for this chapter. They are presented here for your convenience without footnotes or other explanatory text. If you have a question about a term used here, please check the Glossary.

Note: *A revised standard numbering system is being used with the reformatted standards. This revised numbering system will allow for more flexibility to add standards while maintaining the current label for each standard.*

Resident-Specific Information

MM.1.10 Resident-specific information is readily accessible to those involved in the medication management system.

Selection and Procurement

MM.2.10 Medications available for dispensing or administration (including stock medications) are selected, listed, and procured based on criteria.

Storage

MM.2.20 Medications are properly and safely stored.

MM.2.30 Emergency medications and/or supplies, if any, are consistently available, controlled, and secured.

MM.2.40 A process is established to safely manage medications brought into the organization by residents or their families.

Ordering and Transcribing

MM.3.10 Only medications needed to treat the resident's condition are ordered, provided, or administered.

MM.3.20 Medication orders are written clearly and transcribed accurately.

Preparing and Dispensing

MM.4.10 All prescriptions or medication orders are reviewed for appropriateness.

MM.4.20 Medications are prepared safely.

MM.4.30 Medications are labeled.

MM.4.40 Medications are dispensed safely.

MM.4.50 The organization has a system for safely providing medications to meet resident needs when the pharmacy is closed.

MM.4.60 If the organization does not operate a pharmacy but routinely administers medications, the organization has a process for obtaining medications from a pharmacy.

MM.4.70 Medications dispensed by the organization are retrieved when recalled or discontinued by the manufacturer or the Food and Drug Administration for safety reasons.

MM.4.80 The organization has a process to address medications that are returned to the pharmacy or the organization.

Administration

MM.5.10 Medications are safely and accurately administered.

MM.5.20 Self-administered medications are safely and accurately administered.

MM.5.30 Not applicable

Monitoring

MM.6.10 The effects of medication(s) on residents are monitored.

MM.6.20 The organization responds to actual or potential adverse drug events and medication errors.

High-Risk Medications

MM.7.10 The organization develops processes for managing high-risk or high-alert medications.

MM.7.20 Psychotropic medication use is monitored.

MM.7.30 Not applicable

MM.7.40 Investigational medications are safely controlled and administered.

Evaluation

MM.8.10 The organization evaluates its medication management system.

Standards, Rationales, Elements of Performance, and Scoring

Resident-Specific Information

Standard MM.1.10

Resident-specific information is readily accessible to those involved in the medication management system.

Rationale for MM.1.10

A major cause of medication-related sentinel events and medication errors is a lack of information. Licensed independent practitioners and health care staff who participate in the medication management system need access to important information about each resident in order to do the following:

- Facilitate continuity of care, treatment, and services
- Create an accurate medication history and a current list of medications (also known as a drug profile)
- Safely order, prepare, dispense, administer, and monitor medications, as appropriate

Elements of Performance for MM.1.10

A 1. A written policy describes the minimum amount of information about the resident that is to be available to those involved in medication management.

Note: *The organization defines who has access to this information;* see *standard IM.2.10.*

A 2. At a minimum, the information includes the following:

- The resident's age
- The resident's sex
- The resident's current medications
- The resident's diagnoses, comorbidities, and concurrently occurring conditions
- The resident's relevant laboratory values
- The resident's allergies and past sensitivities

As appropriate to the resident, the organization also includes information regarding the following:

- Weight and height
- Pregnancy and lactation status
- Any other information required by the organization for safe medication management

C Ⓜ 3. The information is accessible when needed (except in emergency situations when time does not permit) to licensed independent practitioners and other health care staff.

Selection and Procurement

Standard MM.2.10

Medications available for dispensing or administration (including stock medications) are selected, listed, and procured based on criteria.

Note: *This standard is applicable to all on-site pharmacies and pharmacies contracted by the long term care facility to provide medications to its residents.*

Note: *The formulary is synonymous with the list of medications available for use.*

Elements of Performance for MM.2.10

A 1. Licensed independent practitioners and health care staff involved in ordering, dispensing, administering, and/or monitoring effects of medications, including the medical director, develop criteria for determining what medications are available for dispensing or administration.

A 2. At a minimum, the criteria include the indication for use, effectiveness, risks (including propensity for medication errors, abuse potential, and sentinel events), and costs.

A 3. A list of medications for dispensing or administration (including strength and dosage form) is maintained and readily available.

Note: *Sample medications are not required to be on this list.*

A 4. Processes and mechanisms are established to monitor resident responses to a newly added medication before the medication is made available for dispensing or administration within the organization.

A 5. Medications designated as available for dispensing or administration are reviewed at least annually based on emerging safety and efficacy information.

A 6. The organization has processes to approve and procure medications that are not on the organization's medication list.

A 7. The organization has processes to address medication shortages and outages, including the following:

- Communicating with prescribers and staff who participate in the medication management system
- Developing approved substitution protocols

- Educating licensed independent practitioners and health care staff who participate in medication management systems about these protocols
- Obtaining medications in the event of a disaster

Storage

Standard MM.2.20

Medications are properly and safely stored.

Rationale for MM.2.20

Appropriate medication storage increases resident safety. Medication storage is designed to assist in maintaining medication integrity, promote the availability of medications when needed, minimize the risk of medication diversion, and reduce potential dispensing errors.

Note: *The following EPs also apply to emergency medications. Additional requirements for emergency medications are addressed at standard MM.2.30.*

Elements of Performance for MM.2.20

A Ⓜ 1. Only approved medications are routinely stocked or stored.*

A Ⓜ 2. Medications are stored under conditions suitable for product stability.

A 3. There is a written policy addressing the storage of medication between receipt of a medication by an individual health care provider and medication administration. At a minimum, the policy addresses the following:
- Safe storage
- Safe handling
- Security and
- Disposition of these medications, including return to the medication storage area at the end of the individual's shift

C Ⓜ 4. The policy addressing the storage of medication between receipt of a medication by an individual health care provider and medication administration is implemented.

A 5. Unauthorized persons, in accordance with the organization's policy and law or regulation, cannot obtain access to medications.

A 6. Controlled substances are stored to prevent diversion and according to state and federal laws and regulations.

A 7. All expired, damaged, and/or contaminated medications are segregated until they are removed from the organization.

---

* **Note:** See *standard MM.2.40 for the exception to this EP: The organization has a process to safely manage medications brought in by the resident or the resident's family.*

8. Identify and, at a minimum, annually review a list of look-alike/sound-alike drugs used in the organization, and take action to prevent errors involving the interchange of these drugs.

   Note: *The preceding requirement is not scored here. It is scored at NPSG.03.03.01.*

A 9. Medications and chemicals used to prepare medications are accurately labeled with contents, expiration dates, and warnings.

A 10. Standardize and limit the number of drug concentrations available in the organization.

A Ⓜ 11. Concentrated electrolytes are removed from care units or areas (unless resident safety is at risk if the concentrated electrolyte is not immediately available on a specific care unit or area; in such situations, specific precautions are taken to prevent inadvertent administration). ⚠3

12. Not applicable

13. Not applicable

14. Not applicable

C Ⓜ 15. All medication storage areas are periodically inspected according to the organization's policy to make sure medications are stored properly.

Standard MM.2.30

Emergency medications and/or supplies, if any, are consistently available, controlled, and secured.

Note: *The following requirements for emergency medications are in addition to the requirements at Standard MM.2.20, which are also applicable to emergency medications.*

Elements of Performance for MM.2.30

A 1. Organization leadership, in conjunction with licensed independent practitioners and other health care staff whose scope of practice includes the dispensing or administration of emergency medications, decides which emergency medications and/or supplies, if any, will be readily available in care areas.

2. Not applicable

A 3. Emergency medications are available in unit-dose, age-specific, and ready-to-administer forms whenever possible. ⚠3

A Ⓜ 4. Emergency medications are sealed or stored in containers (for example, crash carts, tackle boxes, emergency drug kits, closed bags that are clearly labeled, and so forth) in such a way that staff can readily determine that the contents are complete and have not expired.

5. Not applicable

A Ⓜ 6. Emergency medications are stored in sealed or in locked containers; in a locked room; or under constant supervision in accordance with law or regulation.

A 7. Emergency medications and supplies are replaced as soon as possible after their use, in accordance with the organization's policies and procedures.

Standard MM.2.40

A process is established to safely manage medications brought into the organization by residents or their families.

Rationale for MM.2.40

A number of valid reasons exist for allowing residents to use their own medications in a health care organization, including the need for continuous therapy; a resident's use of a nonformulary medication; or a lack of alternatives to a resident's personal medication. The organization defines its responsibilities for the safe use of these medications.

Elements of Performance for MM.2.40

A 1. The organization addresses the use of medications brought into the organization by residents or their families, including defining when such medications can be used or administered.

A 2. The organization addresses the use of medications brought into the organization by residents or their families, including identifying the medication and visually evaluating its integrity, when medications brought in by the resident or family are allowed.

A 3. The organization addresses the use of medications brought into the organization by residents or their families, including informing the prescriber and resident if medications brought into the organization by residents or their families are not permitted.

Ordering and Transcribing

Standard MM.3.10

Only medications needed to treat the resident's condition are ordered, provided, or administered.

Element of Performance for MM.3.10

C Ⓜ 1. There is a documented diagnosis, condition, or indication-for-use for each medication ordered.

Standard MM.3.20

Medication orders are written clearly and transcribed accurately.

Rationale for MM.3.20

Many medication errors occur while communicating or transcribing medication orders. The organization is responsible for taking steps to reduce the potential for error or misinterpretation when orders are written or verbally communicated. The required elements of all orders must be specified. To reinforce the skills and judgments needed for safe medication ordering, the organization offers education to care providers. Clear understanding and communication between staff involved in the medication process is essential. Best practices, external and internal data, and medication risks are considered when the organization develops medication policies and procedures.

Elements of Performance for MM.3.20

A 1. Written policy(ies) address the following: The required elements of a complete medication order.

A 2. Written policy(ies) address the following: When generic or brand names are acceptable or required as part of a medication order.

A 3. Written policy(ies) address the following: Whether or when indication for use is required on a medication order.

A 4. Written policy(ies) address the following: Special precautions or procedures for ordering drugs with look-alike or sound-alike names.

A 5. Written policy(ies) address the following: Actions to take when medication orders are incomplete, illegible, or unclear.

A 6. The organization specifies the required elements of the following types of orders that it deems acceptable for use:
- "As needed" (PRN) orders—orders acted upon based on the occurrence of a specific indication or symptom
- Standing orders—written instruction to administer a medication to a person in circumstances specified in instructions without a prescription
- Hold orders—instruction to temporarily suspend (place medication orders on hold) under specified conditions and to alert users at specified times while a medication is on hold
- Automatic stop orders—a date or time to discontinue a medication
- Resume orders—restart an order which was previously held
- Titrating orders—orders in which the dose is either progressively increased or decreased in response to the resident's status
- Taper orders—orders in which the dose is decreased by a particular amount with each dosing interval
- Range orders—orders in which the dose or dosing interval varies over a prescribed range, depending on the situation or resident's status
- Orders for compounded drugs or drug mixtures not commercially available

- Orders for medication-related devices (for example, nebulizers and catheters)
- Orders for investigational medications
- Orders for herbal products
- Orders for medications at discharge or transfer

7. Not applicable

A 8. In addition, the organization reviews and updates preprinted order sheets as needed to support clarity, accuracy, and safety.

A 9. In addition, the organization specifies that blanket reinstatement of previous orders—a summary order to resume all previous orders—for medications are not acceptable.

10. Not applicable

11. Not applicable

12. Not applicable

C Ⓜ 13. Policies and procedures regarding medication orders are implemented.

A 14. Influenza and pneumococcal polysaccharide vaccines are administered according to a physician order, or, as permitted by law and regulation, according to physician-approved, organization-specific protocol(s).

Preparing and Dispensing

Standard MM.4.10

All prescriptions or medication orders are reviewed for appropriateness.

Note: *This standard is applicable to all on-site pharmacies and pharmacies contracted by the long term care facility to provide medications to its residents.*

Elements of Performance for MM.4.10

C Ⓜ 1. Before dispensing, removal from floor stock, or removal from an automated storage and distribution device, a pharmacist reviews all prescription or medication orders unless a licensed independent practitioner controls the ordering, preparation, and administration of the medication; or in urgent situations when the resulting delay would harm the resident, including situations in which the resident experiences a sudden change in clinical status (for example, new onset of nausea). ⚠3

2. Not applicable

3. Not applicable

4. Not applicable

A 5. The organization has a process to review all prescriptions for the following:
- The appropriateness of the drug, dose, frequency, and route of administration
- Therapeutic duplication
- Real or potential allergies or sensitivities
- Real or potential interactions between the prescription and other medications or food
- Current or potential impact as evidenced by laboratory values
- Other contraindications
- Variation from organizational criteria for use
- Other relevant medication-related issues or concerns

A 6. All concerns, issues, or questions are clarified with the individual prescriber before dispensing the medication. ⚠3

Standard MM.4.20

Medications are prepared safely.

Elements of Performance for MM.4.20

A 1. When an on-site, licensed pharmacy is available, only the pharmacy compounds or admixes all sterile medications, intravenous admixtures, or other drugs except in emergencies or when not feasible (for example, when the product's stability is short). ⚠3

A 2. The organization has a written policy that addresses the safety and use of medications acquired by a practitioner from sources other than the organization for use in resident care in that organization. The policy addresses the following:
- Whether such medications are allowed to be used
- If allowed, a process to evaluate the integrity of medications brought in by a practitioner prior to use in resident care

A 3. The written policy that addresses the safety and use of medications acquired by a practitioner from sources other than the organization for use in resident care is implemented.

C Ⓜ 4. Wherever medications are prepared, staff uses safety materials and equipment while preparing hazardous medications.

C Ⓜ 5. Wherever medications are prepared, staff uses techniques to assure accuracy in medication preparation. ⚠3

C Ⓜ 6. Wherever medications are prepared, staff follow techniques to avoid contamination during medication preparation including, but not limited to the following:
- Using clean or sterile techniques
- Maintaining clean, uncluttered, and functionally separate areas for product preparation to minimize the possibility of contamination

- Using a laminar airflow hood or other class 100 environment while preparing any intravenous (IV) admixture in the pharmacy, any sterile product made from nonsterile ingredients, or any sterile product that will not be used within 24 hours
- Visually inspecting the integrity of the medications △3

Standard MM.4.30

Medications are labeled.

Rationale for MM.4.30

A standardized method for labeling all medications will minimize errors.

Elements of Performance for MM.4.30

A 1. Medications are labeled in a standardized manner according to law or regulation and standards of practice. △3

A 2. Any time one or more medications or solutions are prepared but are not administered immediately, the medication container* must be labeled. △3

A 3. At a minimum, all medications prepared in the organization are labeled with the following:
- Drug name, strength, amount (if not apparent from the container)
- Expiration date† when not used within 24 hours
- Expiration time when expiration occurs in less than 24 hours
- The date prepared and the diluent for all compounded IV admixtures and parenteral nutrition solutions △3

A 4. When preparing individualized medications for multiple specific residents, or when the person preparing the individualized medications is not the person administering the medication, the label also includes the following:
- Resident name
- Resident location
- Directions for use and any applicable cautionary statements either on the label or attached as an accessory label (for example, "requires refrigeration," "for IM use only") △3

A 5. Organizations that do not operate a pharmacy validate that all medications coming into the organization are appropriately labeled. △3

A 6. If not labeled, action is taken to have the medications correctly labeled. △3

Standard MM.4.40

Medications are dispensed safely.

---

* A container can be any storage device such as a plastic bag, syringe, bottle, or box, medicine cup or basin.

† Expiration date, also called the "beyond use date," refers to the last date that the product should be used by the resident.

Note: *This standard is applicable to all on-site pharmacies and pharmacies contracted by the long term care facility to provide medications to its residents.*

Elements of Performance for MM.4.40

A 1. Quantities of medications are dispensed and minimize diversion yet are still consistent with the resident's needs.

A 2. Dispensing adheres to law, regulation, licensure, and professional standards of practice, including record keeping.

C Ⓜ 3. Medications are dispensed in a timely* manner to meet resident needs.

C Ⓜ 4. Medications are dispensed in the most ready-to-administer forms available from the manufacturer or if feasible, in unit-doses that have been repackaged by the pharmacy or licensed repackager. ⚠3

A 5. The organization consistently uses the same dose packaging system, or if a different system is used, provides education about the use of the dose packaging system to the residents impacted by the change.

Standard MM.4.50

The organization has a system for safely providing medications to meet resident needs when the pharmacy is closed.

Note: *This standard only applies when an organization has an on-site pharmacy and residents present in the organization.*

Rationale for MM.4.50

If an urgent or emergent resident need occurs, the organization is able to provide medications to the residents in its facility.

Element of Performance for MM.4.50

A 1. The organization has a process for providing medications to meet resident needs when the pharmacy is closed.

Standard MM.4.60

If the organization does not operate a pharmacy but routinely administers medications, the organization has a process for obtaining medications from a pharmacy.

Elements of Performance for MM.4.60

A 1. If the organization does not operate a pharmacy, the organization has a process for obtaining medications from a pharmacy for residents.

A 2. If the organization obtains medications from a pharmacy that is not open 24 hours a day, 7 days a week, the organization has a process for obtaining

* **Timely** Defined by organization policy and based on the intended use of the information.

medications from another source for urgent or emergent conditions when the pharmacy is closed. ⚠3

Standard MM.4.70

Medications dispensed by the organization are retrieved when recalled or discontinued by the manufacturer or the Food and Drug Administration for safety reasons.

Note: *This standard is applicable to all on-site pharmacies, and pharmacies contracted by the long term care facility to provide medications to its residents.*

Elements of Performance for MM.4.70

A 1. When the organization has been informed of a medication recall or discontinuation by the manufacturer or the Food and Drug Administration (FDA) for safety reasons, medications within the organization are retrieved* and handled per organization policy and law or regulation.

A 2. The organization notifies all those ordering, dispensing, and/or administering active† medications of any manufacturer or FDA recall or discontinuance.

A 3. When the organization has been informed of a medication recall or discontinuation by the manufacturer or the FDA for safety reasons, residents who are actively receiving the medication are identified and informed of the recall or discontinuation.

Standard MM.4.80

The organization has a process to address medications that are returned to the pharmacy or the organization.

Rationale for MM.4.80

Medications may be returned when allowed under law or regulation and organization policy. Previously dispensed but unused, expired, or returned medications in the organization must be accounted for, controlled, and disposed of. The pharmacy is responsible for controlling and accounting for all unused medications returned to the pharmacy.

Elements of Performance for MM.4.80

A 1. The organization has a process in place that addresses if and when unused, expired, or returned medications will be managed by the pharmacy or by the organization.

---

* Although recalls are generally by lot number, an organization may retrieve all lots of a recalled medication instead of recording and identifying medications by their lot number.

† Dispensed medications that have not passed expiration date and prescriptions that can be refilled without an additional physician order.

A 2. The organization has a process in place that addresses how medications are returned to the pharmacy's or organization's control, including procedures that address preventing diversion of medications and account for all unused, expired, or returned medications.

A 3. The organization has a process in place that addresses how outside sources, if any, are used for destruction of medications.

C Ⓜ 4. These processes for addressing medications returned to the pharmacy or organization are implemented.

Administration

Standard MM.5.10

Medications are safely and accurately administered.

Elements of Performance for MM.5.10

A 1. Policies and procedures address: Health care staff who are allowed to administer medications, with or without supervision, consistent with law or regulation and organization policy.

C Ⓜ 2. Before administering a medication, the licensed independent practitioner or qualified individual administering the medication does the following: Verifies that the medication selected for administration is the correct one based on the medication order and product label. ⚠3

C Ⓜ 3. Before administering a medication, the licensed independent practitioner or qualified individual administering the medication does the following: Verifies that the medication is stable based on visual examination for particulates or discoloration and that the medication has not expired. ⚠3

C Ⓜ 4. Before administering a medication, the licensed independent practitioner or qualified individual administering the medication does the following: Verifies that there is no contraindication for administering the medication. ⚠3

C Ⓜ 5. Before administering a medication, the licensed independent practitioner or qualified individual administering the medication does the following: Verifies that the medication is being administered at the proper time, in the prescribed dose, and by the correct route. ⚠3

C Ⓜ 6. Before administering a medication, the licensed independent practitioner or qualified individual administering the medication does the following: Advises the resident or if appropriate, the resident's family about any potential clinically significant adverse reaction or other concerns about administering a new medication.*

* Please refer to PC.6.10, EP3 for additional information addressing the education of patients regarding medication use.

C Ⓜ 7. Before administering a medication, the licensed independent practitioner or qualified individual administering the medication does the following: Discusses any unresolved, significant concerns about the medication with the resident's physician, prescriber (if different from the physician), and/or relevant staff involved with the resident's care, treatment, and service. ⚠3

A 8. Policies and procedures address guidelines for prescriber notification in the event of an adverse drug reaction or medication error.

Standard MM.5.20

Self-administered medications are safely and accurately administered.

Elements of Performance for MM.5.20

A 1. If self administration is allowed, procedures guide the safe and accurate self administration* of medications or administration of medications by a person who is not a staff member and address training, supervision, and administration documentation.

C Ⓜ 2. Persons who administer medications but are not staff members (for example, the resident if self-administering) receive information about the following:
- The nature of the medications to be administered
- How to administer medications, such as the frequency, route of administration, and dose
- The expected actions and side effects of the medications to be administered
- How to monitor the effects of the medications on the resident

C Ⓜ 3. Persons who administer medications but are not staff members (including the resident, if self-administering) are determined to be competent at medication administration before being allowed to administer medications.

Standard MM.5.30

Not applicable

Monitoring

Standard MM.6.10

The effects of medication(s) on residents are monitored.

* Self administration includes those instances where a resident independently uses a medication, including medications that may be held by the organization for the independent use by the resident.

Rationale for MM.6.10

Monitoring the effects of medications on residents helps to assure that medication therapy is appropriate and minimizes the occurrence of adverse events.

Elements of Performance for MM.6.10

C Ⓜ 1. Each resident's response to his or her medication is monitored according to the clinical needs of the resident and addresses the resident's response to the prescribed medication and actual or potential medication-related problems. ⚠3

C Ⓜ 2. Monitoring a medication's effect on a resident includes the following:
- Gathering the resident's own perceptions about side effects, and when appropriate, perceived efficacy
- Referring to information from the resident's clinical record, relevant laboratory results, clinical response, and medication profile

A 3. The organization has a process for monitoring the resident's response to the first dose(s) of a medication new to a resident when he or she is under the direct care of the organization.

4. Not applicable

C Ⓜ 5. The consultant pharmacist reviews each resident's medication regimen at least monthly.

C Ⓜ 6. The findings, conclusions, and recommendations of medication monitoring are documented in the clinical record and communicated to the physician, prescriber (if different from the physician), and those involved in the resident's care.

Standard MM.6.20

The organization responds to actual or potential adverse drug events and medication errors.

Elements of Performance for MM.6.20

A 1. The organization has a process to respond to actual or potential adverse drug events and medication errors.

C Ⓜ 2. Action is taken when an actual or potential adverse drug event is identified (depending on the organization's services, this may be limited to calling for outside assistance, for example, community-sponsored 911 service). ⚠3

C Ⓜ 3. The organization or responsible individual complies with internal and external reporting requirements for actual or potential adverse drug events (for example, to the United States Pharmacopoeia [USP], the FDA, and the Institute for Safe Medication Practices [ISMP]).

High-Risk Medications

High-risk or high-alert drugs are those drugs involved in a high percentage of medication errors and/or sentinel events and medications that carry a higher risk for abuse, errors, or other adverse outcomes. Lists of high-risk or high-alert drugs are available from such organizations as the ISMP, the USP, and so forth, based on national data about medication use. However, the organization needs to develop its own list of high-risk or high-alert drugs based on its unique utilization patterns or drugs and its own internal data about medication errors and sentinel events. Examples of high-risk drugs include investigational drugs, controlled medications, medications not on the approved FDA list, medications with a narrow therapeutic range, psychotherapeutic medications, and look-alike/sound-alike medications. Organizations determine whether medications that are new to the market or new to the organization are high risk.

Standard MM.7.10

The organization develops processes for managing high-risk or high-alert medications.

Elements of Performance for MM.7.10

A 1. The organization identifies the high-risk or high-alert medications used within the organization, if any. ⚠3

A 2. Based on the services provided, the organization develops processes for procuring, storing, ordering, transcribing, preparing, dispensing, administering, and/or monitoring high-risk or high-alert medications.

C Ⓜ 3. The processes for managing high-risk or high-alert medications are implemented. ⚠3

Standard MM.7.20

Psychotropic medication use is monitored.

Rationale for MM.7.20

The ongoing monitoring of the use of psychotropic medication* helps to do the following:

- Determine the resident's continued need for the current psychotropic dosing regimen
- Identify, as early as possible, when the resident has achieved the optimal benefit from the drug dose
- Identify when the drug dose can be lowered or the drug discontinued or replaced with another, less potent prescription
- Identify adverse side effects
- Evaluate the effectiveness of PRN orders in managing behavior

---

* **Psychotropic medication** Any medication whose intended purpose is to alter perception, mental status, or behavior. These include, but are not limited to, those medications that produce drug dependence. Some examples of drug classes that are considered psychotropic medications include, but are not limited to, hypnotics, antipsychotics, long- and short-acting benzodiazepines, sedatives/anxiolytics, and antidepressants.

Elements of Performance for MM.7.20

A 1. The organization uses an interdisciplinary process that includes the physician, pharmacist, nurse, and other members of the health care team involved in the resident's care to monitor psychotropic medications.

A 2. The organization specifies that psychotropic medications are used only during the following circumstances:
- When indicated by assessment and medical necessity
- After other nonpharmacological interventions or alternatives have been considered or used
- At the lowest effective therapeutic dose

A 3. The use of PRN orders for psychotropic medications is periodically reviewed to determine the appropriateness and effectiveness of these PRN orders, with the objective of decreasing their use as much as possible.

A 4. The organization's compliance with its own monitoring process is evaluated regularly.

Standard MM.7.30

Not applicable

Standard MM.7.40

Investigational medications are safely controlled and administered.

Rationale for MM.7.40

The organization protects the safety of residents participating in investigational or clinical medication studies by controlling and monitoring the use of these medications. In addition, the organization addresses the use of specific populations for experimentation and research, and reviews all investigational medications to evaluate safety (*see* standard RI.2.180).

Elements of Performance for MM.7.40

A 1. Procedures for the use of investigational medications specify a written process for reviewing, approving, supervising, and monitoring investigational medications use.

A 2. When the organization operates a pharmacy, procedures specify the pharmacy controls the storage, dispensing, labeling, and distribution of the investigational medication.

A 3. Procedures specify that when a patient is involved in an investigational protocol that is independent of the organization, the organization will review and accommodate the resident's continued participation in the protocol (*see* standard RI.2.180).

A 4. The procedures for the use of investigational medications are implemented.

Evaluation

Standard MM.8.10

The organization evaluates its medication management system.

Elements of Performance for MM.8.10

A 1. The organization evaluates its medication management system for risk points and identifies areas to improve safety.

A 2. The organization identifies opportunities for improvement by routinely evaluating the literature for new technologies or successful practices that have been demonstrated to enhance safety in other organizations to determine if it can improve its own medication management system.

3. The organization reviews internally generated reports to identify trends or issues in its medication management system (*see* standards PI.2.10 and PI.2.20).

A 4. The organization acts to implement improvements based on the following:
- Evaluation of its medication management system
- Review of new technologies
- External data
- Successful practices that have been demonstrated to enhance safety

A 5. The performance of new and modified medication management processes is measured.

A 6. The organization uses information from data analysis to identify subsequent changes to improve its medication management system.

A 7. The pharmacy and long term care facility collaborate to determine whether the medication management system is effective.

A 8. When a pharmacy is the primary provider of pharmaceutical services to a long term care facility, the pharmacy collaborates with the long term care facility to implement a medication management system to control all medications.

A 9. When a pharmacy is the primary provider of pharmaceutical services to a long term care facility or consultant pharmacist services are provided, the pharmacy or pharmacist participates in educating the long term care facility about the following:
- The collection and use of performance measures for medication management
- Techniques to reduce medication errors and minimize waste of medications

2009 SLTC

Surveillance, Prevention, and Control of Infection (IC)

IC

IC

Surveillance, Prevention, and Control of Infection (IC)

Overview

Prevention of health care–associated infections (HAIs) represents one of the major safety initiatives that a long term care organization can undertake. The Centers for Disease Control and Prevention (CDC)* estimates that each year approximately 2 million patients admitted to acute care hospitals in the United States acquire infections that were not related to the condition for which they were hospitalized. Residents of long term care facilities are often transferred to and from hospital settings, making infection prevention and control a priority. Older adults may not present with the typical signs and symptoms of infection, making identification of these residents with infections more challenging.

The design and scope of the long term care organization's infection prevention and control program (hereafter referred to as the "IC program") are based on the risk(s) that the organization faces for the transmission of infectious disease. Therefore, the organization assesses its risk and designs the IC program based on this assessment. Once the organization has designed its IC program, the program must be monitored to ensure that the infection prevention and control activities are implemented.

The goal of an effective IC program is to reduce the risk of acquisition and transmission of HAIs. Long term care organizations must do the following to achieve this goal:

- The organization incorporates its infection program as a major component of its safety and performance improvement programs
- The organization performs an ongoing assessment to identify its risks for the acquisition and transmission of infectious agents
- The organization uses an epidemiological approach that consists of surveillance, data collection, and trend identification
- The organization effectively implements infection prevention and control processes
- The organization educates and collaborates with leaders across the organization to effectively participate in the design and implementation of the IC program
- The organization integrates its efforts with health care and community leaders to the extent practicable, recognizing that infection prevention and control is a communitywide effort
- The organization plans for responding to infections that may potentially overwhelm its resources

* Monitoring hospital-acquired infections to promote patient safety—United States, 1990–1999. *MMWR Morb Mortal Wkly Rep* 49:149–153, Mar. 10, 2000.

Key: 0 = Insufficient compliance; 1 = Partial compliance; 2 = Satisfactory compliance; NA = Not applicable; **A** indicates scoring category A; **C** indicates scoring category C; ▲(2) indicates situational decision rules apply; △(3) indicates direct impact requirements apply; Ⓜ indicates Measure of success is needed

A program with aims of such broad scope and depth requires the direct involvement of organization leaders. Only with the ongoing attention and direction of organization leadership can the appropriate scope of the program be determined and adequately resourced.

The standards in this chapter, which focus on development and implementation of plans to prevent and control infections, are supported by standards in other chapters, such as "Management of the Environment of Care," "Management of Human Resources," "Improving Organization Performance," and "Leadership," to produce a comprehensive approach to infection control.

Standards

The following is a list of all standards for this function. They are presented here for your convenience without footnotes or other explanatory text. If you have a question about a term used here, please check the Glossary.

Note: *A revised standard numbering system is being used with the reformatted standards. The revised numbering system will allow for more flexibility to add standards while maintaining the current label for each standard.*

The IC Program and Its Components

IC.1.10 The risk of development of a health care–associated infection is minimized through an organizationwide infection control program.

IC.2.10 The infection control program identifies risks for the acquisition and transmission of infectious agents on an ongoing basis.

IC.3.10 Based on risks, the organization establishes priorities and sets goals for preventing the development of health care–associated infections within the organization.

IC.4.10 Once the organization has prioritized its goals, strategies must be implemented to achieve those goals.

IC.4.15 Immunization against influenza is offered to staff and licensed independent practitioners.

IC.5.10 The infection control program evaluates the effectiveness of the infection control interventions and, as necessary, redesigns the infection control interventions.

IC.6.10 As part of its emergency management activities, the organization prepares to respond to an influx, or the risk of an influx, of infectious residents.

Structure and Resources for the IC Program

IC.7.10 The infection control program is managed effectively.

IC.8.10 Relevant components/functions within the organization collaborate to implement the infection control program.

IC.9.10 Organization leaders allocate adequate resources for the infection control program.

Standards, Rationales, Elements of Performance, and Scoring

The IC Program and Its Components

Standard IC.1.10

The risk of development of a health care–associated infection is minimized through an organizationwide infection control program.

Rationale for IC.1.10

The risk of HAIs exists throughout the organization. An effective IC program that can systematically identify risks and respond appropriately must involve all relevant programs and settings within the organization.

Elements of Performance for IC.1.10

A 1. An organizationwide IC program is implemented.

A 2. Individuals and/or positions with the authority to take steps to prevent or control the acquisition and transmission of infectious agents are identified.

A 3. All applicable organizational components and functions are integrated into the IC program.

A 4. Systems are in place to communicate with licensed independent practitioners; staff; students/trainees; volunteers; and, as appropriate, visitors, residents, and families about infection prevention and control issues, including their responsibilities in preventing the spread of infection within the organization.

A 5. The organization has systems for reporting infection surveillance, prevention, and control information to the following:

- The appropriate staff within the organization
- Federal, state, and local public health authorities in accordance with law and regulation
- Accrediting bodies (*see* Sentinel Event Reporting, page 104, and National Patient Safety Goals, pages 119 and 130)
- The referring or receiving organization when a resident was transferred or referred and the presence of an infection was not known at the time of transfer or referral

Note: *When a referring organization becomes aware that a resident they have transferred has an active infection for which treatment should start or change, the referring organization communicates this to the receiving organization. If a receiving organization identifies an infection not identified by the referring organization (such as an infected wound), the receiving organi-*

zation should communicate the omission to the referring organization. This action will aid the referring organization's improvement efforts.

A 6. Systems for the investigation of outbreaks of infectious diseases are in place.

A 7. Applicable policies and procedures are in place throughout the organization.

A 8. Written policies and procedures include at least the following, departments' participation in infection prevention and control activities: clinical services, food services, housekeeping, maintenance, and laundry services, hotel service (for example, beauty shops), resident activities, and staff health.

A 9. The organization has a written IC plan* that includes the following:
- A description of prioritized risks
- A statement of the goals of the IC program
- A description of the organization's strategies to minimize, reduce, or eliminate the prioritized risks
- A description of how the strategies will be evaluated

Standard IC.2.10

The infection control program identifies risks for the acquisition and transmission of infectious agents on an ongoing basis.

Rationale for IC.2.10

An organization's risks of infection will vary based on the organization's geographic location, the community environment, the types of programs/services provided, and the characteristics and behaviors of the population served. As these risks change over time—sometimes rapidly—risk assessment must be an ongoing process.

Elements of Performance for IC.2.10

A 1. The organization identifies risks for the transmission and acquisition of infectious agents throughout the organization based on the following factors:
- The geographic location and community environment of the organization, program/services provided, and the characteristics of the population served
- The results of the analysis of the organization's infection prevention and control data
- The care, treatment, and services provided

A 2. The risk analysis is formally reviewed at least annually and whenever significant changes occur in any of the preceding factors.

* **Written plan** A succinct, useful document, formulated beforehand, that identifies needs, lists strategies to meet those needs, and sets goals and objectives. The format of the "plan" may include narratives, policies and procedures, protocols, practice guidelines, clinical paths, care maps, or a combination of these.

A 3. Surveillance activities, including data collection and analysis, are used to identify infection prevention and control risks pertaining to the following:
- Residents
- Licensed independent practitioners, staff, volunteers, and student/trainees
- Visitors and families, as warranted

Standard IC.3.10

Based on risks, the organization establishes priorities and sets goals for preventing the development of health care–associated infections within the organization.

Rationale for IC.3.10

The risks of HAIs within an organization are many, while resources are limited. An effective IC program requires a thoughtful prioritization of the most important risks to be addressed. Priorities and goals related to the identified risks guide the choice and design of strategies for infection prevention and control in an organization. These priorities and goals provide a framework for evaluating the strategies.

Elements of Performance for IC.3.10

A 1. Priorities are established and goals related to preventing the acquisition and transmission of potentially infectious agents are developed based on the risks identified.

These goals include, but are not limited to, the following (EPs 2–5):

A 2. Limiting unprotected exposure to pathogens throughout the organization

A 3. Enhancing hand hygiene

4. Not applicable

A 5. Minimizing the risk of transmitting infections associated with the use of procedures, medical equipment, and medical devices

Standard IC.4.10

Once the organization has prioritized its goals, strategies must be implemented to achieve those goals.

Rationale for IC.4.10

The organization plans and implements interventions to address the IC issues that it finds important based on prioritized risks and associated surveillance data.

Elements of Performance for IC.4.10

A 1. Interventions are designed to incorporate relevant guidelines* for infection prevention and control activities.

* Examples of guidelines include those offered by the CDC, Healthcare Infection Control Practices Advisory Committee (HICPAC), and National Quality Forum (NQF).

Interventions are implemented which include the following (EPs 2–3):

2. An organizationwide hand hygiene program that complies with current World Health Organization (WHO) hand hygiene guidelines or Centers for Disease Control and Prevention (CDC) hand hygiene guidelines*

   Note: *The preceding requirement is not scored here. It is scored at NPSG.07.01.01.*

A 3. Methods to reduce the risks associated with procedures, medical equipment,† and medical devices, including the following:
   - Appropriate storage, cleaning, disinfection, sterilization, and/or disposal of supplies and equipment
   - Reuse of equipment designated by the manufacturer as disposable in a manner that is consistent with regulatory and professional standards
   - The appropriate use of personal protective equipment ⚠3

A 4. Implementation of applicable precautions, as appropriate, is based on the following:
   - The potential for transmission
   - The mechanism of transmission
   - The care, treatment, and services setting
   - The emergence and reemergence of pathogens in the community that could affect the organization ⚠3

Interventions are implemented which include the following (EPs 5–8):

C Ⓜ 5. Screening for exposure and/or immunity to infectious diseases that licensed independent practitioners, staff, student/trainees, and volunteers may come in contact with in their work is available, as warranted

C Ⓜ 6. Referral for assessment, potential testing, immunization and/or prophylaxis/treatment, and counseling, as appropriate, of licensed independent practitioners, staff, students/trainees, and volunteers who are identified as potentially having an infectious disease or risk of infectious disease that may put the population they serve at risk

C Ⓜ 7. Referral for assessment, potential testing, immunization and/or prophylaxis/treatment, and counseling, as appropriate, of residents, students/trainees, and volunteers who have been exposed to infectious disease(s) at the organization and licensed independent practitioners or staff who are occupationally exposed

A 8. Reduction of risks associated with animals brought into the organization (such as management of animal waste)

---

* Organizations are required to comply with all 1A, 1B, 1C CDC or WHO guidelines.

† **Medical equipment** Fixed and portable equipment used for the diagnosis, treatment, monitoring, and direct care of individuals.

Standard IC.4.15

Immunization against influenza is offered to staff* and licensed independent practitioners.

Rationale for IC.4.15

Transmission of influenza from staff and licensed independent practitioners to residents can create serious health care problems, especially among those who are at high risk for complications related to influenza. There are multiple effective measures that can reduce the risk of health care– associated influenza, including strict adherence to respiratory precautions, prompt treatment, and restricting ill staff and licensed independent practitioners from providing patient care. However, the most successful measure to prevent health care–associated transmission of influenza is vaccinating staff and licensed independent practitioners.

Since 1981, the Centers for Disease Control and Prevention (CDC) has recommended annual influenza vaccinations for all health care personnel.† The recommendations of the Healthcare Infection Control Practices Advisory Committee (HICPAC) and the Advisory Committee on Immunization Practices (ACIP) concerning influenza vaccination of health care personnel (HCP) in the United States apply to HCP in acute care hospitals, nursing homes, skilled nursing facilities, physician's offices, urgent care centers, and outpatient clinics, and to persons who provide home health care and emer-

* The requirements in standard IC.4.15 do not apply to students.

† The CDC defines health care personnel (HCP) as all paid and unpaid persons working in health care settings who have the potential for exposure to infectious materials, including body substances, contaminated medical supplies and equipment, contaminated environmental surfaces, or contaminated air. HCP might include (but are not limited to) physicians, nurses, nursing assistants, therapists, technicians, emergency medical service personnel, dental personnel, pharmacists, laboratory personnel, autopsy personnel, students and trainees, contractual staff not employed by the health care facility, and persons (e.g., clerical, dietary, housekeeping, maintenance, and volunteers) not directly involved in patient care but potentially exposed to infectious agents that can be transmitted to and from HCP.

gency medical services.* Despite ongoing recommendations, vaccination rates as measured by the CDC remain low. Influenza among health care personnel, especially during an epidemic, might increase transmission to residents, and may compromise the ability of an organization to provide care.

One obstacle to effective vaccination is declination by health care personnel. Health care personnel may decline vaccination for many reasons. They may have been vaccinated elsewhere, have a medical contraindication, or have other personal reasons for declining the vaccine. Vaccination might also be declined because it is offered at inconvenient times or locations. Whatever the reason, it is important for organizations to identify why individuals do not participate in the vaccination program, work to overcome these reasons, and increase vaccination rates.

Optimally, influenza vaccination will be offered to everyone. During periods of influenza vaccine supply disruption, organizations may have to establish priorities for whom they will vaccinate. The CDC recommends the use of vaccination priority groups only in the event of vaccine supply disruptions.

Elements of Performance for IC.4.15

A 1. The organization establishes an annual influenza vaccination program that includes at least staff and licensed independent practitioners.

---

* Summary of the recommendations of the Healthcare Infection Control Practices Advisory Committee (HICPAC) and the Advisory Committee on Immunization Practices (ACIP) concerning influenza vaccination of health care personnel (HCP) in the United States. These recommendations apply to HCP in acute care hospitals, nursing homes, skilled nursing facilities, physician's offices, urgent care centers, and outpatient clinics, and to persons who provide home health care and emergency medical services.

- Educate HCP regarding the benefits of influenza vaccination and the potential health consequences of influenza illness for themselves and their patients, the epidemiology and modes of transmission, diagnosis, treatment, and nonvaccine infection control strategies, in accordance with their level of responsibility in preventing health care–associated influenza (category IB).
- Offer influenza vaccine annually to all eligible HCP to protect staff, patients, and family members and to decrease HCP absenteeism. Use of either available vaccine (inactivated and live, attenuated influenza vaccine [LAIV]) is recommended for eligible persons. During periods when inactivated vaccine is in short supply, use of LAIV is especially encouraged when feasible for eligible HCP (category IA).
- Provide influenza vaccination to HCP at the work site and at no cost as one component of employee health programs. Use strategies that have been demonstrated to increase influenza vaccine acceptance, including vaccination clinics, mobile carts, vaccination access during all work shifts, and modeling and support by institutional leaders (category IB).
- Obtain a signed declination from HCP who decline influenza vaccination for reasons other than medical contraindications (category II).
- Monitor HCP influenza vaccination coverage and declination at regular intervals during influenza season and provide feedback of ward-, unit-, and specialty-specific rates to staff and administration (category IB).
- Use the level of HCP influenza vaccination coverage as one measure of a patient safety quality program (category II).

Evidence Ranking Scheme

Category IA. Strongly recommend for implementation and strongly supported by well-designed experimental, clinical, or epidemiological studies.

Category IB. Strongly recommended for implementation and supported by certain experimental, clinical, or epidemiological studies and a strong theoretic rationale.

Category IC. Required by state or federal regulation, or representing an established association standard.

Category II. Suggested for implementation and supported by suggestive clinical or epidemiologic studies, or a theoretic rationale.

Unresolved Issue. No recommendation is offered. No consensus or insufficient evidence exists regarding efficacy.

A 2. The organization provides access to influenza vaccination on site.

A 3. The organization educates staff and licensed independent practitioners about the following:
- Flu vaccination
- Nonvaccine control measures (such as the use of appropriate precautions)
- The diagnosis, transmission, and potential impact of influenza

A 4. The organization annually evaluates vaccination rates and reasons for nonparticipation in the organization's immunization program.

A 5. The organization implements enhancements to the program to increase participation.

Standard IC.5.10

The infection control program evaluates the effectiveness of the infection control interventions and, as necessary, redesigns the infection control interventions.

Rationale for IC.5.10

The evaluation of the effectiveness of interventions helps to identify which activities of the IC program are effective and which activities need to be changed to improve outcomes.

Elements of Performance for IC.5.10

A 1. The organization formally evaluates and revises the goals and program (or portions of the program) at least annually and whenever risks significantly change.

A 2. The evaluation addresses changes in the scope of the IC program (for example, resulting from the introduction of new services or new sites of care).

A 3. The evaluation addresses changes in the results of the IC program risk analysis.

A 4. The evaluation addresses emerging and reemerging problems in the health care community that potentially affect the organization (for example, highly infectious agents).

A 5. The evaluation addresses the assessment of the success or failure of interventions for preventing and controlling infection.

A 6. The evaluation addresses responses to concerns raised by leadership and others within the organization.

A 7. The evaluation addresses the evolution of relevant infection prevention and control guidelines that are based on evidence or, in the absence of evidence, expert consensus.

Standard IC.6.10

As part of its emergency management activities, the organization prepares to respond to an influx, or the risk of an influx, of infectious residents.

Rationale for IC.6.10

The health care organization is an important resource for the continued functioning of a community. An organization's ability to deliver care, treatment, or services is threatened when it is ill-prepared to respond to an epidemic or infections likely to require expanded or extended care capabilities over a prolonged period. Therefore, it is important for an organization to plan how to prevent the introduction of the infection into the organization, how to quickly recognize that existing residents have become infected, and/or how to contain the risk or spread of the infection.

This planned response may include a broad range of options, including the temporary halting of services and/or admissions, delaying transfer or discharge, limiting visitors within an organization, or fully activating the organization's emergency management plan. The actual response depends upon issues such as the extent to which the community is affected by the epidemic or infection, the types of services the organization offers, and the organization's capabilities.

The concepts included in these standards are supported by standards found elsewhere in the manual, including standard EC.4.10.

Elements of Performance for IC.6.10

A 1. The organization determines its response to an influx or risk of an influx of infectious residents.

A 2. If the organization will continue to accept or treat residents, then the organization has a plan for managing an ongoing influx of potentially infectious residents over an extended period.

A 3. The organization does the following:
- Determines how it will keep abreast of current information about the emergence of epidemics or new infections which may result in the organization activating its response
- Determines how it will disseminate critical information to staff and other key practitioners
- Identifies resources in the community (through local, state, and/or federal public health systems) for obtaining additional information

Structure and Resources for the IC Program

Standard IC.7.10

The infection control program is managed effectively.

Rationale for IC.7.10

The IC program requires management by an individual (or individuals) with knowledge that is appropriate to the level of risks identified by the organization, as well as knowledge of the analysis of infection risks, principles of infection prevention and control, and data analysis. The individual gathering data for the infection control program does not have to be the person analyzing the data and managing the program. The individual may be employed by the organization or the organization may contract with this individual. The number of individuals and their qualifications are based on the organization's size, complexity, and needs.

Elements of Performance for IC.7.10

A 1. The organization assigns responsibility for managing IC program activities to one or more individuals whose number, competency, and skill mix are determined by the goals and objectives of the IC activities.

A 2. Qualifications of the individual(s) responsible for managing the IC program are determined by the risks entailed in the care, treatment, and services provided, the organization's resident population(s), and the complexity of the activities that will be carried out.

Note: *Qualifications may be met through ongoing education, training, experience, and/or certification (such as that offered by the Certification Board for Infection Control [CBIC]) in the prevention and control of infections).*

A 3. This individual(s) coordinates all infection prevention and control activities within the organization.

A 4. This individual(s) facilitates ongoing monitoring of the effectiveness of prevention and/or control activities and interventions.

Standard IC.8.10

Relevant components/functions within the organization collaborate to implement the infection control program.

Rationale for IC.8.10

The successful creation of an organizationwide IC program requires collaboration with all relevant components/functions. This collaboration is vital to successful data gathering and interpretation, design of interventions, and effective implementation of interventions. Individuals within the organization who have the power to implement plans and make decisions about interventions related to infection prevention and control participate in the IC program. In smaller organizations, this may only represent one or two people, while in larger organizations this may require representation by multiple divisions. Whatever the number of components/functions represented, it is important that the components/functions that have a direct impact on infection control are represented. While a formal committee consisting of leadership and other components is not required as evidence of this collaboration, the organization may want to consider this option.

Elements of Performance for IC.8.10

A 1. Organization leaders, with licensed independent practitioners, and other direct and indirect resident care staff, including, when applicable, administration, building maintenance/engineering, food services, housekeeping, and pharmacy collaborate on an ongoing basis with the qualified individual(s) managing the IC program.

A 2. These representatives participate in the following:
- Development of strategies for each components/functions role in the IC program
- Assessment of the adequacy of the human, information, physical, and financial resources allocated to support infection prevention and control activities
- Assessment of the overall failure or success of key processes for preventing and controlling infection
- The review and revision of the IC program, as warranted to improve outcomes

Standard IC.9.10

Organization leaders allocate adequate resources for the infection control program.

Rationale for IC.9.10

Adequate resources are needed to effectively plan and successfully implement a program of this scope.

Elements of Performance for IC.9.10

A 1. The effectiveness of the organization's infection prevention and control activities is reviewed on an ongoing basis, and findings are reported to the integrated resident safety program at least annually.

A 2. Adequate systems to access information are provided to support infection prevention and control activities.

A 3. When applicable, adequate laboratory support is provided to support infection prevention and control activities.

A 4. Adequate equipment and supplies are provided to support infection prevention and control activities.

2009

SLTC

Improving Organization Performance (PI)

PI

PI

Improving Organization Performance (PI)

Overview

Performance improvement (PI) is a continuous process. It involves measuring the functioning of important processes and services, and, when indicated, identifying changes that enhance performance. These changes are incorporated into new or existing work processes, products or services, and performance is monitored to ensure that the improvements are sustained.

PI focuses on outcomes of care, treatment, and services. Leaders establish a planned, systematic, and organizationwide approach(es) to PI. They set priorities for PI and ensure that the disciplines representing the scope of care, treatment, and services across the organization work collaboratively to plan and implement improvement activities. The leaders' responsibilities are described in the "Leadership" chapter of this manual.

An important aspect of improving organization performance is effectively reducing factors that contribute to unanticipated adverse events and/or outcomes. Unanticipated adverse events and/or outcomes may be caused by poorly designed systems, system failures, or errors. Reducing unanticipated adverse events and/or unanticipated outcomes requires an environment in which residents, their families, and organization staff and leaders can identify and manage actual and potential risks to safety. Such an environment encourages the following:

- Recognizing and acknowledging risks and unanticipated adverse events
- Initiating actions to reduce these risks and unanticipated adverse events
- Reporting internally on risk reduction initiatives and their effectiveness
- Focusing on processes and systems
- Minimizing individual blame or retribution for involvement in an unanticipated adverse event
- Investigating factors that contribute to unanticipated adverse events and sharing that acquired knowledge both internally and with other organizations

The leaders are responsible for fostering such an environment through their personal example and by supporting effective responses to actual occurrences of unanticipated adverse events; ongoing proactive reduction of safety risks to residents; and integration of safety priorities into the design and redesign of all relevant organization processes, functions, and services.

Key: 0 = Insufficient compliance; 1 = Partial compliance; 2 = Satisfactory compliance; NA = Not applicable; **A** indicates scoring category A; **C** indicates scoring category C; ▲(2) indicates situational decision rules apply; △(3) indicates direct impact requirements apply; Ⓜ indicates Measure of success is needed

This chapter focuses on the following fundamental components of PI:

- Measuring performance through data collection
- Assessing current performance
- Improving performance

Standards

The following is a list of all standards for this function. They are presented here for your convenience without footnotes or other explanatory text. If you have a question about a term used here, please check the Glossary.

Note: *A revised standard numbering system is being used with the reformatted standards. This revised numbering system will allow for more flexibility to add standards while maintaining the current label for each standard.*

PI.1.10 The organization collects data to monitor its performance.

PI.1.20 Not applicable

PI.2.10 Data are systematically aggregated and analyzed.

PI.2.20 Undesirable patterns or trends in performance are analyzed.

PI.2.30 Not applicable

PI.3.10 Information from data analysis is used to make changes that improve performance and resident safety and reduce the risk of sentinel events.

PI.3.20 Not applicable

Standards, Rationales, Elements of Performance, and Scoring

Standard PI.1.10

The organization collects data to monitor its performance.

Rationale for PI.1.10

Data help determine performance improvement priorities. The data collected for high priority and required areas are used to monitor the stability of existing processes, identify opportunities for improvement, identify changes that lead to improvement, or sustain improvement. Data collection helps identify specific areas that require further study. These areas are determined by considering the information provided by the data about process stability, risks, sentinel events, and priorities set by the leaders. Data may come from internal sources such as staff or external sources such as residents, referral sources, and so on. In addition, the organization identifies those areas needing improvement and identifies desired changes. Performance measures are used to determine whether the changes result in desired outcomes. The organization identifies the frequency and detail of data collection.

Note 1: *The organization also collects data on the following areas that will be scored in their respective chapters:*

- *Evaluation and improvement of conditions in the environment* (see *"Management of the Environment of Care" chapter)*
- *Staffing effectiveness* (see *"Management of Human Resources" chapter)*

Note 2: *For long term care organizations that serve residents with dementia, the organization may measure performance in the following areas: psychotropic drugs, incidents, acute behavioral events, family involvement, do-not-resuscitate orders, appropriate use of services, transfers, programs that meet resident needs, infection control, environmental adaptations, and safety.*

Elements of Performance for PI.1.10

A 1. The organization collects data for priorities identified by leaders (*see* standard LD.4.50).

A 2. The organization considers collecting data in the following areas:
- Staff opinions and needs
- Staff perceptions of risks to individuals and suggestions for improving resident safety
- Staff willingness to report unanticipated adverse events

A 3. The organization collects data on the perceptions of care, treatment, and services* of residents, including the following:
- Their specific needs and expectations
- How well the organization meets these needs and expectations
- How the organization can improve resident safety
- The effectiveness of pain management, when applicable

The organization collects data that measure the performance of each of the following potentially high-risk processes, when provided (EPs 4–8):

A 4. Medication management

A 5. Blood and blood product use

A 6. Restraint use

7. Not applicable

A 8. Behavior management and treatment

9. Through 12. Not applicable

Relevant information developed from the following activities (EPs 13–17) is integrated into performance improvement initiatives. This occurs in a way consistent with any organization policies or procedures intended to preserve any confidentiality or privilege of information established by applicable law.

A 13. Risk management

A 14. Utilization management

A 15. Quality control

A 16. Infection control surveillance and reporting

A 17. Research, as applicable

Standard PI.1.20

Not applicable

Standard PI.2.10

Data are systematically aggregated and analyzed.

Rationale for PI.2.10

Aggregating and analyzing data means transforming data into information. Aggregating data at points in time enables the organization to judge a particular process's stabil-

* The Joint Commission is moving from the phrase *satisfaction with care, treatment, and services* toward the more inclusive phrase *perception of care, treatment, and services* to better measure the performance of organizations meeting the needs, expectations and concerns of residents. By using this term, the organization will be prompted to assess not only residents' and/or families' satisfaction with care, treatment, or services, but also whether the organization meets their needs and expectations.

ity or a particular outcome's predictability in relation to performance expectations. Accumulated data are analyzed in such a way that current performance levels, patterns, or trends can be identified.

Elements of Performance for PI.2.10

A 1. Collected data are aggregated and analyzed.

A 2. Data are aggregated at the frequency appropriate to the activity or process being studied.

A 3. Statistical tools and techniques are used to analyze and display data.

A 4. Data are analyzed and compared internally over time and externally* with other sources of information, when available.

A 5. Comparative data are used to determine if there is excessive variability or unacceptable levels of performance when available.

Standard PI.2.20

Undesirable patterns or trends in performance are analyzed.

Elements of Performance for PI.2.20

A 1. Analysis is performed when data comparisons indicate that levels of performance, patterns, or trends vary substantially from those expected.

A 2. Analysis occurs for those topics chosen by leaders as performance improvement priorities.

A 3. Analysis is performed when undesirable variation occurs which changes priorities.

An analysis is performed for the following (EPs 4–6, 9, 10):

A 4. All confirmed transfusion reactions, if applicable to the organization

A 5. All serious adverse drug events, if applicable and as defined by the organization

A 6. All significant medication errors, if applicable and as defined by the organization

7. Not applicable

8. Not applicable

A 9. Hazardous conditions

A 10. Staffing effectiveness issues

---

* External sources of information include recent scientific, clinical, and management literature, including sentinel event alerts; well-formulated practice guidelines or parameters; performance measures; reference databases; other organizations with similar processes; and standards that are periodically reviewed and revised.

Standard PI.2.30

Not applicable

Standard PI.3.10

Information from data analysis is used to make changes that improve performance and resident safety and reduce the risk of sentinel events.

Elements of Performance for PI.3.10

A 1. The organization uses the information from data analysis to identify and implement changes that will improve the quality of care, treatment, and services.

A 2. The organization identifies and implements changes that will reduce the risk of sentinel events.

A 3. The organization uses the information from data analysis to identify changes that will improve resident safety.

A 4. Changes made to improve processes or outcomes are evaluated to ensure that they achieve the expected results.

A 5. Appropriate actions are undertaken when planned improvements are not achieved or sustained.

Standard PI.3.20

Not applicable

2009 SLTC

Leadership (LD)

LD

LD

Leadership (LD)

Overview

The safety and quality of care, treatment, or services depend on many factors, including the following:

- A culture that fosters safety as a priority for everyone who works in the organization
- The planning and provision of services that meet the needs of residents
- The availability of resources—human, financial, and physical—for providing care, treatment, or services
- The existence of competent staff and other care providers
- Ongoing evaluation of and improvement in performance

Management of these important functions is the direct responsibility of leaders; they are, in effect, responsible for the care, treatment, or services that the organization provides to its residents. In organizations with a governing body, governance has ultimate responsibility for this oversight. In larger organizations, different individuals or groups may be assigned different responsibilities, and they bring with them different skills, experience, and perspectives. In these situations, the way the leaders interact with each other and manage their assigned accountabilities can affect overall organization performance. In smaller organizations, these responsibilities may be handled by just one or two individuals. This chapter addresses the role of leaders in managing their diverse and, at times, complex responsibilities.

Leaders shape the organization's culture, and the culture, in turn, affects how the organization accomplishes its work. A healthy, thriving culture is built around the organization's mission and vision, which reflect the core values and principles that the organization finds important. Leaders must ask some basic questions in order to provide this focus: How does the organization plan to meet the needs of its population? By what ethical standards will the organization operate? What does the organization want to accomplish through its work? Once leaders answer these questions, the culture of the organization will begin to take shape. Leaders also have an obligation to set an example of how to work together to fulfill the organization's mission.

On a more practical level, leaders oversee operations and guide the organization on a day-to-day basis. They keep operations running smoothly so that the important work of the organization—serving its residents—can continue.

To meet their obligations effectively, leaders must collaborate, which means working together in a spirit of collegiality to achieve a common end. In smaller organizations, this may mean that a single leader or small group of leaders works closely with staff in order to meet the organization's managerial needs. In this case, key staff members share governance and decision making with senior leadership in order to direct the

Key: 0 = Insufficient compliance; 1 = Partial compliance; 2 = Satisfactory compliance; NA = Not applicable; **A** indicates scoring category A; **C** indicates scoring category C; ▲2 indicates situational decision rules apply; △3 indicates direct impact requirements apply; Ⓜ indicates Measure of success is needed

day-to-day operations, assess needs, secure resources, and plan for the future. Senior managers direct the day-to-day operations of the organization; governance determines what resources the organization needs and then secures those resources.

About This Chapter

This chapter is divided into four sections: Leadership Structure, Leadership Relationships, Organization Culture and System Performance Expectations, and Operations. The organization's culture, systems, and leadership structure and relationships all come together to shape and drive its operations.

The standards in the Leadership Structure section identify and define the various leadership groups and their responsibilities. The standards in Leadership Relationships address the development of the organization's mission, vision, and goals and communication among leaders. The standards in the Organization Culture and System Performance Expectations section focus on the framework for the organization's culture and systems. The standards also demonstrate how leaders help shape the culture of an organization and how culture, in turn, affects important systems within the organization (for example, data use, planning, communication, changing performance, staffing). The standards in the Operations section address the functions that are important to resident safety and high-quality care, treatment, or services. Some leaders may not be directly involved in the day-to-day operations of the organization, but the decisions they make and the initiatives they implement do affect operations.

Chapter Outline

I. Leadership Structure
   A. Leadership Structure (revised LD.01.01.01)
   B. Not applicable to long term care (revised LD.01.02.01)
   C. Governance Accountabilities (revised LD.01.03.01)
   D. The Chief Executive Responsibilities (revised LD.01.04.01)
   E. Not applicable to long term care (revised LD.01.05.01)
   F. Medical Director Oversees Care to Residents (revised LD.01.06.01)
   G. Leaders' Knowledge (revised LD.01.07.01)

II. Leadership Relationships
   A. Mission, Vision, and Goals (revised LD.02.01.01)
   B. Not applicable to long term care (revised LD.02.02.01)
   C. Communication Among Leaders (revised LD.02.03.01).
   D. Not applicable to long term care (revised LD.02.04.01).

III. Organization Culture and System Performance
   A. Culture of Safety and Quality (revised LD.03.01.01)
   B. Using Data and Information (revised LD.03.02.01)
   C. Organization-wide Planning (revised LD.03.03.01)
   D. Communication (revised LD.03.04.01)
   E. Change Management and Performance Improvement (revised LD.03.05.01)
   F. Staffing (revised LD.03.06.01)

IV. Leadership Operations
   A. Administration (revised LD.04.01.01, LD.04.01.03, LD.04.01.05, LD.04.01.07, LD.04.01.11) *(revised LD.04.01.09 is not applicable to long term care)*
   B. Ethical Issues (revised LD.04.02.01, LD.04.02.03, LD.04.02.05)
   C. Meeting Patient Needs (revised LD.04.03.01, LD.04.03.07, LD.04.03.09) *(revised LD.04.03.03, LD.04.03.05, and LD.04.03.11 are not applicable to long term care)*
   D. Managing Safety and Quality (revised LD.04.04.01, LD.04.04.03, LD.04.04.05) *(revised LD.04.04.07 and LD.04.04.09 are not applicable to long term care)*
   E. Not applicable to long term care (revised LD.04.05.01 through LD.04.05.15)

Standards, Rationales, Elements of Performance, and Scoring

Introduction to Leadership Structure, Standards LD.01.01.01 through LD.01.07.01

Each organization, regardless of its complexity, has a structured leadership. Many leadership responsibilities directly affect the provision of care, treatment, or services, as well as the day-to-day operations of the organization. In some cases, these responsibilities will be shared among leaders, and, in other cases, a particular leader has primary responsibility. Individual leaders may have several different roles. Regardless of the organization's structure, it is important that leaders carry out all their responsibilities.

A variety of individuals may work in the organization, including licensed independent practitioners, staff, volunteers, students, and independent contractors. These standards describe the overall responsibility of the governance for the safety and quality of care, treatment, or services provided by all of these individuals.

How well the leaders work together is key to effective organization performance, and the standards emphasize this. Leaders with different responsibilities—governance, management, and the clinical staff—bring different skills, experiences, and perspectives to the organization. Working together means that leaders have the opportunity to participate in discussions and have their opinions heard. Depending upon the topic and the organization, individuals may participate in decision making, and the governing body may delegate decision making to certain leaders. Final decisions, however, are always the ultimate responsibility of governance; this key principle is assumed in any standard that describes how leaders work together.

Standard LD.01.01.01

The organization has a leadership structure.

Rationale for LD.01.01.01

Every organization has a leadership structure to support operations. Many functions need to be carried out, including governance, administration, and overseeing care, treatment, or services. In some organizations leaders have distinct roles in carrying out these functions; in others a single individual may perform all leadership functions

Elements of Performance for LD.01.01.01

A 1. The organization identifies those responsible for governance.

A 2. Governance identifies those responsible for planning, management, and operational activities.

A 3. Governance identifies those responsible for the provision of care, treatment or services.

Standard LD.01.03.01

Governance is ultimately accountable for the safety and quality of care, treatment, or services.

Rationale for LD.01.03.01

Governance's ultimate responsibility for safety and quality derives from its legal responsibility and operational authority for organization performance. In this context, governance provides for internal structures and resources, including staff, that support safety and quality.

Elements of Performance for LD.01.03.01

A 1. Governance defines in writing its responsibilities.

A 2. Governance provides for organization management and planning.

A 3. Governance approves the organization's written scope of services.

A 4. Governance selects the administrator.

A 5. Governance provides for the resources needed to maintain safe, quality care, treatment, or services. ⚠3

A 6. Governance works with other leaders to annually evaluate the organization's performance in relation to its mission, vision, and goals.

A 11. If the organization has an organized medical staff, the governance approves its bylaws, rules, and regulations.

Standard LD.01.04.01

An administrator manages the organization.

Elements of Performance for LD.01.04.01

The administrator provides for the following (EPs 1–3):

A 1. Information and support systems

A 2. Recruitment and retention of staff

A 3. Physical and financial assets

A 6. The administrator identifies a registered nurse, qualified by education and experience, to direct nursing services.

A 7. When the director of nursing is responsible for more than one organization or specialty program, an appropriately qualified registered nurse is assigned responsibility for the nursing staff activities in each setting.

A 8. When the director of nursing is absent, responsibility for continuity and supervision of nursing care is delegated to a registered nurse.

A 9. The individual with the authority to address administrative issues is accessible to the organization on a full-time basis.

A 11. When the administrator is absent from the organization, a qualified individual is designated to perform the duties of this position.

Standard LD.01.06.01

A medical director oversees the care, treatment or services provided to residents.

Elements of Performance for LD.01.06.01

A 1. The medical director is appointed by the chief executive or is designated by the medical staff.

A 2. The responsibilities of the medical director are defined in a written agreement with the governing body.

A 3. The medical director does the following:
- Directs and coordinates medical care in the organization
- Participates in establishing policies, procedures, and guidelines for comprehensive services
- Helps develop emergency treatment procedures for residents
- Helps develop resident transfer procedures
- Participates in the resident care management system
- Participates in in-service training programs

A 4. The medical director advises the administration, the governance, and other professionals on the following:
- Credentialing and privileging recommendations
- The development and maintenance of the clinical record system
- The organization's ability to meet residents' needs
- Adequacy and appropriateness of the organization's scope of services, medical equipment, and its professional and support staff
- Future resident care programs
- Hazards to health and safety identified in environmental incident reports (or summaries of incident reports)
- Improving the performance of medical services as an integral part of improving organization performance
- Employees' health status and employee health policies
- Policies requiring health care professionals to practice within the scope of their licenses

A 5. The medical director serves as a liaison for the organization in the following ways:
- By helping to arrange and communicate physician availability and coverage
- By communicating medical staff responsibilities and medical care policies, procedures, and guidelines to all licensed independent practitioners providing or ordering care
- By serving as a member of the organized medical staff if the organization has one

- By collaborating with the administrator and the organized medical staff, if the organization has one, to formulate the bylaws and the rules and regulations
- By being responsible, when there is no medical staff, for the written rules and regulations for all licensed independent practitioners who attend residents in the organization
- By being familiar with the policies and programs of public health agencies that affect resident care programs
- By acting as the organization's medical representative in the community

Note: *This standard does not require the creation of a medical staff where one does not exist. That is entirely the decision of the long term care organization.*

Standard LD.01.07.01

Individual leaders have the knowledge needed for their roles in the organization, or they seek guidance to fulfill their roles.

Elements of Performance for LD.01.07.01

C Ⓜ 2. Leaders are oriented to all of the following:
- The organization's mission and vision
- The organization's safety and quality goals
- The organization's structure and the decision-making process
- The development of the budget as well as the interpretation of the organization's financial statements
- The population(s) served by the organization and any issues related to that population(s)
- The individual and interdependent responsibilities and accountabilities of leaders as they relate to supporting the mission of the organization and to providing safe and quality care
- Applicable law and regulation

A 3. Governance provides leaders with access to information and training in areas where they need additional skills or expertise.

A 4. If the facility's medical director does not have the expertise to direct specialty programs, another physician with that expertise is identified to direct the medical care provided, and the relationship between these two positions is clearly defined.

Introduction to Leadership Relationships, Standards LD.02.01.01 through LD.02.03.01

How well leaders work together and manage conflict affects an organization's performance. In fulfilling its role, the governance involves senior managers and leaders of the clinical staff in governance and management functions.

Good relationships thrive when leaders work together to develop the mission, vision, and goals of the organization; encourage honest and open communication; and address conflicts of interest.

Standard LD.02.01.01

The mission, vision, and goals of the organization support the safety and quality of care, treatment, or services.

Rationale for LD.02.01.01

The primary responsibility of leaders is to provide for the safety and quality of care, treatment or services. The purpose of the organization's mission, vision, and goals is to define how the organization will achieve safety and quality. The leaders are more likely to be aligned with the mission, vision and goals when they create them together. The common purpose of the organization is most likely achieved when it is understood by all who work in or are served by the organization.

Elements of Performance for LD.02.01.01

A 1. Leaders work together to create the organization's mission, vision, and goals.

A 2. The organization's mission, vision, and goals guide the actions of leaders.

A 3. Leaders communicate the mission, vision, and goals to staff and the population(s) the organization serves.

Standard LD.02.03.01

Leaders regularly communicate with each other on issues of safety and quality.

Rationale for LD.02.03.01

Leaders, who provide for safety and quality, must communicate with each other on matters affecting the organization and those it serves. The safety and quality of care, treatment, or services depend on open communication. Ideally, this will result in trust and mutual respect among those who work in the organization.

Elements of Performance for LD.02.03.01

A 1. Leaders discuss issues that affect the organization and the population it serves, including the following:

- Performance improvement activities
- Reported safety and quality issues
- Proposed solutions and their impact on the organization's resources
- Reports on key quality measures and safety indicators
- Safety and quality issues specific to the population(s) served
- Input from the population(s) served

A 2. The organization establishes time frames for the discussion of issues that affect the organization and the population(s) it serves.

Introduction to Organization Culture and System Performance, Standards LD.03.01.01 through LD.03.06.01

An organization's culture reflects the beliefs, attitudes, and priorities of its members, and it influences the effectiveness of performance. Although there may be a dominant culture, in many larger organizations diverse cultures exist that may or may not share the same values. In fact, diverse cultures can exist even in smaller organizations. Organization performance can be effective in either case. Successful organizations will work to develop a culture of safety and quality.

In a culture of safety and quality, all individuals are focused on maintaining excellence in performance. They accept the safety and quality of resident care, treatment, or services as personal responsibilities and work together to minimize any harm that might result from unsafe or poor quality of care, treatment, or services. Leaders create this culture by demonstrating their commitment to safety and quality and by taking actions to achieve the desired state. In a culture of this kind, one finds teamwork, open discussions of concerns about safety and quality, and the encouragement of and reward for internal and external reporting of safety and quality issues. The focus of attention is on the performance of systems and processes instead of the individual, although reckless behavior and a blatant disregard for safety are not tolerated. Organizations are committed to ongoing learning and have the flexibility to accommodate changes in technology, science, and the environment.

The leaders provide for the effective functioning of the organization, with a focus on safety and quality. Leaders plan, support, and implement key systems critical to this effort. The Joint Commission has identified five key systems that influence the effective performance of an organization. They are:

- Using data
- Planning
- Communicating
- Changing performance
- Staffing

Leadership provides the foundation for effective performance. The five key systems serve as pillars that are based on the foundation set by leadership and in turn support the many organization-wide processes (such as medication management) that are important to individual care, treatment, or services. Culture permeates the entire structure.

The five key systems are interrelated and need to function well together. The integration of these systems throughout the organization will facilitate the effective performance of the organization as a whole. Leaders develop a vision and goals for the performance of these systems and evaluate their performance. Leaders use results to develop strategies for future improvements.

Performance of many aspects of these systems may be directly observable. But in many cases, organizations demonstrate compliance through performance in standards located in other sections of this manual. These leadership standards are cited when patterns of performance suggest organization-wide issues.

The effective performance of these systems results in a culture in which safety and quality are priorities. The organization demonstrates this through a proactive, nonpunitive culture that is monitored and sustained by related reporting systems and improvement initiatives.

Many of the concepts in the following section have long existed in the standards.

Standard LD.03.01.01

Leaders create and maintain a culture of safety and quality throughout the organization.

Rationale for LD.03.01.01

Safety and quality thrive in an environment that supports teamwork and respect for other people, regardless of their position in the organization. Leaders demonstrate their commitment to quality and set expectations for those who work in the organization. Leaders evaluate the culture on a regular basis, using a variety of methods, such as formal surveys, focus groups, staff interviews, and data analysis.

Leaders encourage teamwork and create structures, processes, and programs that allow this positive culture to flourish. Disruptive behavior that intimidates others and affects morale or staff turnover can be harmful to resident care. Leaders must address disruptive behavior of individuals working at all levels of the organization, including management, clinical and administrative staff, licensed independent practitioners, and governing body members.

Elements of Performance for LD.03.01.01

A 1. Leaders regularly evaluate the culture of safety and quality.

A 2. Leaders prioritize and implement changes identified by the evaluation.

A 3. Leaders provide opportunities for all individuals who work in the organization to participate in safety and quality initiatives.

A 4. The organization has a code of conduct that defines acceptable, disruptive, and inappropriate behaviors.

A 5. Leaders create and implement a process for managing disruptive and inappropriate behaviors. ⚠3

A 6. Leaders provide education that focuses on safety and quality for all individuals. (*See also* LD.04.04.05, EP 6)

A 7. Leaders establish a team approach among all staff at all levels.

A 8. All individuals who work in the organization, including staff and licensed independent practitioners, are able to openly discuss issues of safety and quality.

A 9. Literature and advisories relevant to resident safety are available to all individuals who work in the organization.

A 10. Leaders define how members of the population(s) served can help identify and manage issues of safety and quality within the organization.

Standard LD.03.02.01

The organization uses data and information to guide decisions and to understand variation in the performance of processes supporting safety and quality.

Rationale for LD.03.02.01

Data help organizations make the right decisions. When decisions are supported by data, organizations are more likely to move in directions that help them achieve their goals. Successful organizations measure and analyze their performance. When data are analyzed and turned into information, this process helps organizations see patterns and trends and understand the reasons for their performance. Many types of data are used to evaluate performance, including data on outcomes of care, performance on safety and quality initiatives, resident satisfaction, process variation, and staff perceptions.

Elements of Performance for LD.03.02.01

A 1. Leaders set expectations for using data and information to improve the safety and quality of care, treatment, or services.

A 2. Leaders are able to describe how data and information are used to create a culture of safety and quality.

A 3. The organization uses processes to support systematic data and information use.

A 4. Leaders provide the resources needed for data and information use, including staff, equipment, and information systems.

A 5. The organization uses data and information in decision making that supports the safety and quality of care, treatment, or services.

A 6. The organization uses data and information to identify and respond to internal and external changes in the environment.

A 7. Leaders evaluate how effectively data and information are used throughout the organization.

Standard LD.03.03.01

Leaders use organizationwide planning to establish structures and processes that focus on safety and quality.

Rationale for LD.03.03.01

Planning is essential to the following:

- The achievement of short- and long-term goals
- Meeting the challenge of external changes
- The design of services and work processes

- The creation of communication channels
- The improvement of performance
- The introduction of innovation

Planning includes contributions from the populations served, from those who work for the organization, and from other interested groups or individuals.

Elements of Performance for LD.03.03.01

A 1. Planning activities focus on improving resident safety and health care quality.

A 2. Leaders can describe how planning supports a culture of safety and quality.

A 3. Planning is systematic, and it involves designated individuals and information sources.

A 4. Leaders provide the resources needed to support the safety and quality of care, treatment, or services. ⚠3

A 5. Safety and quality planning is organizationwide.

A 6. Planning activities adapt to changes in the environment.

A 7. Leaders evaluate the effectiveness of planning activities.

Standard LD.03.04.01

The organization communicates information related to safety and quality to those who need it, including staff, residents, families, and external interested parties.

Rationale for LD.03.04.01

Effective communication is essential among individuals and groups within the organization and between the organization and external parties. Poor communication often contributes to adverse events and can compromise safety and quality of care, treatment, or services. Effective communication is timely, accurate, and usable by the audience.

Elements of Performance for LD.03.04.01

A 1. Communication processes foster the safety of the resident and the quality of care.

A 2. Leaders are able to describe how communication supports a culture of safety and quality.

A 3. Communication is designed to meet the needs of internal and external users.

A 4. Leaders provide the resources required for communication, based on the needs of resident, staff, and administration.

A 5. Communication supports safety and quality throughout the organization. (*See also* LD.04.04.05, EPs 6 and 12)

A 6. When changes in the environment occur, the organization communicates those changes effectively.

A 7. Leaders evaluate the effectiveness of communication methods.

Standard LD.03.05.01

Leaders implement changes in existing processes to improve the performance of the organization.

Rationale for LD.03.05.01

Change is inevitable, and agile organizations are able to manage change and rapidly execute new plans. The ability of leaders to manage change is necessary for performance improvement, for successful innovation, and to meet environmental challenges. The organization integrates change into all relevant processes so that its effectiveness can be sustained, assessed, and measured.

Elements of Performance for LD.03.05.01

A 1. Structures for managing change and performance improvements exist that foster the safety of the resident and the quality of care, treatment, or services.

A 2. Leaders are able to describe how the organization's approach to performance improvement and its capacity for change support a culture of safety and quality.

A 3. The organization has a systematic approach to change and performance improvement.

A 4. Leaders provide the resources required for performance improvement and change management, including sufficient staff, access to information, and training.

A 5. The management of change and performance improvement supports both safety and quality throughout the organization.

A 6. The organization's internal structures can adapt to changes in the environment.

A 7. Leaders evaluate the effectiveness of processes for the management of change and performance improvement.

Standard LD.03.06.01

Those who work in the organization are focused on improving safety and quality.

Rationale for LD.03.06.01

The safety and quality of care, treatment, or services are highly dependent on the people who work in the organization. The mission, scope, and complexity of services define the design of work processes and the skills and number of individuals needed. In a successful organization, work processes and the environment make safety and quality paramount. This standard, therefore, applies to all those who work in or for the organization, including staff and licensed independent practitioners.

Elements of Performance for LD.03.06.01

A 1. Leaders design work processes to focus individuals on safety and quality issues.

A 2. Leaders are able to describe how those who work in the organization support a culture of safety and quality.

A 3. Leaders provide for a sufficient number and mix of individuals to support safe, quality care, treatment, or services. ⚠3

A 4. Those who work in the organization are competent to complete their assigned responsibilities. ⚠3

A 5. Those who work in the organization adapt to changes in the environment.

A 6. Leaders evaluate the effectiveness of those who work in the organization to promote safety and quality.

Introduction to Leadership Operations, Standards LD.04.01.01 through LD.04.04.05

Although some leaders may not be involved in the day-to-day, hands-on operations of the organization, their decisions and work affect, either directly or indirectly, every aspect of operations. They are the driving force behind the culture of the organization. Leaders establish the ethical framework in which the organization operates, create policies and procedures, and secure resources and services that support resident safety and quality care, treatment, or services. Policies, procedures, resources, and services are all influenced by the culture of the organization, and, in turn, they influence the culture.

Standard LD.04.01.01

The organization complies with law and regulation.

Elements of Performance for LD.04.01.01

A 1. The organization is licensed, certified, or has a permit, in accordance with law and regulation, to provide the care, treatment, or services for which the organization is seeking accreditation from The Joint Commission. ▲2

Note 1: *Applicable law and regulation include, but are not limited to, individual and facility licensure, certification, Food and Drug Administration regulations, Drug Enforcement Agency regulations, Centers for Medicare & Medicaid Services regulations, Occupational Safety and Health Administration regulations, Department of Transportation regulations, Health Insurance*

Portability and Accountability Act, and other local, state, and federal laws and regulations.

Note 2: *Each service location that performs laboratory testing (waived or non waived) must have a Clinical Laboratory Improvement Amendments of 1988 (CLIA '88) certificate, as specified by the federal CLIA regulations (42 CFR 493.55 and 493.3) and applicable state law.* *

A 2. The organization provides care, treatment, or services in accordance with licensure requirements, laws, and rules and regulations.

A 3. Leaders act on or comply with reports or recommendations from external authorized agencies, such as accreditation, certification, or regulatory bodies.

Standard LD.04.01.03

The organization develops an annual operating budget and, when needed, a long-term capital expenditure plan.

Elements of Performance for LD.04.01.03

A 1. Leaders solicit comments from those who work in the organization when developing the operational and capital budgets.

A 3. The operating budget reflects the organization's goals and objectives.

A 4. The governance approves an annual operating budget and, when needed, a long-term capital expenditure plan.

A 5. The leaders monitor the implementation of the budget and long-term capital expenditure plan.

A 6. An independent public accountant conducts an annual audit of the organization's finances, unless otherwise provided by law.

Standard LD.04.01.05

The organization effectively manages its programs, services, sites, or departments.

Rationale for LD.04.01.05

Leaders at the program, service, site, or department level create a culture that enables the organization to fulfill its mission and meet its goals. They support staff and instill in them a sense of ownership of their work processes. Leaders may delegate work to qualified staff, but the leaders are responsible for the care, treatment, or services provided in their areas.

Elements of Performance for LD.04.01.05

A 1. Leaders of the program, service, site, or department oversee operations.

---

* For more information on how to obtain a CLIA certificate, *see* http://www.cms.hhs.gov/CLIA/downloads/HowObtainCLIACertificate.pdf.

2009

SLTC

Management of the Environment of Care (EC)

EC

EC

Management of the Environment of Care (EC)

Overview

The **goal** of this function is to provide a safe, functional, supportive, and effective environment for residents, staff members, and other individuals in the organization. This is crucial to providing quality resident care, achieving good outcomes, and improving resident safety. Achieving this goal depends on performing the following processes:

- Performing strategic and ongoing master planning by organization leaders for the space, clear circulation of occupants, equipment, supportive environment, and resources needed to safely and effectively support the services provided. Planning and designing of the environment is consistent with the organization's mission and vision and the resident's physical condition/health, cultural background, age, and cognitive abilities.
- Educating staff about the role of the environment in safely, sensitively, and effectively supporting resident care. The organization educates staff about the physical characteristics necessary for attaining such an environment and the processes for monitoring, maintaining, and reporting on the organization's environment of care.
- Developing standards to measure staff and organization performance in managing and improving the environment of care.
- Implementing plans to create and manage the organization's environment of care. An Information Collection and Evaluation System (ICES) is developed and used to continuously measure, assess, and improve the status of the environment of care.

The "environment of care" consists of three basic components: building(s), equipment, and people. A variety of key elements and issues can contribute to creating the way the space feels and works for residents, families, staff, and others experiencing the health care delivery system. In addition, the key elements and issues can be significant in their ability to positively influence resident outcomes and satisfaction and improve resident safety. These elements include the following:

- Light (both natural and artificial)
- Privacy (visual and auditory)
- Space size and configuration that are appropriate and consistent with the clinical philosophy
- Security
- Orientation and access to nature and the outside
- Clarity of access (both exterior and interior circulation)
- Color
- Efficient layouts that support staffing and overall functional operation

Key: 0 = Insufficient compliance; 1 = Partial compliance; 2 = Satisfactory compliance; NA = Not applicable; **A** indicates scoring category A; **C** indicates scoring category C; ▲(2) indicates situational decision rules apply; △(3) indicates direct impact requirements apply; Ⓜ indicates Measure of success is needed

When appropriately designed into and managed as part of the physical environment, these elements create safe, welcoming, and comfortable environments that support and maintain resident dignity and personhood, allow ease of interaction, reduce stressors, and encourage family participation in the delivery of care.

Effective management of the environment of care includes using processes and activities to do the following:

- Reduce and control environmental hazards and risks
- Prevent accidents and injuries
- Maintain safe conditions for residents, staff, and others coming to the organization's facilities
- Maintain an environment that is sensitive to resident needs for comfort, social interaction, and positive distraction
- Maintain an environment that minimizes unnecessary environmental stresses for residents, staff, and others coming to the organization's facilities

The standards in this chapter focus on how everyone in the organization participates in the processes and activities that make the care environment safe and effective. They also address department leaders' responsibility for identifying and communicating the care environment needs to the organization and allocating appropriate space, equipment, and resources to safely and effectively support the organization's services.

Note 1: *The standards in this chapter do not prescribe any particular structure (such as a safety committee), specific individual (such as one employee hired to be a safety officer), or format for the required designs and planning activities.*

Note 2: *The standards do not require the Statement of Conditions™ compliance document to be completed by anyone other than an employee of the organization. This statement is the basis for corrective actions needed to make the environment compliant with the requirements of the* Life Safety Code® (LSC), *NFPA 101®.*

Note 3: *The standards in this chapter require each organization to develop a written plan for the following:*

- *Safety management (EC.1.10)*
- *Security management (EC.2.10)*
- *Hazardous materials and waste management (EC.3.10)*
- *Emergency management (EC.4.10)*
- *Fire safety (EC.5.10)*
- *Medical equipment management (EC.6.10)*
- *Utilities management (EC.7.10)*

If an organization has multiple sites, it may have separate management plans for each of its locations, or it may choose to have one comprehensive set of plans. In either case, the organization must address specific risks and the unique conditions at each of its sites.

Standards

The following is a list of all standards for this function. They are presented here for your convenience without footnotes or other explanatory text. If you have a question about a term used here, please check the Glossary.

Note: *A revised standard numbering system is being used with the reformatted standards. The revised numbering system will allow for more flexibility to add standards while maintaining the current label for each standard.*

Planning and Implementation Activities

EC.1.10 The organization manages safety risks.

EC.1.20 The organization maintains a safe environment.

EC.1.25 Not applicable

EC.1.27 Not applicable

EC.1.30 The organization develops and implements a policy to prohibit smoking except in specified circumstances.

EC.2.10 The organization identifies and manages its security risks.

EC.3.10 The organization manages its hazardous materials and waste risks.

EC.4.10 Not applicable

Emergency Management

EC.4.11 The organization plans for managing the consequences of emergencies.

EC.4.12 The organization develops and maintains an Emergency Operations Plan.

EC.4.13 The organization establishes emergency communications strategies.

EC.4.14 The organization establishes strategies for managing resources and assets during emergencies.

EC.4.15 The organization establishes strategies for managing safety and security during emergencies.

EC.4.16 The organization defines and manages staff roles and responsibilities.

EC.4.17 The organization establishes strategies for managing utilities during emergencies.

EC.4.18 The organization establishes strategies for managing resident clinical and support activities during emergencies.

EC.4.20 The organization regularly tests its emergency management plan.

EC.5.10 The organization manages fire safety risks.

EC.5.20 Not applicable

EC.5.30 The organization conducts fire drills regularly.

EC.5.40 The organization maintains fire-safety equipment and building features.

EC.5.50 Not applicable

EC.6.10 The organization manages medical equipment risks.

EC.6.20 Medical equipment is maintained, tested, and inspected.

EC 6.30 Through EC 6.130 Not applicable

EC.7.10 The organization manages its utility risks.

EC.7.20 The organization provides a reliable emergency electrical power source.

EC.7.30 The organization maintains, tests, and inspects its utility systems.

EC.7.40 The organization maintains, tests, and inspects its emergency power systems.

EC.7.50 The organization maintains, tests, and inspects its medical gas and vacuum systems.

EC.8.10 The organization establishes and maintains an appropriate environment.

EC.8.20 The organization establishes and maintains an appropriate dining environment.

EC.8.30 The organization manages the design and building of the environment when it is renovated, altered, or newly created.

Measuring and Improving Activities

EC.9.10 The organization monitors conditions in the environment.

EC.9.20 The organization analyzes identified environment issues and develops recommendations for resolving them.

EC.9.30 The organization improves the environment.

Standards, Rationales, Elements of Performance, and Scoring

Planning and Implementation Activities

No organization can ensure that residents, staff, and others coming to the organization's facilities will never suffer an accidental injury. However, organizations can minimize avoidable risks and injuries through sound planning, resource allocation (*see* "Leadership" chapter), effective training (*see* "Management of Human Resources" chapter), implementation, and ongoing monitoring and improvement of risk reduction activities. These activities can be accomplished through the management process, staff activities, and/or technology.

Standard EC.1.10

The organization manages safety risks.

Rationale for EC.1.10

Each organization has inherent safety risks associated with providing services for residents, the performance of daily activities by staff, and the physical environment in which services occur. It is important that each organization identifies these risks and plans and implements processes to minimize the likelihood of those risks causing incidents.

Elements of Performance for EC.1.10

A 1. The organization develops and maintains a written management plan describing the processes it implements to effectively manage the environmental safety of residents, staff, and other people coming to the organization's facilities.

A 2. The organization identifies a person(s), as designated by leadership, to coordinate the development, implementation, and monitoring of the safety management activities.

A 3. The organization identifies a person(s) to intervene whenever conditions immediately threaten life or health or threaten damage to equipment or buildings.

A 4. The organization conducts comprehensive, proactive risk assessments that evaluate the potential adverse impact of buildings, grounds, equipment, occupants, and internal physical systems on the safety and health of residents, staff, and other people coming to the organization's facilities.

C Ⓜ 5. The organization uses the risks identified to select and implement procedures and controls to achieve the lowest potential for adverse impact on the safety and health of residents, staff, and other people coming to the organization's facilities.

C Ⓜ 6. The organization establishes safety policies and procedures that are practiced and reviewed as frequently as necessary, but at least every three years.

7. Not applicable

A 8. The organization ensures that a process exists for responding to product safety recalls by appropriate organization staff.

A 9. The organization ensures that all grounds and equipment are maintained appropriately.

Standard EC.1.20

The organization maintains a safe environment.

Rationale for EC.1.20

It is essential that the organization conduct periodic environmental tours to determine if its current processes for managing resident, public, and staff safety risks are being practiced correctly and are effective. These tours can also be used to assess staff knowledge and behaviors, identify new or altered risks in areas where construction or changes in services have occurred, and identify opportunities to improve the environment.

Elements of Performance for EC.1.20

A 1. The organization conducts environmental tours to identify environmental deficiencies, hazards, and unsafe practices.

C Ⓜ 2. The organization conducts environmental tours at least every six months in all areas where residents are served.

C Ⓜ 3. The organization conducts environmental tours at least annually in areas where residents are not served.

Standard EC.1.25

Not applicable

Standard EC.1.27

Not applicable

Standard EC.1.30

The organization develops and implements a policy to prohibit smoking except in specified circumstances.

Rationale for EC.1.30

This standard is intended to reduce the following risks:

- To people who smoke, including possible adverse effects on care, treatment, and services
- Of passive smoking for others
- Of fire

The standard prohibits smoking in all areas of all building(s) under the organization's control, except for residents in circumstances specified in the EPs.

Elements of Performance for EC.1.30

A 1. The organization develops a policy regarding smoking in all areas of all building(s) under the organization's control.

A 2. The organization's policy prohibits smoking in all areas of all building(s) under the organization's control (no medical exceptions allowed) for the following:

- All children or youth residents

A 3. The organization's policy may permit residents to smoke in the organization's buildings under the following circumstance:

- A resident meets criteria developed and approved by the organization's leaders

C Ⓜ 4. When residents are permitted to smoke in the organization's buildings, they smoke only under the following circumstances:

- In designated locations environmentally separate from care, treatment, and services areas*
- After the organization has taken measures to minimize fire risks ⚠3

C Ⓜ 5. Residents who do smoke in the organization's buildings are provided education, including information about options for smoking cessation.

A 6. The organization identifies and implements a process(es) for monitoring compliance with the policy.

A 7. The organization develops strategies to eliminate the incidence of policy violations when identified.

Standard EC.2.10

The organization identifies and manages its security risks.

Rationale for EC.2.10

It is essential that an organization manages the physical and personal security of residents, staff (including the potential for violence to residents and staff in the work-

---

* **Note:** *This does not require that a designated smoking area be a specific distance from care, treatment, and services areas. A physically separate, well-ventilated room (a designated area for authorized smoking by residents that is exhausted to the outside) is acceptable.*

place), and individuals coming to the organization's buildings. In addition, security of the established environment, equipment, supplies, and information is also important.

Elements of Performance for EC.2.10

A 1. The organization develops and maintains a written management plan describing the processes it implements to effectively manage the security of residents, staff, and other people coming to the organization's facilities.

A 2. The organization identifies a person(s), as designated by leadership, to coordinate the development, implementation, and monitoring of the security management activities.

A 3. The organization conducts proactive risk assessments that evaluate the potential adverse impact of the external environment and the services provided on the security of residents, staff, and other people coming to the organization's facilities.*

C Ⓜ 4. The organization uses the risks identified to select and implement procedures and controls to achieve the lowest potential for adverse impact on security.

A 5. The organization identifies, as appropriate, residents, staff, and other people entering the organization's facilities.

C Ⓜ 6. The organization controls access to and egress from security-sensitive areas, as determined by the organization. △3

A 7. The organization identifies and implements security procedures that address actions taken in the event of a security incident.

8. Not applicable

A 9. The organization identifies and implements security procedures that address handling of situations involving VIPs or the media.

Standard EC.3.10

The organization manages its hazardous materials and waste† risks.

* The potential for workplace violence and for resident elopement or wandering is considered during the risk assessment.

† **Hazardous materials (HAZMAT) and waste** Materials whose handling, use, and storage are guided or regulated by local, state, or federal regulation. Examples include the Occupational Safety and Health Administration Regulations for Bloodborne Pathogens (regarding blood, other infectious materials, contaminated items that would release blood or other infectious materials, or contaminated sharps); the Nuclear Regulatory Commission regulations for handling and disposal of radioactive waste; management of hazardous vapors (such as glutaraldehyde, ethylene oxide, and nitrous oxide); chemicals regulated by the Environmental Protection Agency; Department of Transportation requirements; and hazardous energy sources (for example, ionizing or nonionizing radiation, lasers, microwaves, and ultrasound).

Rationale for EC.3.10

Organizations must identify materials they use that need special handling and implement processes to minimize the risks of their unsafe use and improper disposal.

Elements of Performance for EC.3.10

A 1. The organization develops and maintains a written management plan describing the processes it implements to effectively manage hazardous materials and waste.

A 2. The organization creates and maintains an inventory that identifies hazardous materials and waste used, stored, or generated using criteria consistent with applicable law and regulation (for example, the EPA and OSHA).

The organization establishes and implements processes for selecting, handling, storing, transporting, using, and disposing of hazardous materials and waste from receipt or generation through use and/or final disposal, including managing the following (EPs 3–6):

C Ⓜ 3. Chemicals

A 4. Chemotherapeutic materials ⚠3

A 5. Radioactive materials ⚠3

C Ⓜ 6. Infectious and regulated medical wastes, including sharps ⚠3

A 7. The organization provides adequate and appropriate space and equipment for safely handling and storing hazardous materials and waste.

8. Not applicable

A 9. The organization identifies and implements emergency procedures that include the specific precautions, procedures, and protective equipment used during hazardous materials and waste spills or exposures. ⚠3

A 10. The organization maintains documentation, including required permits, licenses, and adherence to other regulations.

C Ⓜ 11. The organization maintains required manifests for handling hazardous materials and waste.

C Ⓜ 12. The organization properly labels hazardous materials and waste.

A 13. The organization effectively separates hazardous materials and waste storage and processing areas from other areas of the facility.

Standard EC.4.10

Not applicable

Emergency Management

Introduction

Catastrophic emergencies are a threat to any health care organization, regardless of size, scope, or location. A single emergency* can temporarily affect demand for services; however, multiple emergencies that occur concurrently or sequentially can adversely impact patient safety and the organization's ability to provide care, treatment, and services for an extended length of time. This is especially true in situations where the community cannot adequately support the organization. Power failures, water and fuel shortages, flooding, and communication breakdowns are just a few of the hazards that can disrupt patient care, and pose risks to staff and the organization.

No organization can predict the nature of a future emergency, nor can it predict the date of its arrival. However, organizations can plan for managing six critical areas of emergency response in order to assess their needs and prepare staff to respond to events most likely to occur regardless of the cause(s) of an emergency situation. The six critical areas of emergency management are as follows:

1. **Communication (*see* EC.4.13).** In the event that community infrastructure is damaged and/or an organization's power or facilities experience debilitation, communication pathways, whether dependent on fiber optic cables, electricity, satellite, or other conduits, are likely to fail. Organizations must develop a plan to maintain communication pathways both within the organization and to critical community resources.
2. **Resources and assets (*see* EC.4.14).** A solid understanding of the scope and availability of an organization's resources and assets is as important, and perhaps more important, during an emergency than during times of normal operation. Materials and supplies, vendor and community services, as well as state and federal programs, are some of the essential resources that organizations must know how to access in times of crisis in order to ensure patient safety and sustain care, treatment, and services.
3. **Safety and security (*see* EC.4.15).** The safety and security of residents is the prime responsibility of the organization during an emergency. As emergency situations develop and parameters of operability shift, organizations must provide a safe and secure environment for their residents and staff.
4. **Staff responsibilities (*see* EC.4.16).** During an emergency, the probability that staff responsibilities will change is high. As new risks develop along with changing conditions, staff will need to adapt their roles to meet new demands on their ability to care for patients. If staff cannot anticipate how they may be called to perform during an emergency, the likelihood that the organization will not sustain itself during an emergency increases.

---

* **Emergency** A natural or manmade event that significantly disrupts the environment of care (for example, damage to the organization's building[s] and grounds due to severe winds, storms, or earthquakes); that significantly disrupts care, treatment, and services (for example, loss of utilities such as power, water, or telephones due to floods, civil disturbances, accidents, or emergencies within the organization or in its community); or that results in sudden, significantly changed, or increased demands for the organization's services (for example, bioterrorist attack, building collapse, plane crash in the organization's community). Some emergencies are called "disasters" or "potential injury creating events" (PICEs).

5. **Utilities management (*see* EC.4.17).** An organization is dependent on the uninterrupted function of its utilities during an emergency. The supply of key utilities, such as power or potable water, ventilation, and fuel must not be disrupted, or adverse events may occur as a result.
6. **Patient clinical and support activities (*see* EC.4.18).** The clinical needs of patients during an emergency are of prime importance. The organization must have clear, reasonable plans in place to address the needs of patients during extreme conditions when the organization's infrastructure and resources are taxed.

When organizations have a sound understanding of their response to these six critical areas of emergency management, they have developed an "all hazards" approach that supports a level of preparedness sufficient to address a range of emergencies, regardless of the cause. Organizations should also identify potential hazards, threats, and adverse events, and assess their impact on the care, treatment, and services they must sustain during an emergency. This assessment is known as a Hazard Vulnerability Analysis (HVA) and is designed to assist organizations in gaining a realistic understanding of their vulnerabilities, and to help focus their resources and planning efforts. Finally, organizations should use the information from their assessments to develop Emergency Operations Plans (EOPs), which should be tested regularly, and use the lessons learned to improve.

Organizations should note that additional standards in other chapters are integral to organization-wide emergency preparedness, including processes for the following:
- Maintaining continuity of information ("Management of Information" chapter)
- Responding to an influx, or the risk of influx, of infectious patients ("Surveillance, Prevention, and Control of Infection" chapter)
- Granting disaster privileges ("Management of Human Resources" chapter)
- Assigning disaster responsibilities ("Management of Human Resources" chapter)

Standard EC.4.11

The organization plans for managing the consequences of emergencies.

Rationale for EC.4.11

An emergency in a health care organization or in its community can suddenly and significantly affect demand for its services or its ability to provide those services. Therefore, it is important that organizations define a comprehensive approach to identifying risks and mobilizing an effective response within the organization as well as in collaboration and coordination with essential response partners in the community.

Elements of Performance for EC.4.11

A 1. The organization's leaders, including the administrator, the medical director, the nursing leader, and other clinical leaders actively participate in emergency management planning.

A 2. The organization conducts a Hazard Vulnerability Analysis (HVA) to identify events that could affect demand for its services or its ability to provide those services, the likelihood of those events occurring, and the consequences of those events.

Note: *The HVA is evaluated at least annually as part of EP 11.*

A 3. The organization prioritizes those hazards, threats and events identified in its HVA.

A 4. When developing its EOP (*see* EC.4.12), the organization communicates its needs and vulnerabilities to community emergency response agencies and identifies the capabilities of its community in meeting their needs.

For each emergency identified in its HVA, the organization defines the following (EPs 5–8):

A 5. Mitigation activities designed to reduce the risk of and potential damage due to an emergency

A 6. Preparedness activities that will organize and mobilize essential resources

A 7. Response strategies and actions to be activated during the emergency

A 8. Recovery strategies and actions designed to help restore the systems that are critical to resuming normal care, treatment, and services

A 9. The organization keeps a documented inventory of the assets and resources it has on site, that would be needed during an emergency (at a minimum, personal protective equipment, water, fuel, staffing, medical, and pharmaceuticals resources and assets).

Note: *The inventory is evaluated at least annually as part of EP 11.*

A 10. The organization establishes methods for monitoring quantities of assets and resources during an emergency.

A 11. The objectives, scope, performance, and effectiveness of the organization's emergency management planning efforts are evaluated at least annually.

Standard EC.4.12

The organization develops and maintains an Emergency Operations Plan.

Rationale for EC.4.12

A successful response relies upon planning around the management of six critical areas: communications; resources and assets; safety and security; staffing; utilities; and clinical activities. It is important for organizations to develop a comprehensive Emergency Operations Plan (EOP) as documentation to help guide the organization in its emergency response and recovery efforts. While the EOP can be formatted in a variety of ways, it must address these six critical areas to serve as a blueprint for managing care and safety during an emergency.

Some emergencies can escalate unexpectedly and strain the organization and the entire community. An organization cannot mitigate risks, plan thoroughly, and sustain an effective response and recovery without preparing its staff and collaborating with the community, suppliers and external response partners as well. Such an approach will aid the organization in developing a scalable response capability and in defining the timing and criteria for decisions that involve sheltering in place, resident transfer, facility closings, or evacuation.

Elements of Performance for EC.4.12

A 1. The organization develops and maintains a written EOP that describes an "all-hazards" command structure for coordinating six critical areas (*see* EC.4.13 through EC.4.18) within the organization during an emergency.

A 2. The EOP establishes an incident command structure.

A 3. The EOP identifies to whom staff report in the organization's incident command structure.

A 4. The EOP describes processes for initiating and terminating the response and recovery phases, including who has the authority to activate the phases.

A 5. The EOP describes processes for initiating and terminating the response and recovery phases, including how the phases are to be activated.

A 6. The EOP identifies the organization's capabilities and establishes response efforts when the organization cannot be supported by the local community for at least 96 hours in the six critical areas.

Note: *Acceptable response efforts could include the following:*
- *Conservation of resources*
- *Curtailment of services*
- *Supplementing of resources from outside the local community*
- *Staged evacuation*
- *Total evacuation*

A 7. The EOP identifies alternative sites for care, treatment, or service that meet the needs of its residents during emergencies.

Standard EC.4.13

The organization establishes emergency communications strategies.

Rationale for EC.4.13

The organization maintains reliable surveillance and communications capability to detect emergencies and communicate response efforts to organization response personnel, residents and their families, and external agencies. The organization plans for back-up communications processes and technologies (e.g., cell phones, land lines, bulletin boards, fax machines, satellite phones, ham radio, text messages) if primary communications systems fail. It is important that responders and incident managers use common terminology; there simply is little or no room for misunderstanding in an emergency situation.

Elements of Performance for EC.4.13

A 1. The organization plans for notifying staff when emergency response measures are initiated.

A 2. The organization plans for ongoing communication of information and instructions to its staff once emergency response measures are initiated.

A 3. The organization defines processes for notifying external authorities when emergency response measures are initiated.

A 4. The organization plans for communicating with external authorities once emergency response measures are initiated.

A 5. The organization plans for communicating with residents and their families during emergencies, including notification when residents are relocated to alternative care sites.

A 6. The organization defines the circumstances and plans for communicating with the community and/or the media during emergencies.

A 7. The organization plans for communicating with purveyors of essential supplies, services, and equipment once emergency measures are initiated.

The organization plans for communicating in a timely manner with other health care organizations that together provide services to a contiguous geographic area (for example, among health care organizations serving a town or borough) regarding the following (EPs 8–11):

A 8. Essential elements of their command structures and control centers for emergency response

A 9. Names and roles of individuals in their command structures and command center telephone numbers

A 10. Resources and assets that potentially could be shared in an emergency response

A 11. Names of residents and deceased individuals brought to their organizations in accordance with applicable law and regulation, when requested

A 12. The organization defines the circumstances and plans for communicating information about residents to third parties (such as other health care organizations, the state health department, police, FBI, etc.).

A 13. The organization plans for communicating with identified alternative care sites.

A 14. The organization establishes back-up communication systems and technologies for the activities identified above.

Standard EC.4.14

The organization establishes strategies for managing resources and assets during emergencies.

Rationale for EC.4.14

During emergencies, health care organizations that continue to provide care, treatment, and services to their residents must sustain essential resources, materials, and facilities. The EOP should identify how resources and assets will be solicited and acquired from a range of possible sources, such as vendors, neighboring health care providers, other community organizations, state affiliates, or a regional parent company. To address emergencies of long duration or broad geographic scope, the organization's plan must proactively identify, locate, acquire, distribute and account for critical resources and supplies. The plan should also recognize the risk that some assets may not be available from planned sources and that contingency plans will be necessary for critical supplies. This situation may occur when multiple organizations are vying for a limited supply from the same vendor.

The infrastructure for supplying and supporting the health care organization is complex, and the HVA will help identify risks to this infrastructure that can be mitigated. Planning must address managing and maintaining the facility, but also must consider evacuation of the entire facility when the environment is no longer deemed safe.

Elements of Performance for EC.4.14

The organization plans for the following (EPs 1–11):

A 1. Obtaining supplies that will be required at the onset of emergency response (medical, pharmaceutical, and non-medical)

A 2. Replenishing medical supplies and equipment that will be required throughout response and recovery, including personal protective equipment where required

A 3. Replenishing pharmaceutical supplies that will be required throughout response and recovery, including access to and distribution of caches (stockpiled by the organization or its affiliates, local, state or federal sources) to which the organization has access

A 4. Replenishing non-medical supplies that will be required throughout response and recovery (for example, food, linens, water, fuel for generators and transportation vehicles, etc.)

A 5. Managing staff support activities (for example, housing, transportation, incident stress debriefing, etc.)

A 6. Managing staff family support needs (for example, child care, elder care, communication, etc.)

A 7. Potential sharing of resources and assets (e.g., personnel, beds, transportation, linens, fuel, PPE, medical equipment and supplies, etc.) with other health care organizations within the community that could potentially be shared in an emergency response

A 8. Potential sharing of resources and assets with health care organizations outside of the community in the event of a regional or prolonged disaster

A 9. Evacuating (both horizontally and, when required by circumstances, vertically) when the environment cannot support care, treatment, and services

A 10. Transporting residents, their medications and equipment, and staff to an alternative care site or sites when the environment cannot support care, treatment, and services

A 11. Transporting pertinent information, including essential clinical and medication-related information, for residents to an alternative care site or sites when the environment cannot support care, treatment, and services

Standard EC.4.15

The organization establishes strategies for managing safety and security during emergencies.

Rationale for EC.4.15

Controlling the movement of individuals into, throughout, and out of the organization during an emergency is essential to the safety of residents and staff, and to the security of critical supplies, equipment, and utilities. The organization determines the type of access and movement to be allowed by staff, residents, visitors, emergency volunteers, vendors, maintenance and repair workers, utility suppliers, and other individuals when emergency measures are initiated. Factors influencing access and movement vary depending upon the type of emergency and local conditions (i.e., the decision by the organization to shelter staff families, the allowance for or prohibition against firearms, mutual aid agreements with nearby facilities or vendors, etc.).

During an emergency, the campus or immediate environment around the organization may be under the authority of the local police or sheriff serving the larger community. Access to and from the organization on local roads and interstates could be subject to local, state or even federal control. As an incident evolves, this responsibility and authority may shift from one agency to another. For this reason, it is important that the EOP includes reference to any existing community command structure to provide for ongoing communication and coordination with this structure. In the absence of such a command structure, the organization maintains direct contact with the agencies charged with community security.

Elements of Performance for EC.4.15

A 1. The organization establishes internal security and safety operations that will be required once emergency measures are initiated.

A 2. The organization identifies the roles of community security agencies (police, sheriff, national guard, etc.) and defines how the organization will coordinate security activities with these agencies.

A 3. The organization identifies a process that will be required for managing hazardous materials and waste once emergency measures are initiated.

4. Not applicable

A 5. The organization identifies residents who might be susceptible to wandering once emergency measures are initiated. ⚠3

The organization establishes processes for controlling the following during emergencies (EPs 6–8):

A 6. Entrance into and out of the health care facility

A 7. The movement of individuals within the health care facility

A 8. Traffic accessing the health care facility

Standard EC.4.16

The organization defines and manages staff roles and responsibilities.

Rationale for EC.4.16

To provide safe and effective resident care during an emergency, staff roles are well defined; staff are oriented and trained in their assigned responsibilities; and staff maintains their competencies over time. Staff roles in emergencies are determined largely by the priority emergencies defined in the HVA, and the reporting relationships in the command and control operations of the organization. As such, staff must stand ready to adjust to changes in resident volume or acuity, work procedures or conditions, and response partners within and outside the organization. (**Note:** *Standards in the Management of Human Resources chapter define the processes for accepting volunteer practitioners during emergencies.*) Staff roles and responsibilities may be documented in the EOP using a variety of formats: job action sheets, checklists, flowcharts, etc.

Elements of Performance for EC.4.16

A 1. Staff roles and responsibilities are defined in the EOP for all critical areas (communication, resources and assets, safety and security, utilities, and clinical activities).

A 2. Staff are trained for their assigned roles during emergencies.

A 3. The organization communicates to licensed independent practitioners their roles in emergency response and to whom they report during an emergency.

A 4. The organization establishes a process for identifying care providers and other personnel (such as identification cards, wrist bands, vests, hats, badges, computer print-outs, etc.) assigned to particular areas during emergencies.

Standard EC.4.17

The organization establishes strategies for managing utilities during emergencies.

Rationale for EC.4.17

Different types of emergencies can have the same detrimental impact on an organization's utility systems. For example, brush fires, ice storms, and industrial accidents can all result in a loss of utilities required for care, treatment, services, related transport and building operations. Organizations, therefore, must have alternative means of providing for essential utilities, whether through negotiated relationships with the primary suppliers; Memoranda of Understanding (MOUs) with other organizations in the community; alternative equipment at the organization; or provision through a parent entity, etc. Organizations should determine how long they expect to remain open to care for residents, and plan for their utilities accordingly. Because some emergencies may be regional in scope or of long duration, organizations should not rely solely on single source providers in the community. Where possible, organizations should identify other suppliers outside of the local community in case the communities' infrastructure is severely compromised and unable to support the organization.

Elements of Performance for EC.4.17

The organization identifies an alternative means of providing for the following utilities in the event that their supply is compromised or disrupted (EPs 1–5):

A 1. Electricity

A 2. Water needed for consumption and essential care activities

A 3. Water needed for equipment and sanitary purposes

A 4. Fuel required for building operations or essential transport activities

A 5. Other essential utility needs (for example, ventilation, medical gas/vacuum systems, etc.)

Standard EC.4.18

The organization establishes strategies for managing resident clinical and support activities during emergencies.

Rationale for EC.4.18

The fundamental goal of emergency management planning is to protect life and prevent disability. The manner in which care, treatment, and services are provided may vary by type of emergency. However, certain clinical activities are so fundamental to safe and effective care that the organization should determine how it will re-schedule or manage resident clinical needs even under the most dynamic situations or in the most austere care environments.

The emergency triage process will typically result in residents being quickly treated and discharged, admitted for a longer stay, or transferred to a more appropriate source of care. It is especially important to identify and triage residents whose clinical needs are outside of the usual scope of service of the organization. A catastrophic emergency may result in the decision to keep all residents on the premises in the interest of safety or, conversely, in the decision to evacuate all residents because the facility is no longer safe. Planning for clinical services must address these situations accordingly.

Elements of Performance for EC.4.18

The organization plans to manage the following during emergencies (EPs 1–5):

A 1. The clinical activities required as part of resident scheduling, triage, assessment, treatment, admission, transfer, discharge, and evacuation

A 2. Clinical services for vulnerable populations served by the organization, including residents who are pediatric, geriatric, disabled, or have serious chronic conditions or addictions

A 3. Personal hygiene and sanitation needs of its residents

A 4. The mental health service needs of its residents

A 5. Mortuary services

A 6. The organization plans for documenting and tracking residents' clinical information.

Emergency Management Drills

Introduction

Periodic testing of an emergency management plan enables organizations to assess the plan's appropriateness, adequacy, and the effectiveness of logistics, human resources, training, policies, procedures, and protocols. Exercises should stress the limits of the organization's emergency management system. The goal of this testing is to assess the organization's preparedness capabilities and performance when systems are stressed during an actual emergency or a simulated situation.

Exercises should be developed using plausible scenarios that are realistic and relevant to the organization. Events should be based on each organization's hazard vulnerability analysis (HVA), and should validate the effectiveness of the plan and identify opportunities to improve.

This standard will assist health care organizations to test their emergency management plans, identify deficiencies, and take corrective actions to continuously improve the effectiveness of their emergency management plan. Only a thorough and objective evaluation of performance during an emergency management event or a planned exercise will demonstrate how effective the organization's planning efforts have been.

It is important to communicate the strengths and weaknesses of the performance revealed by the exercise to all levels of the organization, including administration, clinical staff, governing body, and those responsible for managing the resident safety program.

Standard EC.4.20

The organization regularly tests its emergency management plan.

Elements of Performance for EC.4.20

Number and Types of Exercises

A 1. The organization tests its EOP twice a year, either in response to an actual emergency or in a planned exercise.

Note: *Tabletop sessions, though useful, are not acceptable substitutes for exercises.*

A 2. Organizations that offer emergency services or are community-designated disaster receiving stations conduct at least one exercise a year that includes an influx of actual or simulated residents.

A 3. At least one exercise a year is escalated to evaluate how effectively the organization performs when it cannot be supported by the local community.

Note: *Tabletop sessions are acceptable in meeting the community portion of this exercise.*

A 4. Organizations that have a defined role in the communitywide emergency management program participate in at least one communitywide exercise a year.

Note 1: *"Communitywide" may range from a contiguous geographic area served by the same health care providers, to a large borough, town, city, or region.*

Note 2: *Exercises for EPs 2, 3, and 4 may be conducted separately or simultaneously.*

Note 3: *Table top sessions are acceptable in meeting the community portion of this exercise.*

5. Not applicable

Scope of Exercises

A 6. Planned exercise scenarios are realistic and related to the priority emergencies identified in the organization's HVA.

7. Not applicable

A 8. During planned exercises, an individual whose sole responsibility is to monitor performance and who is knowledgeable in the goals and expectations of the exercise, documents opportunities for improvement.*

During planned exercises the organization monitors, at a minimum, the following six critical areas (EPs 9–14):

A 9. Communication including the effectiveness of communication both within the organization as well as with response entities outside of the organiza-

* This indivdual may be a staff member of the organization who is not participating in the exercise.

tion such as local governmental leadership, police, fire, public health, and other health care organizations within the community

A 10. Resource mobilization and allocation including responders, equipment, supplies, personal protective equipment, and transportation

A 11. Safety and security

A 12. Staff roles and responsibilities

A 13. Utility systems

A 14. Resident clinical and support care activities

A 15. All exercises are critiqued to identify deficiencies and opportunities for improvement based upon all monitoring activities and observations during the exercise.

A 16. Completed exercises are critiqued through a multidisciplinary process that includes administration, clinical, and support staff.

A 17. The organization modifies its emergency management plan in response to critiques of exercises.

A 18. Planned exercises evaluate the effectiveness of improvements that were made in response to critiques of the previous exercise.

Note: *When improvements require substantive resources that cannot be accomplished by the next planned exercise, interim improvements must be put in place until final resolution.*

A 19. The strengths and weaknesses identified during exercises are communicated to the multidisciplinary improvement team responsible for monitoring environment of care issues (*see* EC.9.20).

Standard EC.5.10

The organization manages fire safety risks.

Rationale for EC.5.10

All facilities are designed, constructed, maintained, and operated to minimize the possibility of a fire emergency requiring the evacuation of occupants. Because the safety of occupants cannot be ensured adequately by dependence on evacuation of the building, their protection from fire shall be provided by appropriate arrangement of facilities; adequate, trained staff; and development of operating and maintenance procedures composed of the following:

- Design, construction, and compartmentation
- Provision for detection, alarm, and extinguishment
- Fire prevention and the planning, training, and drilling programs for the isolation of fire, transfer of occupants to areas of refuge, or evacuation of the building

Elements of Performance for EC.5.10

A 1. The organization develops and maintains a written management plan describing the processes it implements to effectively manage fire safety.

A 2. The organization identifies proactive processes for protecting residents, staff, and others coming to the organization's facilities, as well as protecting property from fire, smoke, and other products of combustion.

A 3. The organization identifies processes for regularly inspecting, testing, and maintaining fire protection and fire safety systems, equipment, and components.

A 4. The organization develops and implements a fire response plan that addresses the following:
- Facilitywide fire response
- Area-specific needs, including fire evacuation routes
- Specific roles and responsibilities of staff, licensed independent practitioners, and volunteers at a fire's point of origin
- Specific roles and responsibilities of staff, licensed independent practitioners, and volunteers away from a fire's point of origin
- Specific roles and responsibilities of staff, licensed independent practitioners, and volunteers in preparing for building evacuation △3

A 5. The organization reviews proposed acquisitions of bedding, window draperies, and other curtains, furnishings, decorations, and other equipment for fire safety.

Standard EC.5.20

Not applicable

Standard EC.5.30

The organization conducts fire drills regularly.

Rationale for EC.5.30

The development of a fire response plan is an important part of achieving a fire-safe environment (*see* standard EC.5.10). It is important that this plan be regularly evaluated during implementations (in drill scenarios or actual fire situations) for performance of the fire safety equipment and staff.

Implementation of the plan should be realistic and held at varied times. An implementation held at shift change may present an unrealistic picture as to the number of staff likely available any time a fire occurs. Actual evacuation of residents during the drills is not required.

Elements of Performance for EC.5.30

C Ⓜ 1. Fire drills are conducted quarterly on all shifts in each buildings defined by the *LSC* as the following:
- Health care occupancy

2. Not applicable

3. Not applicable

C Ⓜ 4. At least 50% of the required drills are unannounced.

A 5. Staff in all areas of every building where residents are housed or treated participates in drills to the extent called for in the facility's fire plan. (*See* standard EC.5.10 for required content of fire response plan.)*

A 6. All fire drills are critiqued to identify deficiencies and opportunities for improvement.

A 7. The effectiveness of fire response training according to the fire plan is evaluated at least annually.

A 8. During fire drills, staff knowledge is evaluated, including the following:
- When and how to sound fire alarms (where such alarms are available)
- When and how to transmit for offsite fire responders
- Containment of smoke and fire
- Transfer of residents to areas of refuge
- Fire extinguishment
- Specific fire response duties
- Preparation for building evacuation

Standard EC.5.40

The organization maintains fire-safety equipment and building features.

Note 1: *This standard does not require organizations to have the types of fire-safety equipment and building features discussed here. However, if these types of equipment or features exist within the organization, then the following maintenance, testing, and inspection requirements apply.*

Note 2: *Organizations that offer care, treatment, and services in leased facilities need to communicate maintenance expectations for building equipment not under their control to their landlord through contractual language, lease agreements, memos, and so forth. These organizations are not required to possess maintenance documentation but must only have access to such documentation as needed and during survey. It is also important that the landlord communicate to the organization any building equipment problems identified that could negatively affect the safety or health of residents, staff, and other people coming to the organization, as well as the landlord's plan to resolve such issues.*

---

* When drills are conducted between 9:00 P.M. and 6:00 A.M., a coded announcement will be permitted to be used instead of audible alarms.

Elements of Performance for EC.5.40

C Ⓜ 1. Initiating devices and fire detection and alarm equipment are tested as follows:*
- All supervisory signal devices (except valve tamper switches) are tested at least quarterly
- All valve tamper switches and water flow devices are tested at least semiannually
- All duct detectors, electromechanical releasing devices, heat detectors, manual fire alarm boxes, and smoke detectors are tested at least annually ⚠3

C Ⓜ 2. Occupant alarm notification devices, including all audible devices, speakers, and visible devices, are tested at least annually.† ⚠3

A 3. Off-premises emergency services notification transmission equipment is tested at least quarterly.* ⚠3

C Ⓜ 4. For water-based automatic fire-extinguishing systems, all fire pumps are tested at least weekly under no-flow condition.‡ ⚠3

C Ⓜ 5. For water-based automatic fire-extinguishing systems, all water-storage tank high- and low-water level alarms are tested at least semiannually. ⚠3

C Ⓜ 6. For water-based automatic fire-extinguishing systems, all water-storage tank low-water temperature alarms (during cold weather only) are tested at least monthly. ⚠3

C Ⓜ 7. For water-based automatic fire-extinguishing systems, main drain tests are conducted at least annually at all system risers. ⚠3

C Ⓜ 8. For water-based automatic fire-extinguishing systems, all fire department connections are inspected quarterly. ⚠3

A 9. For water-based automatic fire-extinguishing systems, all fire pumps are tested at least annually under flow. ⚠3

A 10. Kitchen automatic fire-extinguishing systems are inspected for proper operation at least semiannually. (Actual discharge of the fire-extinguishing system is not required.) ⚠3

C Ⓜ 11. Carbon dioxide and other gaseous automatic fire-extinguishing systems are tested for proper operation at least annually. (Actual discharge of the fire-extinguishing system is not required.) ⚠3

C Ⓜ 12. All portable fire extinguishers§ are clearly identified, inspected at least monthly, and maintained at least annually. ⚠3

---

* For additional guidance, see NFPA 72-1999 edition (Table 7-3.2).

† For additional guidance, see NFPA 72-1999 edition (Table 7-3.2).

‡ For additional guidance, see NFPA 25-1998 edition.

§ For additional guidance, see NFPA 10-1998 edition (sections 1-6, 4-3, and 4-4).

C Ⓜ 13. All standpipe occupant hoses are hydrostatically tested five years after installation and at least every three years thereafter,* and systems receive water-flow tests at least every five years.†

C Ⓜ 14. All fire and smoke dampers are operated one year after installation and then at least every four years to verify that they fully close.‡

Note: *The initial test that must occur one year after installation applies only to dampers installed on and after January 1, 2008.*

A 15. All automatic smoke-detection shutdown devices for air-handling equipment are tested at least annually.§ ⚠3

C Ⓜ 16. All horizontal and vertical sliding and rolling fire doors are tested for proper operation and full closure at least annually.|| ⚠3

Standard EC.5.50

Not applicable

Standard EC.6.10

The organization manages medical equipment risks.

Rationale for EC.6.10

Medical equipment is a significant contributor to the quality of care. It is used in treatment, diagnostic activities, and monitoring of the resident. It is essential that the equipment is appropriate for the intended use; that staff, including licensed independent practitioners, be trained to use the equipment safely and effectively; and that the equipment is maintained appropriately by qualified individuals.

Elements of Performance for EC.6.10

A 1. The organization develops and maintains a written management plan describing the processes it implements to manage the effective, safe, and reliable operation of medical equipment.

A 2. The organization identifies and implements a process(es) for selecting and acquiring medical equipment.#

---

* For additional guidance, see NFPA 1962-1998 edition (section 2-3).

† For additional guidance, see NFPA 25-1998 edition.

‡ For additional guidance, see NFPA 80-2007 (19.4.1.1) and NFPA 105-2007 (6.5.2).

§ For additional guidance, see NFPA 90A-1999 edition (section 4-4.1).

|| For additional guidance, see NFPA 80-1999 edition (section 15-2.4).

\# **Note:** *The acquisition process includes initially evaluating the condition and function of the equipment when received and evaluating the training of users before use on residents.*

A 3. The organization establishes and uses risk criteria* for identifying, evaluating, and creating an inventory of equipment to be included in the medical equipment management plan before the equipment is used. These criteria address the following:
- Equipment function (diagnosis, care, treatment, life support, and monitoring)
- Physical risks associated with use
- Equipment incident history

A 4. The organization identifies appropriate inspection and maintenance strategies for all equipment on the inventory for achieving effective, safe, and reliable operation of all equipment in the inventory.†

A 5. The organization defines intervals for inspecting, testing, and maintaining appropriate equipment on the inventory (that is, those pieces of equipment on the inventory benefiting from scheduled activities to minimize the clinical and physical risks) that are based upon criteria such as manufacturers' recommendations, risk levels, and current organization experience.

A 6. The organization identifies and implements processes for monitoring and acting on equipment hazard notices and recalls.

A 7. The organization identifies and implements processes for monitoring and reporting incidents in which a medical device is suspected or attributed to the death, serious injury, or serious illness of any individual, as required by the Safe Medical Devices Act of 1990.

A 8. The organization identifies and implements processes for emergency procedures that address the following:
- What to do in the event of equipment disruption or failure
- When and how to perform emergency clinical interventions when medical equipment fails
- Availability of backup equipment
- How to obtain repair services

Standard EC.6.20

Medical equipment is maintained, tested, and inspected.

Elements of Performance for EC.6.20

C Ⓜ 1. The organization documents a current, accurate, and separate inventory of all equipment identified in the medical equipment management plan, regardless of ownership.

---

* **Note:** *The organization may choose not to use risk criteria to limit the types of equipment to be included in the medical equipment management plan, but rather include all medical equipment.*

† **Note:** *Organizations may use different strategies for different items as appropriate. For example, strategies such as predictive maintenance, interval-based inspections, corrective maintenance, or metered maintenance may be selected to ensure reliable performance.*

A 2. The organization documents performance and safety testing of all equipment identified in the medical equipment management program before initial use.

A 3. The organization documents inspection and maintenance of equipment used for life support* that is consistent with maintenance strategies to minimize clinical and physical risks identified in the equipment management plan (*see* standard EC.6.10). ⚠3

C Ⓜ 4. The organization documents inspection and maintenance of non–life support equipment on the inventory that is consistent with maintenance strategies to minimize clinical and physical risks identified in the equipment management plan (*see* standard EC.6.10).

5. Not applicable

C Ⓜ 6. The organization documents chemical and biological testing of water used in renal dialysis and other applicable tests based upon regulations, manufacturers' recommendations, and organization experience. ⚠3

Standards EC.6.30 Through EC.6.130

Not applicable

Standard EC.7.10

The organization manages its utility risks.

Rationale for EC.7.10

Utility systems† are essential to the proper operation of the environment of care and significantly contribute to effective, safe, and reliable provision of care to residents in health care organizations. It is important that health care organizations establish and maintain a utility systems management program to promote a safe, controlled, and comfortable environment that does the following:

- Ensures operational reliability of utility systems
- Reduces the potential for organization-acquired illness to be transmitted through the utility systems
- Assesses the reliability and minimizes potential risks of utility system failures

Elements of Performance for EC.7.10

1. Through 6. Not applicable

---

* **Life support equipment** Those devices intended to sustain life and whose failure to perform its primary function, when used according to manufacturer's instructions and clinical protocol, is expected to result in imminent death in the absence of immediate intervention (examples include ventilators, anesthesia machines, and heart-lung bypass machines).

† **Utility systems** May include electrical distribution; emergency power; vertical and horizontal transport; heating, ventilating, and air conditioning; plumbing, boiler, and steam; piped gases; vacuum systems; or communication systems, including data-exchange systems.

A 7. The organization develops and maintains a written management plan describing the processes it implements to manage the effective, safe, and reliable operation of utility systems.

A 8. The organization designs and installs utility systems that meet the resident care and operational needs of the services in the organization's buildings.

A 9. The organization establishes risk criteria* for identifying, evaluating, and creating an inventory of operating components of systems before the equipment is used.
These criteria address the following:
- Life support
- Infection control
- Support of the environment
- Equipment support
- Communication

A 10. The organization develops appropriate strategies for all utility systems equipment on the inventory for ensuring effective, safe, and reliable operation of all equipment in the inventory.†

A 11. The organization defines intervals for inspecting, testing, and maintaining appropriate utility systems equipment on the inventory (that is, those pieces of equipment on the inventory benefiting from scheduled activities to minimize the clinical and physical risks) that are based upon criteria such as manufacturers' recommendations, risk levels, and current organization experience.

A 12. The organization identifies and implements emergency procedures for responding to utility system disruptions or failures that address the following:
- What to do if utility systems malfunction
- Identification of an alternative source of organization-defined essential utilities
- Shutting off the malfunctioning systems and notifying staff in affected areas
- How and when to perform emergency clinical interventions when utility systems fail
- Obtaining repair services ⚠3

A 13. The organization maps the distribution of utility systems. ⚠3

C Ⓜ 14. The organization labels controls for a partial or complete emergency shutdown. ⚠3

---

* **Note:** *The organization may choose not to use risk criteria to limit the types of utility systems to be included in the utility management plan, but rather include all utility systems.*

† **Note:** *Organizations may use different strategies as appropriate. For example, strategies such as predictive maintenance, interval-based inspections, corrective maintenance, or metered maintenance may be selected to ensure reliable performance.*

A 15. The organization identifies and implements processes to minimize pathogenic biological agents in cooling towers, domestic hot/cold water systems, and other aerosolizing water systems. ⚠3

A 16. The organization designs, installs, and maintains ventilation equipment to provide appropriate pressure relationships, air-exchange rates, and filtration efficiencies for ventilation systems serving areas specially designed* to control airborne contaminants (such as biological agents, gases, fumes, and dust). ⚠3

Standard EC.7.20

The organization provides an emergency electrical power source.

Rationale for EC.7.20

The organization properly installs an emergency power source that is adequately sized, designed, and fueled, as required by the *LSC* occupancy requirements and the services provided.

Elements of Performance for EC.7.20

The organization provides a reliable emergency power system†, as required by the *LSC* occupancy requirements, that supplies electricity to the following areas when normal electricity is interrupted:

A 1. Alarm systems ⚠3

C Ⓜ 2. Exit route illumination ⚠3

A 3. Emergency communication systems ⚠3

C Ⓜ 4. Illumination of exit signs

The organization provides a reliable emergency power system, as required by the services provided and residents served, that supplies electricity to the following areas when normal electricity is interrupted:

5. Not applicable

6. Not applicable

7. Not applicable

A 8. Elevators (at least one for nonambulatory residents)

A 9. Medical air compressors ⚠3

---

* **Areas specially designed** Include spaces such as rooms for residents diagnosed or suspected of having airborne communicable diseases (for example, pulmonary or laryngeal tuberculosis), residents in "protective isolation" rooms (for example, those receiving bone marrow transplants), laboratories, pharmacies, and sterile supply rooms.

† **Reliable emergency power system** For guidance in establishing a reliable emergency power system (Essential Electrical Distribution System), *see* NFPA 99-2002 edition (chapters 13 and 14).

A 10. Medical and surgical vacuum systems ⚠3

A 11. Areas where electrically powered life-support equipment is used ⚠3

Standard EC.7.30

The organization maintains, tests, and inspects its utility systems.

Note: *Organizations that offer care, treatment, and services in leased facilities need to communicate maintenance expectations for building equipment not under their control to their landlord through contractual language, lease agreements, memos, and so forth. These organizations are not required to possess maintenance documentation but must only have access to such documentation as needed and during survey. It is also important that the landlord communicate to the organization any building equipment problems identified that could negatively affect the safety or health of residents, staff, and other people coming to the organization, as well as the landlord's plan to resolve such issues.*

Elements of Performance for EC.7.30

C Ⓜ 1. The organization maintains documentation of a current, accurate, and separate inventory of utility components identified in the utility management plan.

A 2. The organization maintains documentation of performance and safety testing of each critical component identified in the plan before initial use.

A 3. The organization maintains documentation of maintenance of critical components of life support utility systems/equipment consistent with maintenance strategies identified in the utility management plan (*see* standard EC.7.10).

A 4. The organization maintains documentation of maintenance of critical components of infection control utility systems/equipment for high-risk residents consistent with maintenance strategies identified in the utility management plan (*see* standard EC.7.10).

C Ⓜ 5. The organization maintains documentation of maintenance of critical components of non–life support utility systems/equipment on the inventory consistent with maintenance strategies identified in the utility management plan (*see* standard EC.7.10).

Standard EC.7.40

The organization maintains, tests, and inspects its emergency power systems.

Rationale for EC 7.40

Emergency electrical power supply systems may fail during a power disruption leaving an organization unable to deliver safe care to individuals for whom it is responsible. Testing these systems for sufficient lengths of time at regular frequencies increases the likelihood of detecting reliability problems and reduces the risk of losing this critical resource when it is most needed.

While not all organizations are required to have the types of emergency power systems described below, an organization that has these types of systems must comply with the maintenance, testing, and inspection requirements of this standard.

Elements of Performance for EC.7.40

C Ⓜ 1. The organization tests each generator 12 times a year, with testing intervals not less than 20 days and not more than 40 days apart. These tests shall be conducted for at least 30 continuous minutes under a dynamic load that is at least 30% of the nameplate rating of the generator. ⚠3

Note: *Organizations may choose to test to less than 30% of the emergency generator's nameplate. However, these organizations shall (in addition to performing a test for 30 continuous minutes under operating temperature at the intervals described here) revise their existing documented management plan to conform to NFPA 110 (2005 edition) testing and maintenance activities. These activities shall include inspection procedures for assessing the prime movers' exhaust gas temperature against the minimum temperature recommended by the manufacturer.*

If diesel-powered generators do not meet the minimum exhaust gas temperatures as determined during these tests, they shall be exercised for 30 continuous minutes at the intervals described here with available Emergency Power Supply Systems (EPSS) load and exercised annually with supplemental loads of the following:

- *25% of nameplate rating for 30 minutes, followed by*
- *50% of nameplate rating for 30 minutes, followed by*
- *75% of nameplate rating for 60 minutes for a total of 2 continuous hours*

C Ⓜ 2. The organization tests all automatic transfer switches 12 times a year, with testing intervals not less than 20 days and not more than 40 days apart. ⚠3

C Ⓜ 3. The organization tests all battery-powered lights required for egress. Testing includes (a) a functional test at 30-day intervals for a minimum of 30 seconds and (b) an annual test for a duration of 1.5 hours.

C Ⓜ 4. The organization tests Stored Emergency Power Supply Systems (SEPSS) whose malfunction may severely jeopardize the occupants' life and safety.* Testing includes (a) a quarterly functional test for 5 minutes or as

---

* **Stored Emergency Power Supply Systems (SEPSS)** Are intended to automatically supply illumination or power to critical areas and equipment essential for safety to human life. Included are systems that supply emergency power for such functions as illumination for safe exiting, ventilation where it is essential to maintain life, fire detection and alarm systems, public safety communications systems, and processes where the current interruption would produce serious life safety or health hazards to residents, the public, or staff. **Note:** *Other non-SEPSS battery back-up emergency power systems that an organization has determined to be critical for operations during a power failure (for example, laboratory equipment, electronic medical records) should be properly tested and maintained in accordance with manufacturer's recommendations.*

specified for its class,* whichever is less and (b) an annual test at full load for 60% of the full duration of its class. ⚠3

A 5. Facilities that have a generator providing emergency power for the services listed in elements of performance 8–11 of standard EC.7.20: The organization tests each emergency generator at least once every 36 months for a minimum of four continuous hours. This test shall be conducted under a load (dynamic or static) that is at least 30% of the nameplate rating of the generator.† ⚠3

Note 1: *To be in initial compliance with this element of performance, organizations must have performed this test by July 1, 2007. Organizations that have successfully operated their generator(s) since July 1, 2004, according to the test criteria described above, will be considered to be in initial compliance with this element of performance and are required to retest before the three year anniversary date of such occurrence.*

Note 2: *Organizations that cannot achieve a minimum load of 30% of the emergency generator's nameplate rating, must assess the prime movers' exhaust gas temperature and meet the minimum temperature recommended by the manufacturer.*

A 6. If a test(s) required by EC.7.40 fails, the organization implements interim measures to compensate for the risk to patients, visitors, and staff until necessary repairs or corrections are completed. ⚠3

A 7. If a test(s) required by EC.7.40 fails, the organization performs a retest after making the necessary repairs or corrections. ⚠3

Standard EC.7.50

The organization maintains, tests, and inspects its medical gas and vacuum systems.

Note: *This standard does not require organizations to have the medical gas and vacuum systems discussed here. However, if an organization has these types of systems, then the following maintenance, testing, and inspection requirements apply.*

Elements of Performance for EC.7.50

A 1. The organization inspects, tests, and maintains critical components of piped medical gas systems, including master signal panels, area alarms, automatic pressure switches, shutoff valves, flexible connectors, and outlets. ⚠3

---

* **Class** Defines the minimum time for which the SEPSS is designed to operate at its rated load without being recharged. (For additional guidance, see NFPA 111 [1996 edition] *Standard on Stored Electrical Energy Emergency and Standby Power Systems.*)

† This test may satisfy one of the tests required by EP 1. After the test, the fuel supply should be replenished. Any problems identified during the test shall be resolved promptly. For additional guidance, see *NFPA 110 (2005 edition) Standard for Emergency & Standby Power Systems.*

A 2. The organization tests piped medical gas and vacuum systems when the systems are installed, modified, or repaired, including cross-connection testing, piping purity testing, and pressure testing. ⚠3

A 3. The organization maintains the main supply valve and area shut-off valves of piped medical gas and vacuum systems to be accessible and clearly labeled. ⚠3

Standard EC.8.10

The organization establishes and maintains an appropriate environment.

Rationale for EC.8.10

It is important that the physical environment is functional and promotes caring. It should contribute to relieving loneliness, boredom, and hopelessness.* The environment should also encourage independence and promote quality of life.

Elements of Performance for EC.8.10

A 1. Interior spaces should be the following:
- Appropriate to the care, treatment, and services provided and the needs of the residents related to age and other characteristics
- Include closet and drawer space provided for storing personal property and other items provided for use by residents. Lockers, drawers, or closet space is provided for residents who are in charge of their own personal grooming and who wear street clothes (for example, behavioral health care clients who wear street clothes and are expected to meet their personal grooming needs).
- Allow for good recreational interchange, consider personal preferences when feasible, and accommodate equipment, such as wheelchairs, that are necessary to activities of daily living
- Have equipment for rehabilitation and activities adequate to accomplish goals without compromising the environment's safety

A 2. Furnishings and equipment should do the following:
- Be maintained to be safe and in good repair
- Reflect the resident's level of ability and needs

A 3. Outside areas are the following:
- Appropriate and safe considering the care, treatment, and services provided and the needs of the residents related to age and other characteristics
- Used during appropriate seasons

C Ⓜ 4. Areas used by the residents are safe, clean, functional, and comfortable.

* A powerful tool for improving the quality of life for the elderly is "**The Eden Alternative**™". Part of its mission statement is to relieve loneliness, boredom, and hopelessness. Additional information about its concepts can be found at http://www.edenalt.com.

A 5. Lighting is suitable for care, treatment, and services and the specific activities being conducted. ⚠3

6. Not applicable

A 7. Ventilation provides for acceptable levels of temperature and humidity and eliminates odors. ⚠3

8. Not applicable

9. Not applicable

10. Not applicable

A 11. Door locks and other structural restraints used are consistent with the needs of residents, program policy, law, and regulation.

A 12. Emergency access provision is provided to all locked, occupied spaces. ⚠3

13. Not applicable

14. Not applicable

A 15. Spaces are accessible for safe wandering and exploring.

A 16. A sufficient number of electrical outlets with sufficient capacities are present to accommodate medically complex services offered to residents.

Standard EC.8.20

The organization establishes and maintains an appropriate dining environment.

Elements of Performance for EC.8.20

C Ⓜ 1. The dining environment encourages eating and socialization, for instance, by minimizing distractions and providing small group settings.

C Ⓜ 2. Dining areas are free from loud and distracting noises according to the residents' needs.

3. Not applicable

4. Not applicable

5. Not applicable

C Ⓜ 6. Dining areas have adequate space for residents with equipment such as ventilators and cardiac monitors.

C Ⓜ 7. Dining areas have the following characteristics:
- Offer residents a selection of seating
- Include tables with height(s) to facilitate independent eating
- Have staff that help residents sit in a regular dining chair, when possible

Standard EC.8.30

The organization manages the design and building of the environment when it is renovated, altered, or newly created (*see also* standard EC.5.50).

Elements of Performance for EC.8.30

A 1. When planning for the size, configuration, and equipping of the space of renovated, altered, or new construction, the organization uses one of the following: applicable state rules and regulations; *Guidelines for Design and Construction of Hospitals and Health Care Facilities,* 2001 edition, published by the American Institute of Architects; or standards or guidelines that provide design criteria.

A 2. When planning demolition, construction, or renovation, the organization conducts a proactive risk assessment using risk criteria to identify hazards that could potentially compromise care, treatment, and services in occupied areas of the organization's buildings. The scope and nature of the activities should determine the extent of risk assessment.

A 3. When planning demolition, construction, or renovation, the organization uses risk criteria that address the impact of demolition, renovation, or new construction on air quality requirements, infection control, utility requirements, noise, vibration, and emergency procedures. ⚠3

A 4. When planning demolition, construction, or renovation, the organization selects and implements proper controls, as required, to reduce risk and minimize impact of these activities. ⚠3

Measuring and Improving Activities

Standard EC.9.10

The organization monitors conditions in the environment.

Elements of Performance for EC.9.10

A 1. The organization establishes and implements process(es) for reporting and investigating the following:*
- Injuries to residents or others coming to the organization's facilities, as well as incidents of property damage
- Occupational illnesses and injuries to staff
- Security incidents involving residents, staff, or others coming to the organization's facilities or property
- Hazardous materials and waste spills, exposures, and other related incidents

---

* Organizations have the flexibility to develop a single reporting method that addresses one or more of the items listed.

- Fire-safety management problems, deficiencies, and failures
- Equipment-management problems, failures, and user errors
- Utility systems management problems, failures, or user errors

A 2. The organization's leaders assign a person(s) (hereafter referred to as the "assigned person[s]") to monitor and respond to conditions in the organization's environment. The assigned individual performs the following tasks:
- Coordinates the ongoing, organizationwide collection of information about deficiencies and opportunities for improvement in the environment of care
- Coordinates the ongoing collection and dissemination of other sources of information, such as published hazard notices or recall reports
- Coordinates the preparation of summaries of deficiencies, problems, failures, and user errors related to managing the environment of care*
- Coordinates the preparation of summaries on findings, recommendations, actions taken, and results of performance improvement (PI) activities
- Participates in hazard surveillance and incident reporting
- Participates in developing safety policies and procedures

A 3. The organization establishes and implements a process(es) for ongoing monitoring of performance regarding actual or potential risk(s) in each of the environment of care management plans.†

A 4. Each of the environment of care management plans is evaluated at least annually.

A 5. The objectives, scope, performance, and effectiveness of each of the environment of care management plans are evaluated at least annually.

6. Through 9. Not applicable

A 10. Environmental safety monitoring and response activities are communicated to the resident safety program required in the "Leadership" chapter of this book.

Standard EC.9.20

The organization analyzes identified environment issues and develops recommendations for resolving them.

---

* **Notes:** *Incidents involving residents may be reported to appropriate staff such as staff in quality assessment, improvement, or other functions. However, at least a summary of incidents is shared with the person designated to coordinate safety management activities (see standard EC.1.10). Review of incident reports often requires that various legal processes be followed to preserve confidentiality. Opportunities to improve care, treatment, and services or to prevent future similar incidents are not lost as a result of the legal process followed.*

† The environment of care plans are for managing safety, security, hazardous materials and waste, emergency management, fire safety, medical equipment, and utilities.

Elements of Performance for EC.9.20

A 1. The organization establishes an ongoing process for resolving environment of care issues that involves representatives from clinical, administrative, and support services.

C Ⓜ 2. A multidisciplinary improvement team meets at least bimonthly to address environment of care issues.*

A 3. The organization analyzes environment of care issues in a timely manner.

A 4. Recommendations are developed and approved as appropriate.

A 5. Appropriate staff establishes measurement guidelines.

A 6. Environment of care issues are communicated to the organization's leaders and person(s) responsible for PI activities.

7. Not applicable

A 8. A recommendation for one or more PI activities is communicated at least annually to the organization's leaders based on the ongoing performance monitoring of the environment of care management plans.

A 9. Recommendations for resolving environmental safety issues are communicated, when appropriate, to those responsible for managing the resident safety program required in the "Leadership" chapter of this book.

Standard EC.9.30

The organization improves the environment.

Elements of Performance for EC.9.30

A 1. Appropriate staff participates in implementing recommendations.

A 2. Appropriate staff monitors the effectiveness of the recommendation's implementation.

A 3. Monitoring results are reported through appropriate channels, including the organization's leaders.

A 4. Monitoring results are reported to the multidisciplinary improvement team responsible for resolving environment of care issues.

A 5. Results of monitoring are reported (when appropriate) to those responsible for managing the resident safety program required in the "Leadership" chapter of this book.

---

* **Note:** *Meetings held less frequently than bimonthly are acceptable when supported by current organization experience and the multidisciplinary improvement team's approval. Ongoing justification of meeting frequency depends on a satisfactory annual evaluation of performance as required by standard EC.9.10.*

2009

SLTC

Life Safety (LS)

LS

LS

Chapter Outli

I. Administrative Activ
   A. Statement of Cor
   B. Interim Life Safe

II. Health Care Occupa
   A. All Health Care (
      1. General Buil(
      2. Means of Egr
      3. Protection (I
         a. Fire Alarr
         b. Extinguis
      4. Special Prov
      5. Building Ser
      6. Operating Fe

III. Ambulatory Health
   A. All Ambulatory
      1. Not applicat
      2. Not applicat
      3. Not applicat
         a. Not appli
         b. Not appl
      4. Not applicat
      5. Not applicat
      6. Not applicat

IV. Residential Occupa
   A. Lodging or Roo
      1. Not applical
      2. Not applical
      3. Not applical
   B. Hotels and Dor
      1. Not applica
      2. Not applica
      3. Not applica
      4. Not applica

Life Safety (LS)

Overview

Applicability of the Standards

The standards in this chapter are based on the National Fire Protection Association's (NFPA) *Life Safety Code*®* and address protection of individuals from fire. Long term care organizations must meet the health care occupancy requirements. Health care occupancies include hospitals, nursing homes, and limited care facilities.

About This Chapter

Fire is a concern for everyone, but it is a special concern in long term care organizations because residents are often unable to move to safety by themselves. The *Life Safety Code* considers several options for fire protection: creating safe areas (smoke compartments) that allow people to remain in their locations and "defend in place"; moving people to safe areas within the building; and, as a last resort, moving people out of a building. Health care facility design and related features help prevent, detect, and suppress fires. The measures that organizations must take to protect occupants from the dangers of fire constitute the content of this chapter. These standards focus on the importance of a fire-safe environment and buildings; however, The Joint Commission recognizes that people are equally important in reducing the risk of fire. The responsibilities of managing a safe environment (for example, identifying fire risks, conducting fire drills, maintaining fire protection equipment) by those who work in the organization are addressed in the "Management of the Environment of Care" (EC) chapter.

From time to time, building codes are updated to incorporate new technology that often cannot be introduced easily into older buildings. These settings tend to rely more on passive systems (such as doors and walls) for fire protection. In new buildings, fire protection is more often provided by active systems, such as fire alarms and automatic sprinkler systems. This chapter addresses both existing and new health care occupancies. Buildings are considered existing health care occupancies if final plans for additions, renovations, or changes in occupancy were approved by the local authority having jurisdiction before March 1, 2003. Existing health care occupancy requirements are found in Chapter 19 of the *Life Safety Code* (101–2000). Buildings with final plans for new construction, additions, renovations, or changes in occupancy approved by the local authority having jurisdiction after March 1, 2003, are considered new health care occupancies. New health care occupancy requirements are found in Chapter 18 of the *Life Safety Code*.

---

* *Life Safety Code*® is a registered trademark of the National Fire Protection Association, Quincy, MA.

Key: 0 = Insufficient compliance; 1 = Partial compliance; 2 = Satisfactory compliance; NA = Not applicable; **A** indicates scoring category A; **C** indicates scoring category C; ▲2 indicates situational decision rules apply; △3 indicates direct impact requirements apply; Ⓜ indicates Measure of success is needed

The Joint Commission
source for the key stru
element of performan
also provided in those
source. The *Life Safety*
ter. Compliance with t
and is acceptable to T

This chapter addresses
the following:

- General life safety d
- The means of egres
  and signage
- Protection providec
  ings; corridors; smc
- Fire alarm notificati
- Suppression of fires
- Building services, ir
- Decorations, furnisl

Managing Compli

The Joint Commission
Life Safety Code canno
unpredictable situatio
ciency immediately or

- A management pro
  situation within 45 c
- A *Life Safety Code* E
  are used when an o
  cannot be correctec
  may ask The Joint C
  by submitting docu
  that comply with th
  approve equivalenc
  alency or granted a
  details.)
- A Plan for Improven
  (e-SOC). The Joint C
  organization uses it
  uses the e-SOC to dc
  LS.01.02.01), and is
  will not consider th
  tation process. All c
  jected completion d

2009

SLTC

Management of Human Resources (HR)

HR

HR

Management of Human Resources (HR)

Overview

The goal of the human resources function is to ensure that the organization determines the qualifications and competencies for staff* positions based on its mission, population(s), and care, treatment, and services. Organizations must also provide the right number of competent staff to meet residents' needs. To meet this goal, the organization carries out the following processes and activities:

- **Planning.** The planning process defines the qualifications, competencies, and staffing necessary to provide for the organization's care, treatment, and services.
- **Providing competent staff.** The organization provides for competent staff either through traditional employer-employee arrangements or through contractual arrangements with other entities or persons.
- **Orienting, training, and educating staff.** The organization provides ongoing in-service and other education and training to increase staff knowledge of specific work-related issues.
- **Assessing, maintaining, and improving staff competence.** Ongoing, periodic competence assessment evaluates staff members' continuing abilities to perform throughout their association with the organization.
- **Promoting self-development and learning.** Staff is encouraged to pursue ongoing professional development goals and provide feedback about the work environment.

---

* **Staff** As appropriate to their roles and responsibilities, all people who provide care, treatment, and services in the organization, including those receiving pay (e.g., permanent, temporary, and part-time personnel, as well as contract employees), volunteers, and health profession students. The definition of staff does not include licensed independent practitioners who are not paid staff or who are not contract employees.

Key: 0 = Insufficient compliance; 1 = Partial compliance; 2 = Satisfactory compliance; NA = Not applicable; **A** indicates scoring category A; **C** indicates scoring category C; ▲(2) indicates situational decision rules apply; △(3) indicates direct impact requirements apply; Ⓜ indicates Measure of success is needed

Standards

The following is a list of all standards for this function. They are presented here for your convenience without footnotes or other explanatory text. If you have a question about a term used here, please check the Glossary.

Note: *A revised standard numbering system is being used with the reformatted standards. The revised numbering system will allow for more flexibility to add standards while maintaining the current label for each standard.*

Planning

HR.1.10 The organization provides an adequate number and mix of staff and licensed independent practitioners consistent with the organization's staffing plan.

HR 1.15 Not applicable

HR.1.20 Staff qualifications are consistent with his or her job responsibilities.

HR.1.25 The organization may assign disaster responsibilities to volunteer practitioners

HR.1.30 The organization uses data from clinical/service screening indicators and human resource screening indicators to assess and continuously improve staffing effectiveness.

Orientation, Training, and Education

HR.2.10 The organization provides initial orientation.

HR.2.20 Staff and licensed independent practitioners, as appropriate, can describe or demonstrate their roles and responsibilities relative to safety.

HR.2.30 Ongoing education, including in-services, training, and other activities, maintains and improves staff competence.

Assessing Competence

HR.3.10 Staff competence to perform job responsibilities is assessed, demonstrated, and maintained.

HR.3.20 The organization periodically conducts performance evaluations.

HR.3.25 Through HR 3.60 Not applicable

Credentialing and Granting of Privileges of Licensed Independent Practitioners

HR.4.10 There is a process for ensuring the competence of all practitioners permitted by law and the organization to practice independently.

HR.4.20 Individuals permitted by law and the organization to practice independently are granted clinical privileges.

HR.4.30 The organization has a process for granting temporary clinical privileges, when appropriate.

HR 4.32 Not applicable

HR 4.33 Not applicable

HR 4.34 Not applicable

HR.4.35 The organization may grant disaster privileges to volunteers eligible to be licensed independent practitioners.

HR.4.40 There are mechanisms, including a fair hearing and appeal process, for addressing adverse decisions regarding reappointment denial, reduction, suspension, or revocation of clinical privileges that may relate to quality of care, treatment, and service issues.

HR.4.50 Clinical privileges and appointments/reappointments are reviewed and revised at least every two years.

HR.4.60 Through HR.5.40 Not applicable

Standards, Rationales, Elements of Performance, and Scoring

Planning

Standard HR.1.10

The organization provides an adequate number and mix of staff and licensed independent practitioners consistent with the organization's staffing plan.

Rationale for HR.1.10

An organization must provide appropriate types and numbers of qualified staff necessary to furnish the care, treatment, and services offered by the organization. This can be done either through traditional employer-employee arrangements or through contractual arrangements.

Elements of Performance for HR.1.10

1. Not applicable

A 2. Nursing care and services are provided 24 hours a day, 7 days a week, including relief personnel during vacation periods, sick leaves, emergencies, and holidays. ⚠3

A 3. Except when waived by the state, a registered nurse supervises nursing care at least 8 consecutive hours a day, 7 days a week. ⚠3

A 4. If any resident(s) requires a registered nurse's services, at least one registered nurse, who is currently licensed by the state in which he or she practices, is on duty* on each shift, 7 days a week.[†] ⚠3

Standard HR.1.15

Not applicable

Standard HR.1.20

Staff qualifications are consistent with his or her job responsibilities.

* The use of a registered nurse "on call" instead of "on duty" should be the exception and must not adversely affect resident care.

[†] If none of the residents requires a registered nurse's services, registered nurse coverage on each shift is optional; however, a licensed practical (vocational) nurse, who is currently licensed by the state in which he or she practices, is assigned to each shift seven days a week. Supervision is provided on all shifts.

Elements of Performance for HR.1.20

A 1. The organization defines the required competence and qualifications of staff in each program(s) or service(s).

C Ⓜ 2. When the organization requires current licensure, certification, or registration, but these credentials are not required by law or regulation, the organization verifies these credentials at the time of hire and upon expiration of the credentials.

A 3. When current licensure, certification, or registration are required by law or regulation to practice a profession,* the organization verifies these credentials with the primary source at the time of hire and upon expiration of the credentials.

Note 1: *It is acceptable to verify current licensure, certification, or registration with the primary source via a secure electronic communication or by telephone, if this verification is documented. For additional information, see "primary source verification" in the Glossary.*

Note 2: *A primary source of information may designate another agency to communicate credentials information. The designated agency then can be used as a primary source.*

Note 3: *An external organization (for example, a credentials verification organization [CVO]) may be used to collect credentials information. A CVO must meet the CVO guidelines listed in the Glossary.*

C Ⓜ 4. The organization also verifies the education, experience, and competence appropriate for assigned responsibilities.

C Ⓜ 5. The organization also verifies information on criminal background if required by law and regulation or organization policy.

C Ⓜ 6. The organization also verifies compliance with applicable health screening requirements if required by law and regulation or established by the organization.†

A 7. The information obtained from EPs 2–6 is used in making decisions regarding staff job responsibilities.

A 8. All staff that provide resident care, treatment, and services possess a license, certification, or registration as required by law and regulation. ▲2

9. Not applicable

10. Not applicable

* **Profession** is a specialized work function within society, generally performed by a professional. It often refers specifically to fields that require extensive study and mastery of specialized knowledge and skills.

† Organizations should consider the applicability of the Americans with Disabilities Act (ADA), and if applicable, review policies and procedures. Federal entities are required to comply with the Rehabilitation Act of 1974.

C Ⓜ 11. Prior to the provision of care, treatment, or services, the qualifications and competence of a non-employee individual, brought into the organization by a licensed independent practitioner to provide care, treatment, or services within the scope of the organization's services are assessed by the organization and determined to be commensurate with the qualifications and competence required if the individual were to be employed by the organization to perform the same or similar services. ⚠3

Note: *When the service to be provided by the individual is not currently performed by anyone employed by the organization, it is leadership's responsibility to consult the appropriate professional organization guidelines with respect to expectations for credentials and competence.*

C Ⓜ 12. The organization reviews the qualifications, performance, and competence of each non-employee individual brought into the organization by a licensed independent practitioner to provide care, treatment, or services at the same frequency as individuals employed by the organization.

13. Not applicable

A 14. Staff supervises students when they provide resident care, treatment, and services as part of their training.

Disaster Responsibilities

Standard HR.1.25

The organization may assign disaster responsibilities to volunteer practitioners.

Rationale for HR.1.25

When the disaster plan has been implemented (*see* standard EC.4.10 for a description of emergency management planning requirements) and the immediate needs of the residents cannot be met, the organization may implement a modified process for determining qualifications and competence of volunteer practitioners* (*see* EPs 5–8). The volunteer practitioners that are addressed by this standard only include those practitioners that are required by law and regulation to have a license, certification, or registration to practice their profession. The usual process to determine the qualifications and competence of these practitioners would not allow a volunteer practitioner to provide immediate care, treatment, and services in the event of a disaster (refer to the Glossary for definitions of disaster and emergency) due to the length of time it would take to complete the process. A similar modified process for the assignment of disaster privileges for volunteer licensed independent practitioners exists at standard HR.4.35.

While this standard allows for a method to streamline the process for determining qualifications and competence, safeguards must be in place to assure that the volun-

* Individuals who are qualified to practice a health care profession (for example, a nurse) and are engaged in the provision of care and services. Practitioners are often required to be licensed as defined by law.

teer practitioners are competent to provide safe and adequate care, treatment, and services. Even in a disaster, the integrity of the following two parts of the usual process for determining qualifications and competence must be maintained:

1. Verification of licensure, certification, or registration required to practice a profession
2. Oversight of the care, treatment, and services provided

This option to assign disaster responsibilities to volunteer practitioners is made on a case-by-case basis in accordance with the needs of the organization and its residents, and on the qualifications of its volunteer practitioners.

There are a number of state and federal systems engaged in pre-event verification of qualifications that may facilitate the assigning of disaster responsibilities to volunteer practitioners at the time of a disaster. Examples of such systems include the Medical Reserve Corps (MRC*) and the Emergency System for Advance Registration of Volunteer Health Professionals (ESAR-VHP†). It is expected that additional programs will emerge and evolve.

Elements of Performance for HR.1.25

A 1. Disaster responsibilities are assigned only when the following two conditions are present: the emergency management plan has been activated, and the organization is unable to meet immediate resident needs.

A 2. The organization identifies in writing the individual(s) responsible for assigning disaster responsibilities.

A 3. The organization describes in writing a mechanism (for example, direct observation, mentoring, and clinical record review) to oversee the professional performance of volunteer practitioners who are assigned disaster responsibilities.

A 4. The organization has a mechanism to identify volunteer practitioners that have been assigned disaster responsibilities.

A 5. For volunteer practitioners to be assigned disaster responsibilities, the organization obtains for each volunteer practitioner at a minimum, a valid government-issued photo identification issued by a state or federal agency (e.g., driver's license or passport) and at least one of the following:

---

* **MRC** Medical Reserve Corps units comprised of locally based medical and public health volunteers who can assist their communities during emergencies, such as an influenza epidemic, a chemical spill, or an act of terrorism. The MRC Program was formed in 2002, in cooperation with the White House's USA Freedom Corps, as one of the charter programs of Citizen Corps. Pre-identifying, training, and organizing medical and public health professionals to strengthen their communities through volunteerism is at the core of the MRC concept. MRC volunteers offer their expertise throughout the year by supporting local public health initiatives, such as immunization and prevention activities. When an emergency community need occurs, MRC volunteers can work in coordination with existing local emergency response programs.

† **ESAR-VHP** The Emergency System for Advance Registration of Volunteer Health Professionals (ESAR-VHP) program, created by the Health Resources and Services Administration (HRSA), allows for the advance registration and credentialing of health care professionals needed to augment a hospital or other medical facility to meet increased patient/victim care and increased surge capacity needs.

- A current health care organization [such as a long term care, ambulatory care, laboratory, or hospital] picture identification card that clearly identifies professional designation
- A current license, certification, or registration
- Primary source verification of licensure, certification, or registration (if required by law and regulation to practice a profession)
- Identification indicating that the individual is a member of a Disaster Medical Assistance Team (DMAT*), or MRC, ESAR-VHP, or other recognized state or federal organizations or groups
- Identification indicating that the individual has been granted authority to render resident care, treatment, and services in disaster circumstances (such authority having been granted by a federal, state, or municipal entity)
- Identification by current organization member(s) who possesses personal knowledge regarding the volunteer practitioner's qualifications

A 6. Primary source verification of licensure, certification, or registration (if required by law and regulation to practice a profession) begins as soon as the immediate situation is under control, and is completed within 72 hours from the time the volunteer practitioner presents to the organization.

Note: *In the extraordinary circumstance that primary source verification of licensure, certification, or registration (if required by law and regulation to practice a profession) cannot be completed in 72 hours (for example, no means of communication or a lack of resources), it is expected that it be done as soon as possible. In this extraordinary circumstance, there must be documentation of the following: why primary source verification could not be performed in the required time frame; evidence of a demonstrated ability to continue to provide adequate care, treatment, and services; and an attempt to rectify the situation as soon as possible. Primary source verification of licensure, certification, or registration (if required by law and regulation to practice a profession) would not be required if the volunteer practitioner has not provided care, treatment, and services under the disaster responsibilities.*

A 7. The organization oversees the professional practice of volunteer practitioners.

A 8. The organization makes a decision (based on information obtained regarding the professional practice of the volunteer practitioner) within 72 hours related to the continuation of the disaster responsibilities initially assigned.

Introduction to Staffing Effectiveness

Staffing effectiveness is defined as the number, competency, and skill mix of staff in relation to the provision of needed care and treatment. Effective staffing has been

* **DMAT** A group of medical and support personnel designed to provide emergency medical care during a disaster or other unusual event. The DMAT is a component of the National Disaster Medical System (NDMS). The Department of Health and Human Services in partnership with other Federal Agencies such as Department of Defense, Department of Veterans Affairs, and the Federal Emergency Management Agency administer the program.

linked to positive resident outcomes and improved quality and safety of care. This standard is designed to help health care organizations determine and continuously improve the effectiveness of their nurse staffing (including registered nurses, licensed practical nurses, and nursing assistants or aides) through an objective, evidence-based approach. Other types of practitioners may be included if the organization chooses to do so. The described goal relies on the use of relevant clinical/service outcome and human resource screening indicators to monitor for, identify, and trigger nursing-related improvement opportunities in the provision of resident care. In its simplest conception, the standard reflects the application of continuous quality improvement methods to the performance of staffing effectiveness.

This staffing standard requires health care organizations to collect data on relevant human resource and clinical/service screening indicators for a minimum of two populations/settings,* determine the desired performance for each indicator, trend the data over time, and analyze variation from desired performance. It may be appropriate to rotate the populations/settings being monitored over time, after sufficient data have been reviewed to conclude that care on these units is stable. The use of multiple indicators increases the likelihood that existing problems will be identified and appropriately characterized. The use of nursing-sensitive measures makes it likely that problems identified will be staffing-related. However, this will not be universally true—the types of root causes may be identified and will need to be addressed.

Many organizations will find that they are already collecting the types of data contemplated by this standard. Since indicators selected are organization specific and part of internal performance improvement activities and are not designed for comparison with other health care organizations, it may be appropriate to rotate indicator selection, after sufficient data have been reviewed to conclude that performance is stable and acceptable.

Methods of data collection and tools for data analysis do not need to be sophisticated, and may vary based on the availability of resources. Simple control charts or other graphics to display data may be sufficient.

The purpose of collecting data for these indicators is to screen for possible nurse staffing issues and then to analyze underlying causes when the data do not meet performance expectations. Identification of statistical correlations among measure results is not required; however, identified relationships among results may provide clues to underlying causes.

The data for each screening indicator are analyzed to identify any variations from desired performance by individual measure. Variations in performance trigger further analysis to determine the causes of the variation and whether staffing effectiveness issues might be affecting outcomes of care. When variation from desired performance is detected in one indicator, other indicator results are reviewed to identify information that may assist in clarifying the potential cause of variation.

* **Populations/settings** refers to level in which staffing is planned and is provided within the organization. For example, staffing may be provided for individual populations or settings or may be planned for a group of settings or populations.

The organization drills down to determine the cause(s) of variation when data varies from what is expected; the organization then undertakes steps leading to appropriate actions that are likely to remedy identified problems. For example, analysis of the data may indicate the need for evaluation of the organization's staffing practices. If so, the organization takes specific actions to improve its performance. Examples of strategies that may be used to address identified staffing issues include the following:

- Staff recruitment
- Education/training
- Service curtailment
- Increased technology support
- Reorganization of work flow
- Provision of additional ancillary or support staff
- Adjustment of skill mix

Standard HR.1.30

The organization uses data from clinical/service screening indicators and human resource screening indicators to assess and continuously improve staffing effectiveness.

Rationale for HR.1.30

Significant changes in nurse staffing level and the skill mix of nursing personnel in health care organizations raise questions about potential adverse effects on the quality and safety of resident care related to staffing effectiveness. The Joint Commission has developed a comprehensive approach to the management of staffing effectiveness that looks at staffing as more than just "numbers." The approach relies on data driven quality improvement principles and is objective and methodologically sound. Since the causes and consequences of diminished staffing effectiveness differ from organization to organization, the approach allows flexibility to reflect characteristics unique to individual heath care settings.

Elements of Performance for HR.1.30

A 1. The organization identifies no fewer than two inpatient populations/settings for which data on staffing effectiveness are to be collected.

Note: *If the organization has only one population/setting, the organization may collect data for that single population/setting.*

A 2. The organization identifies the populations/settings (no less than two) based on assessment of relevant information or risk, including the following:

- Knowledge about staffing issues likely to impact resident safety or quality of care
- Resident population served
- Type of setting
- Review of existing data (e.g., incident logs, sentinel event data, performance improvement reports)
- Input from clinical staff who provide resident care

Note: *If the organization has only one population/setting, the organization need not apply these criteria.*

A 3. A minimum set of four indicators are selected for each of the identified inpatient populations/settings.

Note: *Organizations are free to choose the same set, the same set in part or completely different measure sets for each identified population/setting.*

A 4. The organization determines the indicators for each population/setting based on assessment of relevant information or risk, including the following:

- Knowledge about staffing issues likely to impact resident safety or quality of care
- Resident population served
- Type of setting
- Review of existing data (e.g., incident logs, sentinel event data, performance improvement reports)
- Input from clinical staff who provide resident care

A 5. Of the four indicators required for each population/setting, two must be clinical/service indicators and two must be human resource indicators.

A 6. One of the human resource indicators and one of the clinical/service indicators must be selected from The Joint Commission's list of approved indicators.*

Note: *Additional indicators may be selected from among the organization's own indicators.*

A 7. The human resource indicators for all identified populations/settings include all nursing staff (including registered nurses, licensed practical nurses, and nursing assistants or aides)

Note: *Decisions regarding stratification of data by discipline are left to the organization.*

A 8. When the organization chooses to include other practitioner groups (in addition to nursing staff in the human resource indicators for the identified populations/settings, this decision is based on the impact the absence of such care/service providers would be expected to have on resident outcomes.

A 9. The organization does the following:

- Defines the numerator and denominator for indicators chosen
- Standardizes the data element definitions for each indicator, including those indicators applied in more than one setting
- Determines acceptable ranges/parameters/trigger levels† for the indicators

---

* The Joint Commission's list of approved screening indicators consists of National Quality Forum (NQF)–endorsed voluntary consensus standards for nursing home care and Joint Commission consensus measures.

† Acceptable ranges/parameters/trigger levels may be reflective of past performance, expert opinion, expert literature, or a combination of these. The ranges/parameters/trigger levels should be reasonable goals that are possible to attain. When desired ranges/parameters/trigger levels are not met, an investigation into the cause(s) is needed.

A 10. The organization does the following for each populations/settings selected:
- Collects data for all indicators
- Analyzes data for all indicators
- Reviews all indicator data together when analyzing variation from desired performance for additional information that may assist in identifying any potential causes of variation
- Investigates to identify any staffing effectiveness issues when indicator data varies from expected
- Takes appropriate action in response to analyzed data

A 11. The organization reports at least annually to the leaders on the results of data analyses related to staffing effectiveness (*see* PI.1.10 and PI.2.20) and any actions taken to resolve identified problems.

List of Joint Commission Approved Subjects for Screening Indicators for Long Term Care

1. Prevalence of pressure ulcers (Clinical/Service)
2. Resident satisfaction (Clinical/Service)
3. Family satisfaction (Clinical/Service)
4. Prevalence of falls (Clinical/Service)
5. Resident complaints (Clinical/Service)
6. Injuries to residents (Clinical/Service)
7. Family complaints (Clinical/Service)
8. Restraint use (Clinical/Service)
9. Prevalence of unintended weight loss (Clinical/Service)
10. Elopements/wandering of residents (Clinical/Service)
11. Adverse drug events (Clinical/Service)
12. Prevalence of dehydration (Clinical/Service)
13. Pain assessment and management (that is, wait time to receive medications) (Clinical/Service)
14. Urinary tract infection rate (Clinical/Service)
15. Change in resident functioning (Clinical/Service)
16. Prevalence of malnutrition (Clinical/Service)
17. Activities of daily living (ADL) met or unmet (Clinical/Service)
18. Prevalence of urinary catheter use (Clinical/Service)
19. Average time in activities (Clinical/Service)
20. Antibiotic use (Clinical/Service)
21. Unexpected hospital admissions or emergency department visits (Clinical/Service)
22. Prevalence of untreated depression (Clinical/Service)
23. Prevalence of more than eight prescribed medications (Clinical/Service)
24. Pneumonia rate (Clinical/Service)
25. Unnecessary antipsychotic medication usage (Clinical/Service)

Chronic Care Measures

26. Residents whose need for more help with daily activities has increased (Clinical/Service) (National Quality Forum Measure)
27. Residents who lost too much weight (Clinical/Service) (National Quality Forum Measure)

28. Residents who experience moderate to severe pain during the seven-day assessment period (Clinical/Service) (National Quality Forum Measure)
29. Residents who were physically restrained during the seven-day assessment period (Clinical/Service) (National Quality Forum Measure)
30. Residents who spent most of their time in bed or in a chair in their room during the seven-day assessment period (Clinical/Service) (National Quality Forum Measure)
31. Residents with a decline in their ability to move about in their room or the adjacent corridor (Clinical/Service) (National Quality Forum Measure)
32. Residents with a urinary tract infection (Clinical/Service) (National Quality Forum Measure)
33. Residents with worsening of a depressed or anxious mood (Clinical/Service) (National Quality Forum Measure)

Chronic Care Measure Pairs

34. High-risk residents with pressure ulcers AND average-risk residents with pressure ulcers (Clinical/Service) (National Quality Forum Measure)
35. Residents who frequently lose control of the bowel or bladder (low-risk) AND residents who have a catheter in the bladder at any time during the 14-day assessment period (Clinical/Service) (National Quality Forum Measure)

Post-Acute Care Measures

36. Recently hospitalized residents with symptoms of delirium (Clinical/Service) (National Quality Forum Measure)
37. Recently hospitalized residents who experienced moderate to severe pain at any time during the seven-day assessment period (Clinical/Service) (National Quality Forum Measure)
38. Recently hospitalized residents with pressure ulcers (Clinical/Service) (National Quality Forum Measure)

Measures for All Nursing Home Residents

39. Pneumococcal polysaccharide vaccination of residents age 65 or older (Clinical/Service) (National Quality Forum Measure)
40. Influenza vaccination for all nursing home residents (Clinical/Service) (National Quality Forum Measure)
41. Staff vacancy rate (Human Resource)
42. Staff turnover rate (Human Resource)
43. Staff satisfaction (Human Resource)
44. Use of overtime (Human Resource)
45. Staff injury rate (Human Resource)
46. Nursing hours per resident day (registered nurse, licensed practical nurse, certified nursing assistant) compared to baseline such as actual versus planned or budgeted (Human Resource)
47. Staff training hours (Human Resource)
48. Agency usage/contract staff (Human Resource)
49. Understaffing as compared to organization's staffing plan (Human Resource)
50. Use of sick time (Human Resource)
51. Activity staff hours per resident day (Human Resource)

52. Number of dietary staff hours per resident day (Human Resource)
53. Number of housekeeping staff hours per resident day (Human Resource)
54. Average response time for consultation order (Human Resource)
55. Nurse staffing hours (Human Resource) (National Quality Forum Measure)

Note: *Additional information on nursing home care measures can be found at http://www.qualityforum.org.*

Orientation, Training, and Education

Standard HR.2.10

The organization provides initial orientation.

Rationale for HR.2.10

Orientation is a process in which initial job training and information is provided to staff and licensed independent practitioners. Staff and licensed independent practitioner orientation promotes safe and effective job performance. Some elements of orientation need to occur before staff and licensed independent practitioners provide care, treatment, and services. Other elements of orientation can occur when staff and licensed independent practitioners are providing care, treatment, and services.

Elements of Performance for HR.2.10

A 1. The organization determines what key elements of orientation should occur before staff and licensed independent practitioners provide care, treatment, and services.

C Ⓜ 2. The organization orients staff and licensed independent practitioners to the identified key elements prior to the provision of care, treatment, and services.

As appropriate, staff and licensed independent practitioner orientation addresses the following (EPs 3–7):

C Ⓜ 3. The organization's mission and goals

C Ⓜ 4. Organizationwide policies and procedures (including safety and infection control) and relevant unit, setting, or program-specific policies and procedures

C Ⓜ 5. Specific job duties and responsibilities and service, setting, or program-specific job duties and responsibilities related to safety and infection control

6. Not applicable

C Ⓜ 7. Cultural diversity and sensitivity

C Ⓜ 8. Staff orientation includes education about the rights of residents and ethical aspects of care, treatment, and services and the process used to address ethical issues.

C Ⓜ 9. Staff orientation includes education about the effects of psychotropic medications as appropriate.

Standard HR.2.20

Staff and licensed independent practitioners, as appropriate, can describe or demonstrate their roles and responsibilities relative to safety.

Rationale for HR.2.20

The human element is the most critical factor in any process, determining whether the right things are done correctly. The best policies and procedures for minimizing risks in the environment where care, treatment, and services are provided are meaningless if staff and licensed independent practitioners, if applicable, do not know and understand them well enough to perform them properly.

It is important that everyday precautions identified by the health care organization for minimizing various risks, including those related to resident safety and environmental safety,* are properly implemented. It is also important that the appropriate emergency procedures be instituted should an incident or failure occur in the environment.

Elements of Performance for HR.2.20

Staff and licensed independent practitioners, as appropriate, can describe or demonstrate the following (EPs 1–4):

C Ⓜ 1. Risks within the organization's environment

C Ⓜ 2. Actions to eliminate, minimize, or report risks

C Ⓜ 3. Procedures to follow in the event of an incident

C Ⓜ 4. Reporting processes for common problems, failures, and user errors

Standard HR.2.30

Ongoing education, including in-services, training, and other activities, maintains and improves staff competence.

Elements of Performance for HR.2.30

A 1. Staff training occurs when job responsibilities or duties change.

C Ⓜ 2. Staff participate in ongoing in-services, training, or other activities to increase knowledge of work-related issues.

* The "Management of the Environment of Care" chapter of this book identifies risks associated with the following categories: safety, security, hazardous materials and wastes, emergency management, medical equipment, and utility management.

C Ⓜ 3. Ongoing in-services and other education and training of staff are appropriate to the needs of the population(s) served and comply with law and regulation.

C Ⓜ 4. Ongoing in-services, training, or other staff activities emphasize specific job-related aspects of safety and infection prevention and control.

C Ⓜ 5. Ongoing in-services, training, or other staff education incorporate methods of team training, when appropriate.

C Ⓜ 6. Ongoing in-services, training, or other staff education reinforce the need and ways to report unanticipated adverse events.

C Ⓜ 7. Ongoing in-services or other staff education are offered in response to learning needs identified through performance improvement findings and other data analysis (that is, data from staff surveys, performance evaluations, or other needs assessments).

C Ⓜ 8. Ongoing staff education is documented.

9. Not applicable

A 10. Staff are educated, as appropriate to their responsibilities, about psychotropic medications including the following:
- The need for a medication in relation to the resident's documented diagnosis and condition
- The potential for drug–drug and drug–food interactions
- Adverse reactions to psychotropic medications
- The use of a medication for an appropriate duration
- The optimal dose
- Frequent monitoring of the medication's effectiveness
- Nonmedication interventions and alternatives developed through interdisciplinary team assessment
- Reduction and discontinuation of a medication

Assessing Competence

Standard HR.3.10

Staff competence to perform job responsibilities is assessed, demonstrated, and maintained.

Rationale for HR.3.10

Competence assessment is systematic and allows for a measurable assessment of the person's ability to perform required activities. Information used as part of competence assessment may include data from performance evaluations, performance improvement, and aggregate data on competence, as well as the assessment of learning needs.

Elements of Performance for HR.3.10

The competence assessment process for staff is based on the following (EPs 1–7):

A 1. The population(s) served

A 2. The defined competencies to be required

A 3. The defined competencies to be assessed during orientation

A 4. Defined competencies that need to be assessed and reassessed on an ongoing basis, based on techniques, procedures, technology, equipment, or skills needed to provide care, treatment, and services

A 5. A defined time frame for how often competence assessments are performed for each person, minimally, once in the three-year accreditation cycle and in accordance with law and regulation

A 6. The assessment methods (appropriate to determine the skill being assessed)

A 7. The use of qualified individuals to assess competence

Note: *When there is no qualified individual in the organization that performs comparable care, treatment, and services, the organization may:*

- *Utilize qualified staff from other organizations to assist with the assessment of competence*

  or
- *Consult the appropriate professional organization guidelines with respect to expectations for competence and use these guidelines to assess competence*

C Ⓜ 8. The organization assesses and documents staff's ability to carry out assigned responsibilities safely, competently, and in a timely manner upon completion of orientation.

C Ⓜ 9. The organization assesses staff according to its competence assessment process.

A 10. When improvement activities lead to a determination that a person with performance problems is unable or unwilling to improve, the organization takes appropriate action (which may include modifying the person's job assignment).

Standard HR.3.20

The organization periodically conducts performance evaluations.

Rationale for HR.3.20

Performance is evaluated as an ongoing process for providing positive and negative feedback to staff. Formal performance evaluations can be conducted concurrently with competence assessments or can be completed at a separate time.

Elements of Performance for HR.3.20

C Ⓜ 1. The organization conducts performance evaluations periodically at time frames identified by the organization (at a minimum, at least once in the three-year accreditation cycle).

C Ⓜ 2. Performance is evaluated based on the performance expectations described in job descriptions or through the privileging process.

3. Not applicable

C Ⓜ 4. Performance evaluations are documented.

Standards HR.3.25 Through HR.3.60

Not applicable

Credentialing and Privileging of Licensed Independent Practitioners

Introduction

Credentialing

Credentialing involves the collection, verification, and assessment of information regarding four critical parameters: current licensure, relevant training, current competence, and the ability to perform the clinical privileges requested.

The verification of current licensure informs the organization that the individual is appropriately licensed to practice as required by state and/or federal law. The license verification process is conducted prior to initial granting of clinical privileges, at the time of renewal of clinical privileges, and at the time of expiration of the license.

The verification of relevant training informs the organization of the licensed independent practitioner's clinical knowledge and skill set. Verification must be obtained from the original primary source of the specific credential. Primary sources include the specialty certifying boards approved by the American Dental Association for a dentist's board certification, letters from professional schools (for example, medical and dental) and from residency or postdoctoral programs for completion of training. When it is not possible to obtain information from the primary source, reliable secondary sources* may be used.

Designated equivalent sources may be used to verify certain credentials in lieu of using the primary source. *See* the Glossary for the list of designated equivalent sources.

Current competence in performing clinical privileges is verified by peers knowledgeable about the applicant's professional performance.

---

* A reliable secondary source can be another health care organization that has documented primary source verification of the applicant's credentials.

Privileging

The following principles summarize key concepts as they relate to privileging:

1. The organization administrator may substitute for the governing body
2. An organized medical staff and bylaws are not required
3. The medical director is comparable to the Medical Executive Committee (MEC) in settings where no organized medical staff exists
4. In organizations without an organized medical staff, procedures for appointment, reappointment, and granting, renewal, or revision of clinical privileges are established by the medical director and approved by the governing body
5. Privileges may be delineated by category and should address cognitive and technical skills
6. Each organization defines its scope of care in such a way that practitioners can request privileges consistent with the scope of care
7. In hospital-based long term care units, the long term care medical director reviews the credentials file and makes recommendations to the appropriate group or individual
8. The organization's general credentialing process can be applied to determine credentials, but the privileges granted must be program- and category-specific

Standard HR.4.10

There is a process for ensuring the competence of all practitioners permitted by law and the organization to practice independently.

Elements of Performance for HR.4.10

1. Through 4. Not applicable

A 5. The organization has a defined process approved by the leaders for appointing and reappointing licensed independent practitioners. A

A 6. At the time of initial granting of privileges, the organization verifies, by viewing a valid government-issued photo identification issued by a state or federal agency (e.g., drivers license or passport), that the individual being granted (clinical privileges) is the same individual identified in the credentialing documents.

Note: *Any licensed independent practitioner whose only role is to cover for another licensed independent practitioner(s) is exempt from this requirement.*

A 7. The credentialing process requires that the organization does the following:

- Verifies in writing current licensure, from the primary source at time of initial granting , renewal and revision of clinical privileges, and prior to licensure expiration
- Verifies in writing training (required by the organization to perform the clinical privileges) from the primary source at the time of initial granting and renewal and revision of clinical privileges
- Verifies in writing current competence from the primary source at time of initial granting of clinical privileges

- Obtains a statement from the applicant at the time of initial granting, renewal, or revision of clinical privileges that no health problems exist that could effect his or her ability to perform the privileges requested.*

Note 1: *Verification of current licensure with the primary source through a secure electronic communication or by telephone is acceptable, if this verification is documented. For additional information,* see *"primary source verification" in the Glossary.*

Note 2: *An external organization (for example, a credentials verification organization [CVO] or a Joint Commission–accredited health care organization functioning as a CVO) may be used to collect credentialing information. Both of these organizations must meet the CVO guidelines listed in the Glossary section of the accreditation manual.*

Note 3: *A primary source of verified information may designate to an agency the role of communicating credentials information. The delegated agency then becomes acceptable to be used as a primary source.*

A 8. All licensed independent practitioners that provide resident care possess a license, certification, or registration as required by law and regulation.

9. and 10. Not applicable

A 11. The governing body† does the following:
- Reviews recommendations made by the medical director
- Reviews documentation on which recommendations are based
- Reviews records of any hearings or appeals addressing adverse decisions
- Grants appropriate clinical privileges.

12. through 21. Not applicable.

When the attending licensed independent practitioner designates a licensed independent practitioner (who is not privileged in the organization) to cover in his/her absence for a period of no more than 72 consecutive hours, the following requirements are met (EPs 22–25):

A 22. The medical director and the attending licensed independent practitioner determine that the covering licensed independent practitioner can perform those types of care, treatment, and services that are required

A 23. The organization verifies the current licensure of the covering licensed independent practitioner from the primary source prior to his or her provision of care, treatment and services

Note: *It may be more efficient to obtain a list of possible covering licensed independent practitioners ahead of time and verify licensure from the pri-*

---

* Organizations should consider the applicability of the Americans with Disabilities Act (ADA) to their credentialing and privileging activities, and, if applicable, review their policies and procedures. Federal entities are required to comply with the Rehabilitation Act of 1974.

† The organization administrator or a committee of two or more governing body members may substitute for a governing body.

mary source in advance of the licensed independent practitioner actually covering for the attending.

C Ⓜ 24. A documented review of orders issued by the covering licensed independent practitioner is conducted by the attending licensed independent practitioner upon return in the time frame defined by the organization

A 25. The modified process for credentialing and privileging can only be utilized for a covering licensed independent practitioner for up to 12 days* per calendar year but no more than 72 consecutive hours

Note: *If a licensed independent practitioner will be covering for more than 12 days per calendar year or more than 72 consecutive hours, this individual must undergo the full process for credentialing and privileging by the organization.*

Standard HR.4.20

Individuals permitted by law and the organization to practice independently are granted clinical privileges.

Elements of Performance for HR.4.20

A 1. Based on the scope of services provided, the organization establishes criteria for each privilege. These criteria include the following:
- Current licensure and/or certification as appropriate, verified with the primary source
- Successful completion of training specific to each requested privilege, verified with the primary source
- Peer† and or faculty recommendation
- Evidence of the ability to perform the requested privilege

A 2. Before granting, renewing, or revising privileges, the medical director evaluates the following:
- Challenges to any licensure or registration
- Voluntary and involuntary relinquishment of any license or registration
- Voluntary and involuntary termination of medical staff membership at another organization
- Voluntary and involuntary limitation, reduction, or loss of clinical privileges
- Any evidence of an unusual pattern or an excessive number of professional liability actions resulting in a final judgment against the applicant
- Documentation as to the applicant's health status

A 3. The organization queries the National Practitioner Data Bank (NPDB) at the time of initial granting of privileges, as well as at least every two years thereafter for information on physicians and dentists granted clinical privileges.

---

* A day is considered as any portion of the day (whether it is 1 hour or 24 hours).

† *See* Glossary for definition of peer recommendation.

C Ⓜ 4. Clinical privileges for licensed independent practitioners are delineated according to organization policy and based on the licensed independent practitioner's current credentials and competence, as well as the population(s) served and the types of care, treatment, and services provided in the organization.

A 5. The decision by leaders to appoint licensed independent practitioners is based on the credentials information obtained.

C Ⓜ 6. The licensed independent practitioner is notified in writing of the governing body's decision.

A 7. Individuals with clinical privileges practice within the scope of their privileges. ⚠3

Standard HR.4.30

The organization has a process for granting temporary clinical privileges, when appropriate.

Rationale for HR.4.30

There are two circumstances in which temporary clinical privileges may be granted. Each circumstance has different criteria for granting clinical privileges. The two circumstances are to meet the important needs of residents and for new applicants.

Elements of Performance for HR.4.30

A 1. Policies and procedures, rules, or regulations describe the process for granting temporary privileges for meeting the important needs of residents or for new applicants.

A 2. To grant temporary privileges to meet the important needs of residents, there must be verification (which can be done by telephone) of current licensure and current competence.

A 3. To grant temporary privileges for new applicants, there must be verification (which may be done by telephone) of the following:
- Current licensure
- Relevant education, training, or experience
- Current competence
- Ability to perform the privileges requested
- A query and evaluation of the NPDB for physicians or dentists

A 4. To grant temporary privileges for new applicants, the applicant has the following:
- A complete application
- No current or previously successful challenge to licensure or registration
- Not been subject to involuntary termination of professional or medical staff membership at another organization, when applicable to the discipline

- Not been subject to involuntary limitation, reduction, denial, or loss of privileges, when applicable to the discipline

A 5. The administrator or designee grants temporary privileges for meeting important resident needs and for new applicants upon recommendation of clinical leadership or the medical director.

A 6. Temporary privileges for new applicants are granted for no more than 120 days.

Standard HR 4.32

Not applicable

Standard HR 4.33

Not applicable

Standard HR 4.34

Not applicable

Disaster Privileges

Standard HR.4.35

The organization may grant disaster privileges to volunteers eligible to be licensed independent practitioners.

Rationale for HR.4.35

When the disaster plan has been implemented (*see* standard EC.4.10 for a description of emergency management planning requirements) and the immediate needs of the residents cannot be met, the organization may implement a modified credentialing and privileging process for eligible volunteer practitioners (*see* EPs 5–8). The usual process to credential and privilege practitioners would not allow a volunteer practitioner to provide immediate care, treatment, and services in the event of a disaster (refer to the Glossary for definitions of disaster and emergency) due to the length of time it would take to complete the process. A similar modified process for the assignment of disaster responsibilities for volunteers that are not independent practitioners exists at standard HR.1.25.

While this standard allows for a method to streamline the credentialing and privileging process, safeguards must be in place to assure that volunteer practitioners are competent to provide safe and adequate care, treatment, and services. Even in a disaster, the integrity of two parts of the usual credentialing and privileging process must be maintained:

1. Verification of licensure
2. Oversight of the care, treatment, and services provided

This option to grant disaster privileges to volunteer practitioners is made on a case-by-case basis in accordance with the needs of the organization and its residents, and on the qualifications of its volunteer practitioners.

There are a number of state and federal systems engaged in pre-event credentialing that may facilitate the implementation of disaster privileging of volunteers at the time of a disaster. Examples of such systems include the Medical Reserve Corps (MRC*) and the Emergency System for Advance Registration of Volunteer Health Professionals (ESAR-VHP†). It is expected that additional programs will emerge and evolve.

Elements of Performance for HR.4.35

A 1. Disaster privileges are granted only when the following two conditions are present: the emergency management plan has been activated, and the organization is unable to meet immediate resident needs.

A 2. The organization identifies in writing the individual(s) responsible for granting disaster privileges.

A 3. The organization describes in writing a mechanism (for example, direct observation, mentoring, and clinical record review) to oversee the professional performance of volunteer practitioners who receive disaster privileges.

A 4. The organization has a mechanism to identify the volunteer practitioners who have been granted disaster privileges.

A 5. In order for volunteers to be considered eligible to act as licensed independent practitioners, the organization obtains for each volunteer practitioner at a minimum, a valid government-issued photo identification issued by a state or federal agency (e.g., driver's license or passport) and at least one of the following:
- A current health care organization (such as a long term care, ambulatory care, or hospital) picture identification card that clearly identifies professional designation
- A current license to practice
- Primary source verification of the license

* **MRC** Medical Reserve Corps units comprised of locally-based medical and public health volunteers who can assist their communities during emergencies, such as an influenza epidemic, a chemical spill, or an act of terrorism. The MRC Program was formed in 2002, in cooperation with the White House's USA Freedom Corps, as one of the charter programs of Citizen Corps. Pre-identifying, training and organizing medical and public health professionals to strengthen their communities through volunteerism is at the core of the MRC concept. MRC volunteers offer their expertise throughout the year by supporting local public health initiatives, such as immunization and prevention activities. When an emergency community need occurs, MRC volunteers can work in coordination with existing local emergency response programs.

† **ESAR-VHP** The Emergency System for Advance Registration of Volunteer Health Professionals (ESAR-VHP) program, created by the Health Resources and Services Administration (HRSA), allows for the advance registration and credentialing of health care professionals needed to augment a hospital or other medical facility to meet increased patient/victim care and increased surge capacity needs.

- Identification indicating that the individual is a member of a Disaster Medical Assistance Team (DMAT*), or MRC, ESAR-VHP, or other recognized state or federal organizations or groups
- Identification indicating that the individual has been granted authority to render resident care, treatment, and services in disaster circumstances (such authority having been granted by a federal, state, or municipal entity)
- Identification by current organization member(s) who possesses personal knowledge regarding the volunteer's ability to act as a licensed independent practitioner during a disaster

A 6. Primary source verification of licensure begins as soon as the immediate situation is under control, and is completed within 72 hours from the time the volunteer practitioner presents to the organization.

Note: *In the extraordinary circumstance that primary source verification cannot be completed in 72 hours (e.g., no means of communication or a lack of resources), it is expected that it be done as soon as possible. In this extraordinary circumstance, there must be documentation of the following: why primary source verification could not be performed in the required time frame; evidence of a demonstrated ability to continue to provide adequate care, treatment, and services; and an attempt to rectify the situation as soon as possible. Primary source verification of licensure would not be required if the volunteer practitioner has not provided care, treatment, and services under the disaster privileges.*

A 7. The organization oversees the professional practice of volunteer licensed independent practitioners.

A 8. The organization makes a decision (based on information obtained regarding the professional practice of the volunteer) within 72 hours related to the continuation of the disaster privileges initially granted.

Standard HR.4.40

There are mechanisms, including a fair hearing and appeal process, for addressing adverse decisions regarding reappointment denial, reduction, suspension, or revocation of clinical privileges that may relate to quality of care, treatment, and service issues.

Rationale for HR.4.40

Mechanisms for fair hearing and appeals processes are designed to allow the affected individual a fair opportunity to defend herself or himself regarding the adverse deci-

* **DMAT** A group of medical and support personnel designed to provide emergency medical care during a disaster or other unusual event. The DMAT is a component of the National Disaster Medical System (NDMS). The Department of Health and Human Services in partnership with other Federal Agencies such as Department of Defense, Department of Veterans Affairs, and the Federal Emergency Management Agency administer the program.

sion to an unbiased hearing committee, and an opportunity to appeal the decision of the committee to the governance function. The purpose of a fair hearing and appeal is to assure full consideration and reconsideration of quality and safety issues and, under the current structure of reporting to the NPDB, to allow practitioners an opportunity to defend themselves.

Elements of Performance for HR.4.40

The organization has developed a fair hearing and appeals process that does the following (EPs 1–5):

A 1. Is designed to provide a uniform and fair process

A 2. Has a mechanism to schedule a hearing of such requests

A 3. Has identified the procedures for the hearings to follow

A 4. Identifies or defines the composition of the hearing committee

A 5. Provides for a mechanism to appeal an adverse decision through the governance function

Standard HR.4.50

Clinical privileges and appointments/reappointments are reviewed and revised at least every two years.

Elements of Performance for HR.4.50

A 1. Policies and procedures or rules and regulations specify a period of no more than two years between appointments and reappointments and between granting, renewing, and revising clinical privileges.

C Ⓜ 2. Credential files for licensed independent practitioners contain substantive information and indicate that clinical privileges are reviewed or revised at least every two years and are revised as needed; in addition, appointments and reappointments are made for a period of no more than two years.

A 3. A reappraisal is conducted at the time of reappointment or renewal or revision of clinical privileges.

A 4. The reappraisal addresses current competence and includes the following:
- Confirmation of adherence to organization policies and procedures, rules, or regulations
- Relevant information from organization performance improvement activities when evaluating professional performance, judgment, and clinical or technical skills
- Any results of review of the individual's clinical performance
- Clinical performance in the organization that is outside acceptable standards

A 5. Credentials files contain clear evidence that the full range of privileges has been included in the reappraisal.

Standards HR.4.60 Through HR. 5.40

Not applicable

2009

SLTC

Management of Information (IM)

Management of Information (IM)

Overview

The **goal** of the information management function is to support decision making to improve resident outcomes, improve health care documentation, improve resident safety, and improve performance in resident care, treatment, and services, governance, management, and support processes. While efficiency, effectiveness, resident safety, and the quality of resident care can be improved by computerization and other technologies, the principles of good information management apply to paper-based or electronic methods. The standards in this chapter are designed to be equally compatible with paper-based systems, electronic systems, or hybrid systems.

An organization's provision of care, treatment, and services is a complex endeavor that is highly dependent on information. Furthermore, when many individuals and areas throughout the organization are involved in the provision of care, treatment, and services, their work is coordinated and integrated. As a result, organizations treat information as an important resource to be managed effectively and efficiently. Managing information is an active, planned activity. The organization's leaders have overall responsibility for managing information, just as they do for managing the organization's human, material, and financial resources.

The quality of care, treatment, and services is affected by the many transitions in information management that are currently in progress in health care, such as the transition from handwriting and traditional paper-based documentation to electronic information management, as well as the transition from free text* to structured† and interactive text.‡

---

* **Free text** Free-flowing, nonstructured type of speaking, writing, or inputting of information.

† **Structured text** Process that requires authors to put specific information into specific fields with passive guidance by the information system. In paper-based systems, a form encourages a practitioner to fill in fields or boxes. Electronic systems use the same principle for templates or macros, which are guides used to create standardized information documentation. The purpose is to produce data of more consistent quality, make information more usable for decision support, make information more complete and more easily retrievable, and save documentation time.

‡ **Interactive text** A more complex version of structured text, as it interactively prompts and provides feedback to the person using it. Typically, it uses a higher level of computer intelligence that interacts with the person who records information.

Key: 0 = Insufficient compliance; 1 = Partial compliance; 2 = Satisfactory compliance; NA = Not applicable; **A** indicates scoring category A; **C** indicates scoring category C; ▲(2) indicates situational decision rules apply; △(3) indicates direct impact requirements apply; Ⓜ indicates Measure of success is needed

To achieve the goals of this function, the following processes are performed:

- Identifying information needs
- Designing the structure of the information management system
- Capturing,* organizing, storing, retrieving, processing,† and analyzing‡ data and information
- Transmitting,§ reporting, displaying, integrating, and using data and information
- Safeguarding data‖ and information

The standards in this chapter focus on organizationwide information planning and management processes to meet the organization's internal and external information needs. The standards describe a vision for effectively and continuously improving information management in health care organizations. Achieving this vision involves the following:

- Providing for timely and easy access to complete information throughout the organization
- Providing for data accuracy
- Balancing requirements of security# and ease of access
- Producing and using aggregate data to pursue opportunities for improvement
- Providing for data comparability within and among organizations, where possible, by following national, state, and other recognized standards and guidelines on form and content
- Accessing and using external knowledge bases and comparative data to pursue opportunities for improvement
- Redesigning information-related processes to improve efficiency and effectiveness, as well as resident safety and quality of resident care, treatment and services
- Increasing collaboration and information sharing to enhance resident care

---

* **Capturing** The process of recording representations of human thought, perceptions, or actions, as well as device-generated data or information that is gathered and/or computed about a resident as part of a health care encounter or about other matters in an organization.

† **Processing** The process that manipulates data and information by editing and updating.

‡ **Analyzing** The process that interprets the data and transforms it into information.

§ **Transmitting** Sending data and information from one location to another.

‖ **Data** Uninterpreted observations or facts.

Security The protection of data from intentional or unintentional destruction, modification, or disclosure.

Standards

The following is a list of all standards for this chapter. They are presented here for your convenience without footnotes or other explanatory text. If you have a question about a term used here, please check the Glossary.

Note: *A revised standard numbering system is being used with the reformatted standards. This revised numbering system will allow for more flexibility to add standards while maintaining the current label for each standard.*

Information Management Planning

IM.1.10 The organization plans and designs information management processes to meet internal and external information needs.

Confidentiality and Security

IM.2.10 Information privacy and confidentiality are maintained.

IM.2.20 Information security, including data integrity, is maintained.

IM.2.30 Continuity of information is maintained.

Information Management Processes

IM.3.10 The organization has processes in place to effectively manage information, including the capturing, reporting, processing, storing, retrieving, disseminating, and displaying of clinical/service and nonclinical data and information.

Information-Based Decision Making

IM.4.10 The information management system provides information for use in decision making.

Knowledge-Based Information

IM.5.10 Knowledge-based information resources are readily available, current, and authoritative.

Resident-Specific Information

IM.6.10 The organization has a complete and accurate clinical record for residents assessed, cared for, treated, or served.

IM.6.20 Records contain resident-specific information, as appropriate, to the care, treatment, and services provided.

IM.6.30 Not applicable

IM.6.40 Not applicable

IM.6.50 Designated qualified staff accept and transcribe verbal or telephone orders from authorized individuals.

IM.6.60 The organization provides access to relevant information from a resident's record as needed for use in resident care, treatment, and services.

IM.6.70 Clinical record documentation includes the provision of and response to the activities program at least quarterly.

IM.6.80 Clinical record documentation includes the provision of and response to nutrition care services at least quarterly.

IM.6.90 Clinical record documentation includes the provision of and response to nursing care.

IM.6.100 Clinical record documentation includes the provision of and response to medical treatment and care.

IM.6.110 Clinical record documentation includes the provision of and response to rehabilitation services.

IM.6.120 Clinical record documentation includes the provision of and response to social service interventions.

IM.6.130 Clinical record documentation includes the provision of education and its effectiveness.

IM.6.140 Clinical record documentation includes significant changes in the resident's condition, care, and treatment.

IM.6.150 Treatment provided to the resident by off-site sources is documented in the clinical record.

IM.6.160 Effects of medications on residents, and associated pharmacist evaluation and physician consultation, are documented.

IM.6.170 Discharge information provided to the resident or to the family, as appropriate and permissible, and/or to the receiving organization is documented.

IM.6.180 Through IM.6.280 Not applicable

Standards, Rationales, Elements of Performance, and Scoring

Information Management Planning

Standard IM.1.10

The organization plans and designs information management processes to meet internal and external information needs.

Rationale for IM.1.10

Organizations vary in size, complexity, governance, structure, decision-making processes, and resources. Information management systems and processes vary accordingly. Only by first identifying the information needs can one then evaluate the extent to which they are planned for, and at what performance level the needs are being met. Planning for the management of information does not require a formal written information plan, but does require evidence of a planned approach that identifies the organization's information needs and supports its goals and objectives.

Elements of Performance for IM.1.10

A 1. The organization bases its information management processes on an assessment of internal and external information needs:
- The assessment identifies the flow of information throughout an organization, including information storage and feedback mechanisms.
- The assessment identifies the data and information needed: within and among departments, services, or programs; within and among the staff, the administration, and the governance for supporting relationships with outside services and contractors; with licensing, accrediting, and regulatory bodies; with purchasers, payers, and employers; for supporting informational needs between the organization and the residents; and for participating in research and databases.

A 2. To guide development of processes for managing information used internally and externally, the organization assesses its information management needs based on the following:
- Its mission
- Its goals
- Its services
- Staff
- Resident safety considerations
- Quality of care, treatment, and services
- Mode(s) of service delivery
- Resources

- Access to affordable technology
- Identification of barriers to effective communication among caregivers

A 3. The organization bases its management, staffing, and material resource allocations for information management on the scope and complexity of care, treatment, and services provided.

A 4. Identified staff participates in assessment, selection, integration, and use of information management systems for clinical/service and organization information.

A 5. The organization has an ongoing process to assess the needs of the organization, departments, and individuals for knowledge-based information.

A 6. The organization uses the assessment for knowledge-based information as a basis for planning.

Confidentiality and Security

Standard IM.2.10

Information privacy and confidentiality are maintained.

Rationale for IM.2.10

Confidentiality of data and information applies across all systems and to automated, paper, and verbal communications, as well as to clinical/service, financial, and business records and employee-specific information. The capture, storage, and retrieval processes for data and information are performed on a timely* basis without compromising the data and information's confidentiality. Protecting privacy and confidentiality of information is the responsibility of the whole organization. In achieving this responsibility, the organization provides safeguards for resident privacy and information confidentiality. These safeguards are consistent with available technology and legitimate needs for accessibility of the information by authorized individuals for the delivery of care, treatment, and services, effective functioning of the organization, research, and education.

Elements of Performance for IM.2.10

A 1. The organization has a written policy(ies) for addressing the privacy† and confidentiality‡ of information, that is based on and consistent with law or regulation.

---

* Defined by organization policy and based on the intended use of the information.

† **Privacy** An individual's right to limit the disclosure of personal information.

‡ **Confidentiality** The safekeeping of data/information so as to restrict access to individuals who have need, reason, and permission for such access.

A 2. The organization's policy, including changes to the policy, has been communicated to staff.

A 3. The organization implements the policy.

A 4. The organization monitors compliance with the policy.

A 5. The organization improves privacy and confidentiality of information by monitoring information and developments in technology.

C Ⓜ 6. Individuals for whom identifiable health data and information are maintained or collected are made aware of how the data will be used and whether it will be disclosed.

A 7. Personal identifiers are removed to the extent possible for uses and disclosures of health information, consistent with maintaining the usefulness of the information.

C Ⓜ 8. Protected health information* is used for the purposes identified or as required by law or regulation and not further disclosed without resident authorization.

A 9. The organization preserves the privacy and confidentiality of data and information identified as sensitive.

Standard IM.2.20

Information security, including data integrity, is maintained.

Rationale for IM.2.20

Policies and procedures address security procedures that allow only authorized staff to gain access to data and information. These policies range from access to the paper chart to the various security levels and distribution of passwords in an electronic system. The basic premise of the policies is to provide the security and protection for sensitive resident, staff, and other information, while facilitating access to data by those who have a legitimate need. The capture, storage, and retrieval processes for data and information are designed to provide for timely access without compromising the data and information's security and integrity.

Elements of Performance for IM.2.20

A 1. The organization has a written policy(ies) for addressing information security, including data integrity† that is based on and consistent with law or regulation.

A 2. The organization's policy, including changes to the policy, has been communicated to staff.

---

* **Protected health information** Health information that contains information such that an individual person can be identified as the subject of that information.

† **Integrity** In the context of data security, data integrity means the protection of data from accidental or unauthorized intentional change.

A 3. The organization implements the policy.

A 4. The organization monitors compliance with the policy.

A 5. The organization improves information security, including data integrity, by monitoring information and developments in technology.

A 6. The organization develops and implements controls to safeguard data and information, including the clinical record, against loss, destruction, and tampering.

A 7. Controls to safeguard data and information include the following:
- Policies indicating when the removal of records is permitted
- Protection against unauthorized intrusion, corruption, or damage
- Minimization of the risk of falsification of data and information
- Guidelines for preventing the loss and destruction of records
- Guidelines for destroying copies of records
- Protection of records in a manner that minimizes the possibility of damage from fire and water

A 8. Policies and procedures, including plans for implementation, for electronic information systems address the following: data integrity, authentication,* nonrepudiation,† encryption‡ as warranted, and auditability,§ as appropriate to the system and types of information, for example, resident information and billing information.

Standard IM.2.30

Continuity of information is maintained.

Rationale for IM.2.30

The purpose of the business continuity/disaster recovery plan is to identify the most critical information needs for resident care, treatment, and services and business processes, and the impact on the organization if these information systems were severely interrupted. The plan identifies alternative means for processing data, providing for recovery of data, and returning to normal operations as soon as possible.

Elements of Performance for IM.2.30

A 1. The organization has a business continuity/disaster recovery plan for its information systems.

---

* **Authentication** The validation of correctness for both the information itself and the person who is the author or user of information.

† **Nonrepudiation** The inability to dispute a document's content or authorship.

‡ **Encryption** The process of transforming plain text (readable) into cipher text that is unreadable without a special software key.

§ **Auditability** The ability to do a methodical examination and verification of all information activities such as entering and accessing.

A 2. For electronic systems, the business continuity/disaster recovery plan includes the following:
- Plans for scheduled and unscheduled interruptions, which includes end-user training with the downtime procedures
- Contingency plans for operational interruptions (hardware, software, or other systems failure)
- Plans for minimal interruptions as a result of scheduled downtime
- An emergency service plan
- A back-up system (electronic or manual)
- Data retrieval, including retrieval from storage and information presently in the operating system, retrieval of data in the event of system interruption, and back up of data

A 3. The plan is tested periodically, as defined by the organization (or in accordance with law or regulation) to ensure that the business interruption back-up techniques are effective.

A 4. The business continuity/disaster recovery plan is implemented when information systems are interrupted.

Introduction to Managing Information for Clinical/Service and Organization Decision Making

An organization's ability to make decisions depends on having ready access to reliable and accurate information. To support the decision-making process, the organization captures, processes, stores, and retrieves the needed information. It then supplies the information to management and others involved in the decision-making process.

Standards IM.3.10 and IM.4.10 address the procedures involved in information management in support of clinical/service and organization decision making. These procedures are critical to resident care and safety and the organization's efficient management. The procedures also apply in paper-based, electronic, or a hybrid information management environment.

The standards are relevant to organizations transitioning from a paper-based environment to an electronic environment. The first standard addresses the tasks of collecting, processing, storing, retrieving, reporting, and disseminating data and information. The second standard addresses the use of the information.

Information Management Processes

Standard IM.3.10

The organization has processes in place to effectively manage information, including the capturing, reporting, processing, storing, retrieving, disseminating, and displaying of clinical/service and nonclinical data and information.

Rationale for IM.3.10

Records resulting from data capture and report generation* are used for communication and continuity of the resident's care or financial and business operations over time. Records are also used for other purposes, including litigation and risk management activities, reimbursement, and statistics. Improved data capture and report generation systems enhance the value of the records. Potential benefits include improved resident care, quality and safety, improved efficiency, effectiveness and reduced costs in resident care, and financial and business operations. To maximize the benefits of data capture and report generation, these processes exhibit the following characteristics: unique ID, accuracy, completeness, timeliness,† interoperability,‡ retrievability,§ authentication and accountability,|| auditability, confidentiality, and security.

The processing, storing, and retrieving functions are integral to electronic, computerized, and paper-based information systems in organizations. Important considerations for these functions include data elements, data accuracy, data confidentiality, data security, data integrity, permanence of storage (the time a medium safely stores information), ease of retrievability, aggregation of information, interoperability, clinical/service practice considerations, performance improvement, and decision support processing.

A goal for information storage is to be linked or centrally organized and accessible. This could include the organization having an index identifying where the information is stored and how to access it; or, as the organization moves to electronic systems, the organization creates information systems to be interoperable within the enterprise. As more organizations automate various processes and activities, it is important to share critical data among systems. As challenges of interoperability have arisen, standards organizations for the information technology field have stepped in to develop industry standards. It is important that the organization is aware of the standards development organizations and their recommendations.

Internally and externally generated data and information are accurately disseminated to users. Access to accurate information is required to deliver, improve, analyze, and advance resident care and the systems that support health care delivery. Information is accessed and disseminated through electronic information systems or paper-based records and reports. The use of information is considered in developing forms, screen displays, and standard or ad hoc reports.

---

* **Report generation** The process of analyzing, organizing, and presenting recorded information for authentication and inclusion in the resident's health care record or in financial or business records.

† **Timeliness** The time between the occurrence of an event and the availability of data about the event. Timeliness is related to the use of the data.

‡ **Interoperability** Enables authorized users to capture, share, and report information from any system, whether paper- or electronic-based.

§ **Retrievability** The capability of efficiently finding relevant information.

|| **Accountability** All information is attributable to its source (person or device).

Elements of Performance for IM.3.10

A 1. Information technology industry standards or organization policies are used and address the following:
- Uniform data definitions
- Data capture
- Data display
- Data transmission

2. Standardize a list of abbreviations, acronyms, symbols, and dose designations that are not to be used throughout the organization.

Note: *The preceding requirement is not scored here. It is scored at NPSG.02.02.01.*

A 3. Minimum data sets, terminology, definitions, classifications, vocabulary, and nomenclature, including abbreviations, acronyms, symbols, and dose designations are standardized throughout the organization.

A 4. Quality control systems are used to monitor data content and collection activities.
- The method used provides for timely and economical data collection with the degree of accuracy, completeness, and discrimination necessary for their intended use
- The method used minimizes bias in the data and regularly assesses the data's reliability, validity, and accuracy
- Those responsible for collecting and reviewing the data are accountable for information accuracy and completeness

A 5. Storage and retrieval systems are designed to support organization needs for clinical/service and organization-specific information:
- Storage and retrieval systems are designed to balance the ability to retrieve data and information with the intended use for the data and information
- Storage and retrieval systems are designed to balance security and confidentiality issues with accessibility
- Systems for paper and electronic records are designed to reduce disruption or inaccessibility during such times as diminished staffing and scheduled and unscheduled downtimes of electronic information systems

A 6. Data and information are retained for sufficient time to comply with law or regulation.

A 7. Knowledgeable staff and tools are available for collecting, retrieving, and analyzing data and their transformation into information.

A 8. Data are organized and transformed into information in formats useful to decision makers.

A 9. Dissemination of data and information is timely* and accurate.

---

* **Timely** Defined by organization policy and based on the intended use of the information.

A 10. Data and information are disseminated in standard formats and methods to meet user needs and provide for retrievability and interpretation.

Information-Based Decision Making

Standard IM.4.10

The information management system provides information for use in decision making.

Rationale for IM.4.10

Information management supports timely and effective decision making at all organization levels. The information management processes support managerial and operational decisions, performance improvement activities, and resident care, treatment, and service decisions. Clinical and strategic decision making depends on information from multiple sources, including the resident record, knowledge-based information, comparative data/information, and aggregate data/information.

Elements of Performance for IM.4.10

A 1. The organization has the ability to collect and aggregate data and information to support care, treatment, and service delivery and operations, including the following:

- Individual care, treatment, and services and care, treatment, and service delivery
- Decision making
- Management and operations
- Analysis of trends
- Performance comparisons over time throughout the organization and with other organizations
- Performance improvement
- Infection control
- Resident safety

A 2. To support clinical decision making, information found in the resident record is the following:

- Readily accessible
- Accurate
- Complete
- Organized for retrieval of data
- Timely*

A 3. Comparative performance data and information are used for decision making, when available.

---

* **Timely** Defined by organization policy and based on the intended use of the information.

Knowledge-Based Information

Standard IM.5.10

Knowledge-based information resources are readily available, current, and authoritative.

Rationale for IM.5.10

Organization practitioners and staff have access to knowledge-based information* to do the following:

- Acquire and maintain the knowledge and skills needed to maintain and improve competence
- Assist with clinical/service and management decision making
- Provide appropriate information and education to residents and families
- Support performance improvement and resident safety activities
- Support the institution's educational and research needs

Elements of Performance for IM.5.10

1. Not applicable

A 2. The organization provides access to knowledge-based information resources† needed by staff in any of the following forms: print, electronic, Internet, or audio.

A 3. Knowledge-based information resources are available to clinical/service staff, through electronic means, after-hours access to an in-house collection, or other methods.

A 4. The organization has a process for providing access to knowledge-based information resources when electronic systems are unavailable.

Resident-Specific Information

Standard IM.6.10

The organization has a complete and accurate clinical record for residents assessed, cared for, treated, or served.

Rationale for IM.6.10

Resident-specific data and information are contained in the clinical record, to facilitate resident care, treatment, and services; serve as a financial and legal record; aid in

---

* **Knowledge-based information** A collection of stored facts, models, and information that can be used for designing and redesigning processes and for problem solving. In the context of this manual, knowledge-based information is found in the clinical, scientific, and management literature.

† Examples of knowledge-based information resources include current texts; periodicals; indexes; abstracts; reports; documents; databases; directories; discussion lists; successful practices; equipment and maintenance user manuals; standards; protocols; practice guidelines; clinical trials and other resources.

research; support decision analysis; and guide professional and organization performance improvement. This information is maintained as a paper record or as electronic health information.*

Elements of Performance for IM.6.10

A 1. Only authorized individuals make entries in the clinical record.

A 2. The organization defines which entries made by non-independent practitioners require countersigning consistent with law or regulation.

A 3. Standardized formats are used for documenting all care, treatment, and services provided to residents.

C Ⓜ 4. Clinical record entries† are dated, the author identified and, when necessary according to law or regulation or organization policy, authenticated, either by written signature, electronic signature, or computer key or rubber stamp.‡

C Ⓜ 5. The author authenticates either by written signature, electronic signature, or computer key or rubber stamp the following:
- The history and physical examination
- Medication orders
- Practitioner orders
- Discharge summary

C Ⓜ 6. The clinical record contains sufficient information to identify the resident; support the diagnosis/condition; justify the care, treatment, and services; document the course and results of care, treatment, and services; and promote continuity of care among providers. ⚠3

7. Not applicable

A 8. The organization has a policy on the timely entry of information into the resident's clinical record.

A 9. The organization defines a complete record and the time frame within which the record is completed after discharge, not to exceed 30 days after discharge.

10. Not applicable

11. Not applicable

---

* **Electronic health information** A computerized format of the health care information in paper records that is used for the same range of purposes as paper records, namely to familiarize readers with the resident's status; document care, treatment, and services; plan for discharge; document the need for care, treatment, and services; assess the quality of care, treatment, and services; determine reimbursement rates; justify reimbursement claims; pursue clinical or epidemiological research; and measure outcomes of the care, treatment, and service process.

† For paper-based records, countersignatures entered for purposes of authentication after transcription or for verbal orders are dated when required by law or regulations or organization policy. For electronic records, electronic signatures will be date-stamped.

‡ Authentication is shown by written signatures or initials, rubber-stamp signatures, or computer key. Authorized users of signature stamps or computer keys sign a statement assuring that they alone will use the stamp or key.

A 12. Clinical records are reviewed on an ongoing basis at the point of care.

A 13. The review of clinical records is based on organization-defined indicators that address the presence, timeliness, readability (whether handwritten or printed), quality, consistency, clarity, accuracy, completeness, and authentication of data and information contained within the record.

A 14. The retention time of clinical record information is determined by the organization based on law or regulation, and on its use for resident care, treatment, and services, legal, research, operational purposes, and educational activities.

A 15. Clinical records are retained for five years from the resident's discharge date when there is no requirement in state law.

A 16. Clinical records of minors are retained for three years after the resident reaches legal age under the law.

A 17. Original clinical records are not released unless the organization is responding appropriately to laws or regulations, court orders, or subpoenas.

18. Not applicable

A 19. In the event of a change in the organization's ownership, residents' clinical records remain the organization's property and are transferred to the new owner unless otherwise indicated by law.

Standard IM.6.20

Records contain resident-specific information, as appropriate, to the care, treatment, and services provided.

Elements of Performance for IM.6.20

C Ⓜ 1. Clinical records contain, as applicable, the following clinical/case information:

- Care, treatment, and services provided to the resident before his or her arrival, if any
- Documentation and findings of assessments*
- Initial medical assessment and conclusions or impressions drawn from medical history and physical examination
- Diagnosis, diagnostic impression, or conditions
- Reason(s) for admission or care, treatment, and services
- Goals of the care and care plan
- Orders for care treatment and service as required by law or regulation
- Diagnostic and therapeutic orders
- Diagnostic and therapeutic procedures, tests, and results
- Progress notes made by authorized individuals
- Reassessments and plan of care revisions
- Relevant observations

* *See* the "Provision of Care, Treatment, and Services" chapter in this book.

- Consultation reports
- Allergies to foods and medicines
- Medications ordered or prescribed
- Dosages of medications administered (including the strength, dose, or rate of administration), administration devices used, access site or route, known drug allergies, and adverse drug reactions
- Medications dispensed or prescribed on discharge
- Relevant diagnoses/conditions established during the course of care, treatment, and services

C Ⓜ 2. Clinical records contain, as applicable, the following demographic information:
- Resident's name, address, date of birth, religion, marital status, social security number, gender, and the name of any legally authorized representative
- Resident's legal status
- The resident's language and communication needs

C Ⓜ 3. Clinical records contain, as applicable, the following information:
- Evidence of known advance directives
- Evidence of informed consent when required by organization policy
- Orders, renewal of orders, and documentation that resuscitative services are to be withheld or life-sustaining treatment withdrawn
- Discharge plan, or the reason for lack of an ongoing plan when discharge potential does not exist
- Referrals or communications made to external or internal care providers and community agencies
- Physician's summary and the resident's final diagnosis when the resident is admitted from either a hospital or another health care organization

Standard IM.6.30

Not applicable

Standard IM.6.40

Not applicable

Standard IM.6.50

Designated qualified staff accept and transcribe verbal or telephone orders from authorized individuals.

Rationale for IM.6.50

Processes for receiving, transcribing, and authenticating verbal or telephone orders are established to protect the quality of resident care, treatment, and services.

Elements of Performance for IM.6.50

A 1. Qualified personnel are identified, as defined by organization policy and in accordance with law or regulation, and authorized to receive and record verbal or telephone orders.

C Ⓜ 2. Verbal or telephone orders are dated and identifies the names of the individuals who gave, received, and implemented the order.

A 3. When required by law or regulation, verbal or telephone orders are authenticated within the specified time frame.

4. For verbal or telephone orders or for telephonic reporting of critical test results, verify the complete order or test result by having the person receiving the information record and "read-back" the complete order or test result.

Note: *The preceding requirement is not scored here. It is scored at NPSG.02.01.01.*

Standard IM.6.60

The organization provides access to relevant information from a resident's record as needed for use in resident care, treatment, and services.

Rationale for IM.6.60

To facilitate continuity of care, providers have access to information about all previous care, treatment, and services provided to a resident by the organization.

Elements of Performance for IM.6.60

A 1. The organization has a process to track the location of all components of the clinical record.

A 2. The organization uses a system to assemble required information or make available a summary of information relative for resident care, treatment, and services provided.

Standard IM.6.70

Clinical record documentation includes the provision of and response to the activities program at least quarterly.

Elements of Performance for IM.6.70

C Ⓜ 1. The provision of and response to the activities program based on the interdisciplinary care plan are documented at least quarterly in the clinical record.

C Ⓜ 2. The activity providers document in the clinical record and report to the charge nurse changes in the resident's response to the activity program.

Standard IM.6.80

Clinical record documentation includes the provision of and response to nutrition care services at least quarterly.

Elements of Performance for IM.6.80

C Ⓜ 1. The provision of and response to nutrition care services based on the interdisciplinary care plan is documented at least quarterly in the clinical record.

C Ⓜ 2. Documentation includes the current status and changes in the resident's nutritional status, including the following information:
- The resident's acceptance of prescribed diets
- The resident's food and fluid consumption
- Significant weight loss or gain consistent with law or regulation
- Hydration status
- The resident's ability to eat independently
- The resident's ability to use adaptive devices for eating
- Current status and changes in the resident's physical or behavioral condition, including symptoms
- Summary of the resident's condition, which includes the extent to which nutritional goals included in the interdisciplinary care plan are achieved

Standard IM.6.90

Clinical record documentation includes the provision of and response to nursing care.

Elements of Performance for IM.6.90

C Ⓜ 1. The provision of nursing care that is based on the interdisciplinary care plan and the resident's response to this care are documented in the clinical record.

C Ⓜ 2. Documentation includes the following:
- Medications and treatment given and untoward reactions
- Nursing care provided
- Current status and changes in the resident's physical or behavioral condition, including symptoms
- Summary by licensed nursing staff of the resident's condition, which includes the extent to which nursing goals included in the interdisciplinary care plan are achieved, at least quarterly or more often if the resident's condition warrants

Note: *In determining the frequency of preparing a summary of the residents' condition, consideration should be given to residents with complex needs or short lengths of stay.*

Standard IM.6.100

Clinical record documentation includes the provision of and response to medical treatment and care.

Elements of Performance for IM.6.100

C Ⓜ 1. The provision of medical treatment and care and the resident's response to medical treatment and care are documented in the clinical record. ⚠3

C Ⓜ 2. Documentation in the resident's clinical record includes, before or on admission, the submission of the following:
- Admitting diagnosis
- Current medical findings
- Diet prescribed
- The resident's functional status

C Ⓜ 3. Documentation in the resident's clinical record includes medical observations and recommendations made after the initial medical assessment, as well as progress notes that are reported at the time of observation and that describe significant changes in the resident's condition.

C Ⓜ 4. Documentation in the resident's clinical record includes progress notes recorded by the physician at each visit.

C Ⓜ 5. Upon the resident's discharge, documentation in the resident's clinical record includes the completion of the transfer form when appropriate, the discharge summary, and the resident's clinical record.

C Ⓜ 6. If the resident expires in the organization, the course of events leading up to the resident's death is documented.

C Ⓜ 7. Documentation in the resident's clinical record includes evidence that the attending physician has reviewed the consulting physician's orders for consistency with the overall care plan.

Standard IM.6.110

Clinical record documentation includes the provision of and response to rehabilitation services.

Elements of Performance for IM.6.110

C Ⓜ 1. The provision of rehabilitation services that are provided based on the interdisciplinary care plan and the resident's response to these services are documented in the clinical record.

C Ⓜ 2. Documentation describes the following:
- The resident's and family's perception of and involvement in rehabilitation services
- Reason for the referral to rehabilitation services or admission for medically complex services
- Rehabilitation treatments, modalities, or procedures provided

- The resident's response to treatment
- The resident's involvement in rehabilitation services
- The resident's progress toward treatment goals

C Ⓜ 3. Assessment of rehabilitation achievement and estimates of further rehabilitation potential are entered at least weekly.

C Ⓜ 4. Documentation includes a progress report and reassessment, including the following:
- Summary of the resident's condition, which includes the extent to which rehabilitation goals included in the interdisciplinary care plan are achieved, every two weeks for the first quarter, every month for the second quarter, and quarterly thereafter or more frequently when a resident's condition changes
- Estimates of the resident's further rehabilitation potential
- Discharge plan

Standard IM.6.120

Clinical record documentation includes the provision of and response to social service interventions.

Elements of Performance for IM.6.120

C Ⓜ 1. The provision of and the resident's response to social service interventions are documented in the clinical record.

C Ⓜ 2. Documentation of social service interventions includes the following:
- Specified goals related to social services, including discharge planning, that are an integral part of the interdisciplinary care plan
- Services provided and their outcomes
- Summary of the resident's problems, services provided, goals, and condition, which includes the extent to which social services goals included in the interdisciplinary care plan are achieved, at least quarterly or more often if the resident's condition warrants
- Referrals to outside agencies, resources, or individuals, as well as follow-up actions or recommendations of outside agencies, resources, or individuals

Note: *In determining the frequency of preparing a summary, consideration should be given to residents with complex needs or short lengths of stay.*

Standard IM.6.130

Clinical record documentation includes the provision of education and its effectiveness.

Element of Performance for IM.6.130

C Ⓜ 1. The provision of and the resident's response to education are documented in the clinical record.

Standard IM.6.140

Clinical record documentation includes significant changes in the resident's condition, care, and treatment.

Element of Performance for IM.6.140

C Ⓜ 1. Clinical record documentation includes significant changes in the resident's condition, care, and treatment. ⚠3

Standard IM.6.150

Treatment provided to the resident by off-site sources is documented in the clinical record.

Element of Performance for IM.6.150

C Ⓜ 1. Clinical record documentation includes treatment provided to the resident by off-site sources.

Standard IM.6.160

Effects of medications on residents, and associated pharmacist evaluation and physician consultation, are documented.

Element of Performance for IM.6.160

C Ⓜ 1. Clinical records include documentation of the following:
- Resident's response to medications
- Pharmacist's evaluation and consultation with the physician
- The need for additional laboratory monitoring ⚠3

Note: *Documentation can be included in the resident's clinical record or in another location such as the pharmacist's report.*

Standard IM.6.170

Discharge information provided to the resident or to the family, as appropriate and permissible, and/or to the receiving organization is documented.

Elements of Performance for IM.6.170

C Ⓜ 1. Clinical record documentation includes discharge information provided to the resident and/or to the receiving organization.

C Ⓜ 2. Discharge information includes the following:
- Medical findings, diagnosis(es), and treatment orders
- Summary of the care, treatment, and services provided and progress toward achieving goals
- Diet orders and medication orders
- Behavioral status, ambulation status, nutrition status, and rehabilitation potential

- The resident's physical and psychosocial status
- Nursing information useful in resident care
- Advance directives
- Referrals provided to the resident
- The reason for transfer, discharge, or referral
- Physician's orders for the resident's immediate care
- Instructions given to the resident before discharge
- The referring physician's name
- The physician who has agreed to be responsible for the resident's medical care and treatment, if other than the referring physician

Standards IM.6.180 Through IM.6.280

Not applicable

2009

SLTC

Medicare/Medicaid Certification-Based LTC Accreditation Standards (MC)

MC

Medicare/Medicaid Certification–Based LTC Accreditation Standards (MC)

Overview

This chapter contains standards, rationales, elements of performance (EPs), and scoring applicable to those long term care organizations seeking the Joint Commission's Medicare/Medicaid certification–based long term care accreditation. These requirements are pulled directly out of the functional chapters in this book. Introductory language can be referenced in the specific chapters in this book.

This subset of Joint Commission long term care accreditation standards has been identified for on-site review under the Medicare/Medicaid certification–based long term care accreditation option. These standards go beyond the Conditions of Participation for Skilled Nursing Facilities/Nursing Facilities and address areas that are typically not evaluated during the state agency certification survey. This path to long term care accreditation focuses on systems and processes that support organization safety, performance improvement, resident and family education, credentialing and privileging of licensed independent practitioners, pain management, and point-of-care testing (POCT).

An organization is eligible for the Medicare/Medicaid certification–based accreditation option if it is Medicare/Medicaid certified as a Skilled Nursing Facility (SNF) or Nursing Facility (NF). The on-site survey is usually one day (organizations with an average daily census >300 will be scheduled additional time), and the fee is significantly less than the traditional long term care accreditation fee. Certificates reflect that the accreditation award is substantially based on Medicare/Medicaid certification for long term care. For more information, please visit the Joint Commission's Web site at http://www.jointcommission.org.

Key: 0 = Insufficient compliance; 1 = Partial compliance; 2 = Satisfactory compliance; NA = Not applicable; **A** indicates scoring category A; **C** indicates scoring category C; ▲(2) indicates situational decision rules apply; △(3) indicates direct impact requirements apply; Ⓜ indicates Measure of success is needed

Accreditation Participation Requirements

Overview

This section consists of specific requirements for participation in the accreditation process and for maintaining an accreditation award.

For an organization seeking accreditation for the first time, compliance with the Accreditation Participation Requirements (APRs) is assessed during the initial survey, including the Early Survey Policy Option. For an accredited organization, compliance with these requirements is assessed throughout the accreditation cycle through on-site surveys, the Periodic Performance Review (PPR), Evidence of Standards Compliance, and periodic updates of organization-specific data and information. Organizations are either compliant or not compliant with the APRs. When an organization does not comply with an APR, the organization will be assigned a Requirement for Improvement (RFI) in the same context that noncompliance with a standard or element of performance generates an RFI. However, refusal to permit performance of a survey (APR.02.01.01) will lead to a denial of accreditation. Falsification of information (APR.01.02.01) will lead to preliminary denial of accreditation. All RFIs can impact the accreditation decision and follow-up requirements, as determined by established accreditation decision rules. Failure to resolve an RFI can ultimately lead to loss of accreditation.

Requirements, Rationales, Elements of Performance, and Scoring

APR.01.01.01

The organization submits information to The Joint Commission as required.

Element of Performance for APR.01.01.01

A 1. The organization meets all requirements for timely submissions of data and information to The Joint Commission. ▲2

Note: *The Joint Commission will impose the following consequences for failure to comply with this APR:*

- *If the organization does not comply with the requirement after 31 days, the organization will be placed in Provisional Accreditation.*
- *If the organization does not comply with the requirement after 61 days, the organization's accreditation decision will be changed from Provisional Accreditation to Conditional Accreditation.*
- *If the organization does not comply with the requirement after 91 days, the organization's accreditation decision will be changed from Conditional Accreditation to Denial of Accreditation. In accordance with the*

Accreditation Committee policy, such organizations will not be afforded any appeal.

The proposed consequences address only compliance with the requirement itself. They do not address the content of the organization's submissions to The Joint Commission. For example, if information in an organization's electronic application for accreditation (E-App) leads to inaccuracies in the appropriate length of the survey and a longer survey is required, the organization will incur the additional costs of the longer survey. In addition, if there is evidence that the organization has intentionally falsified the information submitted to The Joint Commission, the requirement at APR.01.02.01, EP 1, and its consequences will apply. (See also *APR.01.02.01, EP 1)*

APR.01.02.01

The organization provides accurate information throughout the accreditation process.

Rationale for APR.01.02.01

The Joint Commission requires each organization seeking accreditation to engage in the accreditation process in good faith. Sound business practices require transparency in all reporting procedures to ensure the safety of the public and the people who work in the organization. Any organization that fails to participate in good faith by falsifying information or by failing to exercise due care and diligence to ensure the accuracy of such information may have its accreditation denied or removed by The Joint Commission.

Element of Performance for APR.01.02.01

A 1. The organization provides accurate information throughout the accreditation process. (*See also* APR.01.01.01, EP 1)

Note 1: *Information may be received in any of the following ways:*

- *Provided verbally*
- *Obtained through direct observation by, or in an interview or any other type of communication with, any Joint Commission employee*
- *Derived from documents supplied by the organization to The Joint Commission*
- *Submitted electronically by the organization through a performance measurement system to The Joint Commission*

Note 2: *For the purpose of this requirement,* falsification *is defined as the fabrication, in whole or in part, and through commission or omission, of any information provided by an applicant or accredited organization to The Joint Commission. This includes redrafting, reformatting, or deleting document content. However, the organization may submit supporting material that explains the original information submitted to The Joint Commission. These additional materials must be properly identified, dated, and accompanied by the original documents.*

APR.01.03.01

The organization reports any changes in the information provided in the application for accreditation and any changes made between surveys.

Element of Performance for APR.01.03.01

A 1. The organization notifies The Joint Commission in writing within 30 days of a change in ownership, control, location, capacity, or services offered.

Note: *When the organization changes ownership, control, location, capacity or services offered, it may be necessary for The Joint Commission to survey the organization again. If the organization does not provide written notification to The Joint Commission within 30 days of these changes, the organization could lose its accreditation.*

APR.02.01.01

The organization permits the performance of a survey at The Joint Commission's discretion.

Element of Performance for APR.02.01.01

A 1. The organization permits the performance of a survey. ⚠2

APR.04.01.01

The organization selects and uses performance measures relevant to the services it provides and the population(s) it serves.

Note 1: *Long term care organizations that are not required to collect Minimum Data Set (MDS) data participate in a Joint Commission–accepted performance measurement system.*

Note 2: *Organizations are encouraged to keep up-to-date on any changes in the ORYX® requirements by reviewing recent issues of* The Joint Commission Perspectives *or by going to the "Performance Measurement" area on The Joint Commission Web site, at http://www.jointcommission.org.*

Elements of Performance for APR.04.01.01

A 6. Medicare/Medicaid-certified organizations required to collect and submit Minimum Data Set data to a state agency provide surveyors with the following information: Monthly Facility Quality Indicator reports.

A 7. Medicare/Medicaid-certified organizations required to collect and submit Minimum Data Set data to a state agency provide surveyors with the following information: Quality Measure reports.

A 8. Medicare/Medicaid-certified organizations required to collect and submit Minimum Data Set data to a state agency provide surveyors with the following information: CMS Form 2567 reports.

A 9. Medicare/Medicaid-certified organizations required to collect and submit Minimum Data Set data to a state agency provide surveyors with the following information: Plans of Correction.

A 10. Medicare/Medicaid-certified organizations required to collect and submit Minimum Data Set data to a state agency provide surveyors with the following information: Publicly reported Quality Measure reports.

A 11. Organizations not collecting Minimum Data Set data select a sufficient number of measures from an approved performance measurement system to meet current ORYX requirements.

A 12. The organization notifies The Joint Commission of its performance measures selections by the required date.

A 17. The organization discusses with the surveyor how the data are used to identify, prioritize, and monitor performance improvement activities.

A 18. The organization uses an individual measure for at least four consecutive quarters before replacing it.

A 19. The organization continues to use a measure if the data suggest an unstable pattern of performance or otherwise identify an opportunity for improvement.

A 20. The organization selects a new measure if the data reflect stable and satisfactory performance.

A 21. Organizations participating in a performance measurement system notify The Joint Commission of any changes in its measure selection.

A 25. Organizations participating in a performance measurement system submit aggregate data to The Joint Commission at least quarterly.

APR.05.01.01

The organization allows The Joint Commission to review the results of external evaluations from publicly recognized bodies.

Rationale for APR.05.01.01

In order to conduct a meaningful accreditation survey, The Joint Commission collects information on many aspects of the organization's performance. External bodies other than the Joint Commission evaluate areas related to safety and quality. These evaluations complement accreditation reviews, but may have a different focus or emphasis. These evaluations may contain information The Joint Commission needs to make accreditation decisions.

Elements of Performance for APR.05.01.01

A 1. When requested, the organization provides The Joint Commission with all official records and reports of licensing, examining, reviewing, or planning bodies.

A 3. The organization notifies The Joint Commission when it is designated by the Centers for Medicare and Medicaid Services (CMS) as a Special Focus Facility prior to public announcement of its designation by CMS. ▲2

Note: *If the organization fails to notify The Joint Commission, a recommendation will be made to the Accreditation Committee to place the organization in Conditional Accreditation.*

APR.06.01.01

Applicant or accredited organizations do not use Joint Commission employees to provide accreditation-related consulting services.

Element of Performance for APR.06.01.01

A 1. The organization does not use Joint Commission employees to provide any accreditation-related consulting services. ▲2

Note: *Consulting services include, but are not limited to, the following:*
- *Helping the organization to meet Joint Commission standards.*
- *Helping the organization to complete its Periodic Performance Review (PPR).*
- *Assisting the organization in remedying areas identified in its PPR as needing improvement.*
- *Conducting mock surveys.*
- *Providing the organization with consultation to address Priority Focus Process information.*

APR.07.01.01

The organization accepts the presence of Joint Commission surveyor management staff or a Board of Commissioners member in the role of observer of an on-site survey.

Element of Performance for APR.07.01.01

A 1. The organization allows Joint Commission surveyor management staff or a member of the Board of Commissioners to observe the on-site survey.

Note: *The observer will not participate in the on-site survey process, including the scoring of standards compliance. The organization will not incur any additional survey fees because an observer(s) is present.*

APR.08.01.01

The organization accurately represents its accreditation status and the facilities and services to which Joint Commission accreditation applies.

Elements of Performance for APR.08.01.01

A 1. The organization's advertising accurately reflects the scope of facilities and services that are accredited by The Joint Commission.

A 2. The organization does not engage in any false or misleading advertising about its accreditation award.

APR.09.01.01

The organization notifies its public about how to contact its organization management or The Joint Commission to report concerns about resident safety and quality of care.

Note: *Methods of notice may include, but are not limited to, distribution of information about The Joint Commission, including contact information in published materials such as brochures and/or posting this information on the organization's Web site.*

Elements of Performance for APR.09.01.01

A 1. The organization informs the public it serves about how to contact its management to report concerns about resident safety and quality of care.

A 2. The organization informs the public it serves about how to contact The Joint Commission to report concerns about resident safety and quality of care.

APR.09.02.01

Any individual who provides care, treatment, or services can report concerns about safety or the quality of care to The Joint Commission without retaliatory action from the organization.

Rationale for APR.09.02.01

Any individual who provides care, treatment, or services should be free to raise concerns to The Joint Commission when the organization has not adequately prevented or corrected problems that can have or have had a serious adverse impact on residents. To support this culture of safety, the organization must communicate to staff that such reporting is permitted. Further, the organization must make it clear to staff that no formal disciplinary actions (e.g., demotions, reassignments, change in working conditions or hours) or informal punitive actions (e.g., harassment, isolation, abuse) will be threatened or carried out in retaliation for reporting concerns to The Joint Commission.

Elements of Performance for APR.09.02.01

A 1. The organization educates its staff that any employee or other individual who provides care, treatment, or services or who has concerns about the safety or quality-of-care provided in the organization may report these concerns to The Joint Commission.

A 2. The organization informs its staff that it will take no disciplinary or punitive action because an employee or other individual who provides care, treatment, or services reports safety or quality-of-care concerns to The Joint Commission.

A 3. The organization takes no disciplinary or punitive action against employees or other individuals who provide care, treatment, or services when they report safety or quality-of-care concerns to The Joint Commission.

APR.09.03.01

The organization is truthful and accurate when describing information in its Quality Report to the public.

Element of Performance for APR.09.03.01

A 1. The organization adheres to The Joint Commission's published guidelines for how it describes information in its Quality Report.

APR.10.01.01

The organization notifies The Joint Commission if it has been terminated from the Medicare/Medicaid program.

Element of Performance for APR.10.01.01

A 1. The organization notifies The Joint Commission within 24 hours of learning that its Medicare/Medicaid certification has been terminated. ▲2

APR.10.02.01

The organization implements and maintains plans of correction that are required by state and federal inspections.

Element of Performance for APR.10.02.01

A 1. The organization implements and maintains plans of correction from its most recent state or federal inspection.

National Patient Safety Goals

Overview

This section addresses the requirements of the 2009 National Patient Safety Goals (NPSGs). The purpose of The Joint Commission's NPSGs is to promote specific improvements in patient safety. The goals highlight problematic areas in health care and describe evidence- and expert-based consensus as solutions to these problems. Because sound system design is intrinsic to the delivery of safe, high-quality health care, the goals generally focus on system-wide solutions, whenever possible.

Note: *The term* implementation expectations *has been changed to* elements of performance (EP) *and the numbering system has been modified to be consistent with the method used for the accreditation standards.*

The broadly representative Sentinel Event Advisory Group (SEAG) works with Joint Commission staff on a continuing basis to prioritize and develop goals, requirements, and EPs. As part of this development process, candidate goals, requirements, and EPs are sent to the field for review and comment. The Advisory Group annually recommends selected existing and new goals, requirements, and EPs to The Joint Commission's Board of Commissioners for review and approval.

Organizations providing care, treatment, or services relevant to these goals are responsible for implementing the applicable requirements or effective alternatives. If an organization thinks that an alternative approach to meeting an EP fulfills the intent of the requirement and wishes to implement such an alternative, the organization must obtain Joint Commission approval of the alternative. The SEAG also assists The Joint Commission in evaluating potential alternatives to goal requirements that have been suggested by individual organizations. Compliance with these requirements is assessed throughout the accreditation cycle, through on-site surveys, and the Periodic Performance Review (PPR), when required by The Joint Commission. When an organization does not fully comply with a requirement, the organization will be assigned a Requirement for Improvement (RFI) in the same way that noncompliance with an accreditation EP generates an RFI. All RFIs must be addressed during the Evidence of Standards Compliance process (ESC). Failure to resolve an RFI affects an organization's accreditation status, which could ultimately lead to a loss of accreditation.

The Joint Commission provides guidance on how to comply with each goal's requirements. This guidance includes detailed answers to Frequently Asked Questions (FAQs), which are posted on The Joint Commission Web site (http://www.jointcommission.org).

Requirements, Rationales, Elements of Performance, and Scoring

Goal 1—Improve the accuracy of resident identification.

NPSG.01.01.01

Use at least two resident identifiers when providing care, treatment, or services.

Rationale for NPSG.01.01.01

Wrong-resident errors occur in virtually all stages of diagnosis and treatment. The intent for this goal is two-fold: first, to reliably identify the individual as the person for whom the service or treatment is intended; second, to match the service or treatment to that individual.

Elements of Performance for NPSG.01.01.01

C Ⓜ 1. Prior to any specimen collection, medication administration, transfusion, or treatment, the organization actively involves the resident and, as needed, the family in the identification and matching process. When active resident involvement is not possible or the resident's reliability is in question, the organization will designate the caregiver responsible for identity verification. ⚠3

Note: *The involvement of a single caregiver is acceptable as long as the other components of resident identification are satisfied.*

C Ⓜ 2. Two resident identifiers are used when administering medications, blood, or blood components. ⚠3

A Ⓜ 3. Two resident identifiers are used when collecting blood samples and other specimens for clinical testing. ⚠3

C Ⓜ 4. Two resident identifiers are used when providing other treatments or procedures. ⚠3

A 5. The resident's room number or physical location is not used as an identifier. ⚠3

A Ⓜ 6. Containers used for blood and other specimens are labeled in the presence of the resident. ⚠3

NPSG.01.02.01

Prior to the start of any surgical or invasive procedure, individuals involved in the procedure conduct a final verification process, such as a time-out, to confirm the correct resident, procedure, and site, using active, not passive, communication techniques.

Elements of Performance for NPSG.01.02.01

A 1. The final verification process must be conducted in the location where the procedure will be done, just before starting the procedure. ⚠3

A Ⓜ 2. The final verification process involves the entire team, uses active communication, and includes the following:
- Correct resident identity
- Correct side and site
- Agreement on the procedure to be done
- Correct resident position
- Availability of correct implants and any special equipment or special requirements ⚠3

A 3. The process is briefly documented using a method such as a checklist. ⚠3

Note: *The organization determines the type and amount of documentation.*

A 4. The organization has processes and systems in place for reconciling differences in staff responses during the final verification process. ⚠3

Goal 2—Improve the effectiveness of communication among caregivers.

NPSG.02.01.01

For verbal or telephone orders or for telephone reporting of critical test results, the individual giving the order or test result verifies the complete order or test result by having the person receiving the information record and "read back" the complete order or test result.

Rationale for NPSG.02.01.01

Ineffective communication is the most frequently cited root cause for sentinel events. Effective communication that is timely, accurate, complete, unambiguous, and understood by the recipient reduces error and results in improved resident safety.

Elements of Performance for NPSG.02.01.01

C Ⓜ 1. The individual receiving the information writes down the complete order or test result or enters it into a computer. ⚠3

C Ⓜ 2. The individual receiving the information reads back the complete order or test result. ⚠3

C Ⓜ 3. The individual who gave the order or test result confirms the information that was read back. ⚠3

NPSG.02.02.01

There is a standardized list of abbreviations, acronyms, symbols, and dose designations that are not to be used throughout the long term care organization.

Elements of Performance for NPSG.02.02.01

A 1. The organization develops a standardized list of abbreviations, acronyms, symbols, and dose designations that are not to be used throughout the organization.

A 2. The current list of abbreviations, acronyms, symbols, and dose designations not to be used includes the following:

- U,u
- IU
- Q.D., QD, q.d., qd
- Q.O.D., QOD, q.o.d., qod
- Trailing zero (X.0 mg)
- Lack of leading zero (.X mg)
- MS
- MSO_4
- $MgSO_4$ ⚠3

Note: *A trailing zero may be used only when required to demonstrate the level of precision of the value being reported, such as for laboratory results, imaging studies that report the size of lesions, or catheter/tube sizes. It may not be used in medication orders or other medication-related documentation.*

C Ⓜ 3. The organization implements the "do not use" list of abbreviations, acronyms, symbols, and dose designations and applies it to all orders and all medication-related documentation that is handwritten or entered as free text into a computer. ⚠3

A 4. The organization does not include any abbreviations, acronyms, symbols, and dose designations identified as not to be used on preprinted forms. ⚠3

NPSG.02.03.01

The organization measures, assesses, and, if needed, takes action to improve the timeliness of reporting, and the timeliness of receipt of critical tests and critical results and values by the responsible licensed caregiver.

Elements of Performance for NPSG.02.03.01

A 1. The organization defines critical tests and critical results and values.

A 2. The organization defines the acceptable length of time between the ordering of critical tests and reporting the results of these tests, whether normal or abnormal.

A 3. The organization defines the acceptable length of time for reporting the results of routine tests with critical abnormal values or findings.

A 4. The organization defines the acceptable length of time between the availability of critical tests and critical results and values and receipt by the responsible licensed caregiver.

A 5. The organization collects data on the timeliness of reporting critical test results and critical results and values from routine tests.

A 6. The organization assesses the data on the timeliness of reporting critical test results and critical results and values from routine tests and determines whether a need for improvement exists.

A 7. The organization takes appropriate action to improve the timeliness of reporting critical test results and critical results and values from routine tests and measures the effectiveness of those actions.

NPSG.02.05.01

The organization implements a standardized approach to hand-off communications, including an opportunity to ask and respond to questions.

Rationale for NPSG.02.05.01

Health care has numerous types of resident hand-offs, including, but not limited to, nursing shift changes; physician transfer of complete responsibility for a resident; physician transfer of on-call responsibility; acceptance of temporary responsibility for staff leaving the unit for a short time; nursing and physician hand-off from the emergency department to inpatient units, different hospitals, nursing homes and home health care; and critical laboratory and radiology results sent to physician offices. The primary objective of a hand-off is to provide accurate information about a resident's care, treatment, or services, current condition, and any recent or anticipated changes. The information communicated during a hand-off must be accurate in order to meet resident safety goals.

Elements of Performance for NPSG.02.05.01

C Ⓜ 1. The organization's process for effective hand-off communication includes the following: Interactive communication that allows for the opportunity for questioning between the giver and receiver of resident information. ⚠3

C Ⓜ 2. The organization's process for effective hand-off communication includes the following: Up-to-date information regarding the resident's condition, care, treatment, medications, services, and any recent or anticipated changes. (*See also* NPSG.08.01.01, EP 4) ⚠3

C Ⓜ 3. The organization's process for effective hand-off communication includes the following: A method to verify the received information, including repeat-back or read-back techniques. ⚠3

A 4. The organization's process for effective hand-off communication includes the following: An opportunity for the receiver of the hand-off information to review relevant resident historical data, which may include previous care, treatment, or services. ⚠3

C Ⓜ 5. Interruptions during hand-offs are limited to minimize the possibility that information fails to be conveyed or is forgotten. ⚠3

Goal 3—Improve the safety of using medications.

NPSG.03.03.01

The organization identifies and, at a minimum, annually reviews a list of look-alike/sound-alike medications used by the organization and takes action to prevent errors involving the interchange of these medications.

Elements of Performance for NPSG.03.03.01

A 1. The organization identifies a list of look-alike/sound-alike medications used by the organization. The list includes a minimum of 10 look-alike/sound-alike medication combinations selected from the tables of look-alike/sound-alike medications posted on The Joint Commission Web site at http://www.jointcommission.org.

A 2. Review the list of look-alike/sound-alike drugs used by the organization at least annually.

A 3. The organization takes action to prevent errors involving the interchange of these drugs. ⚠3

NPSG.03.05.01

Reduce the likelihood of resident harm associated with the use of anticoagulant therapy.

Note: *This requirement applies only to organizations that provide anticoagulant therapy and/or long-term anticoagulation prophylaxis (for example, atrial fibrillation) where the clinical expectation is that the resident's laboratory values for coagulation will remain outside normal values. This requirement does not apply to routine situations in which short-term prophylactic anticoagulation is used for venous thromboembolism prevention (for example, related to procedures or hospitalization) and the clinical expectation is that the resident's laboratory values for coagulation will remain within, or close to, normal values.*

Rationale for NPSG.03.05.01

Anticoagulant therapy poses risks to residents and often leads to adverse drug events due to complex dosing, requisite follow-up monitoring, and inconsistent resident compliance. The use of standardized practices for anticoagulant therapy that include resident involvement can reduce the risk of adverse drug events associated with the use of heparin (unfractionated), low molecular weight heparin, and warfarin.

Elements of Performance for NPSG.03.05.01

A 1. The organization implements a defined anticoagulation management program to individualize the care provided to each resident receiving anticoagulant therapy. ⚠3

A 2. To reduce compounding and labeling errors, the organization uses only oral unit-dose products, pre-filled syringes, or pre-mixed infusion bags, when these products are available. ⚠3

Note: *For pediatric patients, pre-loaded syringe products should only be used if specifically designed for children.*

C Ⓜ 3. The organization uses approved protocols for the initiation and maintenance of anticoagulant therapy appropriate to the medication used, to the condition being treated, and to the potential for medication interactions. ⚠3

A 4. For residents started on warfarin, a baseline International Normalized Ratio (INR) is available, and for all residents receiving warfarin therapy, a current INR is available and is used to monitor and adjust this therapy. ⚠3

C Ⓜ 5. When dietary services are provided by the organization, the service is notified of all residents receiving warfarin and responds according to its established food–medication interaction program. ⚠3

A 6. When heparin is administered intravenously and continuously, the organization uses programmable infusion pumps in order to provide consistent and accurate dosing. ⚠3

A 7. The organization has a written policy that addresses baseline and ongoing laboratory tests that are required for heparin and low molecular weight heparin therapies. ⚠3

C Ⓜ 8. The organization provides education regarding anticoagulant therapy to staff, residents, and families. ⚠3

Note: *Resident/family education includes the importance of follow-up monitoring, compliance issues, dietary restrictions, and potential for adverse drug reactions and interactions.*

A 9. The organization evaluates its anticoagulation safety practices, takes appropriate action to improve its practices, and measures the effectiveness of those actions on a regular basis.

Goal 7—Reduce the risk of health care–associated infections.

NPSG.07.01.01

Comply with current World Health Organization (WHO) Hand Hygiene Guidelines or Centers for Disease Control and Prevention (CDC) hand hygiene guidelines.

Rationale for NPSG.07.01.01

Compliance with the WHO or CDC hand hygiene guidelines will reduce the transmission by staff to residents of infectious agents, thereby decreasing the incidence of health care-associated infections.

Element of Performance for NPSG.07.01.01

C Ⓜ 1. The organization complies with current World Health Organization (WHO) or Centers for Disease Control and Prevention (CDC) hand hygiene guidelines. ⚠3

Note: *Organizations are required to comply with 1A, 1B, and 1C of the WHO or CDC guidelines.*

NPSG.07.02.01

Manage as sentinel events all identified cases of unanticipated death or major permanent loss of function related to a health care associated infection.

Rationale for NPSG.07.02.01

A significant percentage of residents who unexpectedly die or suffer major permanent loss of function have health care associated infections. These unanticipated deaths and injuries meet the definition of a sentinel event and, therefore, are required to undergo a root cause analysis. The root cause analysis should attempt to answer the following questions: Why did the resident acquire an infection? Why did the resident die or suffer permanent loss of function?

Elements of Performance for NPSG.07.02.01

C Ⓜ 1. The organization manages all identified cases of unanticipated death or major permanent loss of function associated with a health care associated infection as sentinel events (that is, the organization conducts a root cause analysis). ⚠3

A 2. The root cause analysis addresses the management of the resident before and after the identification of infection.

Goal 8—Accurately and completely reconcile medications across the continuum of care.

NPSG.08.01.01

There is a process for comparing the resident's current medications with those ordered for the resident while under the care of the organization.

Rationale for NPSG.08.01.01

Residents are at high risk for harm from adverse drug events when communication about medications is not clear. The chance for communication errors increases whenever individuals involved in a resident's care change. Communicating about the medication list, making sure it is accurate, and reconciling any discrepancies whenever new medications are ordered or current medications are adjusted are essential to reducing the risk of transition-related adverse drug events.

Elements of Performance for NPSG.08.01.01

C Ⓜ 1. At the time the resident enters the organization or is admitted, a complete list of the medications the resident is taking at home (including dose, route, and frequency) is created and documented. The resident and, as needed, the family are involved in creating this list. ⚠3

C Ⓜ 2. The medications ordered for the resident while under the care of the organization are compared to those on the list created at the time of entry to the organization or admission. ⚠3

C Ⓜ 3. Any discrepancies (that is, omissions, duplications, adjustments, deletions, additions) are reconciled and documented while the resident is under the care of the organization. ⚠3

C Ⓜ 4. When the resident's care is transferred within the organization, the current provider(s) informs the receiving provider(s) about the up-to-date reconciled medication list and documents the communication. ⚠3

Note: *Updating the status of a resident's medications is also an important component of all resident care hand-offs.* (See also *NPSG.02.05.01, EP 2)*

NPSG.08.02.01

When a resident is referred to or transferred from one organization to another, the complete and reconciled list of medications is communicated to the next provider of service, and the communication is documented. Alternatively, when a resident leaves the organization's care to go directly to his or her home, the complete and reconciled list of medications is provided to the resident's known primary care provider, original referring provider, or a known next provider of service.

Note: *When the next provider of service is unknown or when no known formal relationship is planned with a next provider, giving the resident and, as needed, the family the list of reconciled medications is sufficient.*

Rationale for NPSG.08.02.01

The accurate communication of a resident's reconciled medication list to the next provider of service reduces the risk of transition-related adverse drug events. The communication enables the next provider of service to receive thorough knowledge of the resident's medications and to safely order/prescribe other medications that may be needed. This communication is especially important at transitions in care when a resident is referred or transferred from one organization to another.

Elements of Performance for NPSG.08.02.01

C Ⓜ 1. The resident's most current reconciled medication list is communicated to the next provider of service, either within or outside the organization. The communication between providers is documented. ⚠3

C Ⓜ 2. At the time of transfer, the transferring organization informs the next provider of service how to obtain clarification on the list of reconciled medications.

NPSG.08.03.01

When a resident leaves the organization's care, a complete and reconciled list of the resident's medications is provided directly to the resident and, as needed, the family and the list is explained to the resident and/or family.

Rationale for NPSG.08.03.01

The accurate communication of the resident's medication list to the resident and, as needed, the family reduces the risk of transition-related adverse drug events. A thorough knowledge of the resident's medications is essential for the resident's primary care provider or next provider of service to manage the subsequent stages of care for the resident.

Element of Performance for NPSG.08.03.01

C Ⓜ 1. When the resident leaves the organization's care, the current list of reconciled medications is provided and explained to the resident and, as needed, to the family. This interaction is documented.

Note: *Residents and families are reminded to discard old lists and to update any records with all medication providers or retail pharmacies.*

NPSG.08.04.01

In settings where medications are used minimally or prescribed for a short duration, modified medication reconciliation processes are performed.

Note: This requirement does not apply to organizations that do not administer medications. It may be important for health care organizations to know which types of medications their residents are taking because these medications could affect the care, treatment, or services provided.

Rationale for NPSG.08.04.01

A number of resident care settings exist in which medications are not used, are used minimally, or are prescribed for only a short duration. This includes areas such as the emergency department, urgent and emergent care, convenient care, office-based surgery, outpatient radiology, ambulatory care, and behavioral health care. In these settings, obtaining a list of the resident's original, known, and current medications that he or she is taking at home is still important; however, obtaining information on the dose, route, and frequency of use is not required.

Elements of Performance for NPSG.08.04.01

C Ⓜ 1. The organization obtains and documents an accurate list of the resident's current medications and known allergies in order to safely prescribe any setting-specific medications (for example, local anesthesia, antibiotics) and to assess for potential allergic or adverse drug reactions. ⚠3

C Ⓜ 2. When only short-term medications (for example, a pre-procedure medication or a short-term course of an antibiotic) will be prescribed and no changes are made to the resident's current medication list, the resident and, as needed, the family is provided with a list containing the short term medication additions that the resident will continue after leaving the organization. ⚠3

Note: *This list of new short-term medications is not considered to be part of the original, known and current medication list. When residents leave these settings, a list of the original, known, and current medications does not need to be provided unless the resident is assessed to be confused or unable to comprehend adequately. In this case, the resident's family is provided both medication lists, and the circumstances are documented.*

C Ⓜ 3. In these settings, a complete, documented medication reconciliation process is used when: Any new long-term (chronic) medications are prescribed. ⚠3

C Ⓜ 4. In these settings, a complete, documented medication reconciliation process is used when: There is a prescription change for any of the resident's current, known long-term medications. ⚠3

C Ⓜ 5. In these settings, a complete, documented medication reconciliation process is used when: The resident is required to be subsequently admitted to an organization from these settings for ongoing care. ⚠3

C Ⓜ 6. When a complete, documented medication reconciliation is required in any of these settings, the complete list of reconciled medications is provided to the resident and, as needed, the family, and to the resident's known primary care provider or original referring provider or a known next provider of service. ⚠3

Goal 9—Reduce the risk of resident harm resulting from falls.

NPSG.09.02.01

The organization implements a fall reduction program that includes an evaluation of the effectiveness of the program.

Rationale for NPSG.09.02.01

Falls account for a significant portion of injuries in hospitalized patients, long term care residents, and home care recipients. In the context of the population it serves, the services it provides, and its environment of care, the organization should evaluate the resident's risk for falls and take action to reduce the risk of falling as well as the risk of injury, should a fall occur. The evaluation could include a resident's fall history; review of medications and alcohol consumption; gait and balance screening; assessment of walking aids, assistive technologies and protective devices; and environmental assessments.

Elements of Performance for NPSG.09.02.01

A 1. The organization establishes a fall reduction program.

C Ⓜ 2. The fall reduction program includes an evaluation appropriate to the resident populations, settings, and services provided. ⚠3

A 3. The fall reduction program includes interventions to reduce the resident's fall risk factors. ⚠3

C Ⓜ 4. Staff receive education and training for the fall reduction program

C Ⓜ 5. The organization educates the resident and, as needed, the family on the fall reduction program and any individualized fall reduction strategies.

A 6. The organization evaluates the fall reduction program to determine the effectiveness of the program.

Note: *Outcome indicators such as decreased number of falls and decreased number and severity of fall-related injuries could be used.*

Goal 10—Reduce the risk of influenza and pneumococcal disease in institutionalized older adults.

Introduction to NPSG.10.01.01 through NPSG.10.03.01

Influenza and pneumonia combined represent the fifth leading cause of death in the elderly. Along with the Centers for Medicare & Medicaid Services (CMS) and the Centers for Disease Control and Prevention (CDC), The Joint Commission promotes the administration of influenza and pneumococcal vaccines to adult residents in long term care, assisted living facilities, and disease-specific care programs.

NPSG.10.01.01

The organization develops and implements protocols for administration of the influenza vaccine.

Elements for Performance for NPSG.10.01.01

A 1. Appropriate protocols are developed to determine whether to administer the influenza vaccine to a resident. ⚠3

C Ⓜ 2. Protocols are implemented for residents identified as high risk for influenza. ⚠3

NPSG.10.02.01

The organization develops and implements protocols for administration of the pneumococcus vaccine.

Elements of Performance for NPSG.10.02.01

A 1. Protocols are developed to determine whether to administer the pneumococcus vaccine to a resident. ⚠3

C Ⓜ 2. Protocols are implemented for residents identified as high risk for pneumococcus. ⚠3

NPSG.10.03.01

The organization develops and implements protocols to identify new cases of influenza and to manage outbreaks.

Elements of Performance for NPSG.10.03.01

A 1. Protocols are developed to identify new cases of influenza and to manage an outbreak. ⚠3

C Ⓜ 2. Protocols are implemented for residents displaying signs and symptoms of influenza. ⚠3

A 3. Evidence exists that the outbreak was managed (or identified) and tracked.

Goal 13—Encourage residents' active involvement in their own care as a resident safety strategy.

NPSG.13.01.01

Identify the ways in which the resident and his or her family can report concerns about safety and encourage them to do so.

Rationale for NPSG.13.01.01

Communication with the resident and family about all aspects of care, treatment, or services is an important characteristic of a culture of safety. When the resident knows what to expect, he or she is more aware of possible errors and choices. The resident can also be an important source of information about potential adverse events and hazardous conditions.

Elements of Performance for NPSG.13.01.01

C Ⓜ 1. The resident and family are educated on available reporting methods for concerns related to care, treatment, or services, and resident safety issues.

C Ⓜ 2. The organization provides the resident with information regarding infection control measures for hand hygiene practices, respiratory hygiene practices ,and contact precautions, according to the resident's condition. The information is discussed with the resident and his or her family members on the day the resident enters the long term care organization or as soon as possible (for example, within 24-48 hours). The resident's understanding of this information is evaluated and documented.

Note: *The information provided to the resident may be in any form of media.*

C Ⓜ 4. The organization encourages residents and their families to report concerns about safety.

Goal 14—Prevent health care–associated pressure ulcers (decubitus ulcers).

NPSG.14.01.01

Assess and periodically reassess each resident's risk for developing a pressure ulcer (decubitus ulcer) and take action to address any identified risks.

Rationale for NPSG.14.01.01

Pressure ulcers (decubiti) continue to be problematic in all heath care settings. Most pressure ulcers can be prevented, and deterioration at Stage I can be halted. The use of clinical practice guidelines can effectively identify residents and define early intervention for prevention of pressure ulcers.

Elements of Performance for NPSG.14.01.01

A 1. The organization has a written plan for the prediction, prevention, and early treatment of pressure ulcers, which addresses the following: A
- Identifying individuals at risk for pressure ulcers and the specific factors that place them at risk.
- Maintaining and improving tissue tolerance to pressure in order to prevent injury.
- Protecting against the adverse effects of external mechanical forces.
- Reducing the incidence of pressure ulcers through staff educational programs.

C Ⓜ 2. An initial assessment for the risk of pressure ulcers is performed for each resident at admission. ⚠3

C Ⓜ 3. A systematic risk assessment for pressure ulcers is conducted using a validated risk assessment tool such as the Braden Scale or Norton Scale. ⚠3

C Ⓜ 4. Pressure ulcer risk is reassessed at periodic intervals. ⚠3

C Ⓜ 5. The organization takes action to address any identified risks to the resident for pressure ulcers. ⚠3

Standards

The following is a list of all standards for Medicare/Medicaid Certification–Based Long Term Care Accreditation. They are presented here for your convenience without footnotes or other explanatory text. If you have a question about a term used here, please check the Glossary.

Note: *A revised standard numbering system is being used with the reformatted standards. The revised numbering system allows for more flexibility to add standards while maintaining the current label for each standard.*

Ethics, Rights, and Responsibilities

RI.1.10 Not applicable

RI.1.20 Through RI.2.80 Not applicable

RI.2.90 Residents and, when appropriate, their families are informed about the outcomes of care, treatment, and services that have been provided, including unanticipated outcomes.

RI.2.100 Through RI.2.150 Not applicable

RI.2.160 Residents have the right to pain management.

RI.2.170 Through RI.3.10 Not applicable

Provision of Care, Treatment, and Services

PC.1.10 Through PC.4.120 Not applicable

PC.5.10 The organization provides care, treatment, and services for each resident according to the plan for care, treatment, and services.

PC.5.20 Through PC.5.70 Not applicable

PC.6.10 The resident receives education and training specific to the resident's needs and as appropriate to the care, treatment, and services provided.

PC.6.20 Through PC.8.70 Not applicable

PC.9.10 Blood and blood components are administered safely, as appropriate to the setting.

PC.9.20 Through PC.15.50 Not applicable

PC.16.10 The director named on the CLIA certificate establishes policies and procedures that define the context in which waived test results are used in resident care, treatment, and services.

PC.16.20 The director named on the CLIA certificate identifies the staff responsible for performing and supervising waived testing.

PC.16.30 Staff receive specific training and orientation for the tests they perform and demonstrate satisfactory levels of competence.

PC.16.40 Policies and procedures governing specific testing-related processes are current, approved, and readily available.

PC.16.50 Quality control checks are conducted on each procedure.

PC.16.60 Quality control and test result records are maintained.

PC.17.10 Not applicable

PC.17.20 Not applicable

PC.17.30 Not applicable

Medication Management

MM.1.10 Not applicable

MM.2.10 Not applicable

MM.2.20 Medications are properly and safely stored.

MM.2.30 Through MM.8.10 Not applicable

Surveillance, Prevention, and Control of Infection

IC.1.10 Through IC.9.10 Not applicable

Improving Organization Performance

PI.1.10 The organization collects data to monitor its performance.

PI.1.20 Not applicable

PI.2.10 Data are systematically aggregated and analyzed.

PI.2.20 Undesirable patterns or trends in performance are analyzed.

PI.2.30 Not applicable

PI.3.10 Information from data analysis is used to make changes that improve performance and resident safety and reduce the risk of sentinel events.

PI.3.20 Not applicable

Leadership

LD.01.03.01 Governance is ultimately accountable for the safety and quality of care, treatment, and services.

LD.02.01.01 The mission, vision, and goals of the organization support the safety and quality of care, treatment, and services.

LD.03.01.01 Leaders create and maintain a culture of safety and quality throughout the organization.

LD.03.02.01 The organization uses data and information to guide decisions and to understand variation in the performance of processes supporting safety and quality.

LD.03.03.01 Leaders use organization-wide planning to establish structures and processes that focus on safety and quality.

LD.03.04.01 The organization communicates information related to safety and quality to those who need it, including staff, residents, families, and external interested parties.

LD.03.05.01 Leaders implement changes in existing processes to improve the performance of the organization.

LD.03.06.01 Those who work in the organization are focused on improving safety and quality.

LD.04.01.01 The organization complies with law and regulation.

LD.04.01.07 The organization has policies and procedures that guide and support resident care, treatment, or services.

LD.04.02.03 Ethical principles guide the organization's business practices.

LD.04.02.05 When internal or external review results in the denial of care, treatment, and services or payment, the organization makes decisions regarding the ongoing provision of care, treatment, and services and discharge or transfer, based on the assessed needs of the resident.

LD.04.03.09 Care, treatment, and services provided through contractual agreement are provided safely and effectively.

LD.04.04.01 Leaders establish priorities for performance improvement.

LD.04.04.03 New or modified services or processes are well-designed.

LD.04.04.05 The organization has an organization-wide, integrated resident safety program.

Management of the Environment of Care

EC.1.10 The organization manages safety risks.

EC.1.20 The organization maintains a safe environment.

EC.1.25 Not applicable

EC.1.27 Not applicable

EC.1.30 The organization develops and implements a policy to prohibit smoking except in specified circumstances.

EC.2.10 Not applicable

EC.3.10 The organization manages its hazardous materials and waste risks.

EC.4.10 The organization addresses emergency management.

EC.4.20 Through EC.5.50 Not applicable

EC.6.10 The organization manages medical equipment risks.

EC.6.20 Medical equipment is maintained, tested, and inspected.

EC.6.30 Through EC.6.130 Not applicable

EC.7.10 The organization manages its utility risks.

EC.7.20 Not applicable

EC.7.30 The organization maintains, tests, and inspects its utility systems.

EC.7.40 Not applicable

EC.7.50 The organization maintains, tests, and inspects its medical gas and vacuum systems.

EC.8.10 Not applicable

EC.8.20 Not applicable

EC.8.30 Not applicable

EC.9.10 The organization monitors conditions in the environment.

EC.9.20 The organization analyzes identified environment issues and develops recommendations for resolving them.

EC.9.30 The organization improves the environment.

Management of Human Resources

HR.1.10 Not applicable

HR.1.15 Not applicable

HR.1.20 Staff qualifications are consistent with his or her job responsibilities.

HR.1.25 The organization may assign disaster responsibilities to volunteer practitioners.

HR.1.30 The organization uses data from clinical/service screening indicators and human resource screening indicators to assess and continuously improve staffing effectiveness.

HR.2.10 The organization provides initial orientation.

HR.2.20 Staff and licensed independent practitioners, as appropriate, can describe or demonstrate their roles and responsibilities relative to safety.

HR.2.30 Ongoing education, including in-services, training, and other activities, maintains and improves staff competence.

HR.3.10 Staff competence to perform job responsibilities is assessed, demonstrated, and maintained.

HR.3.20 Through HR.3.60 Not applicable

HR.4.10 There is a process for ensuring the competence of all practitioners permitted by law and the organization to practice independently.

HR.4.20 Individuals permitted by law and the organization to practice independently are granted clinical privileges.

HR.4.30 The organization has a process for granting temporary clinical privileges, when appropriate.

HR.4.32 Not applicable

HR.4.33 Not applicable

HR.4.34 Not applicable

HR.4.35 The organization may grant disaster privileges to volunteers eligible to be licensed independent practitioners.

HR.4.40 There are mechanisms, including a fair hearing and appeal process, for addressing adverse decisions regarding reappointment denial, reduction, suspension, or revocation of clinical privileges that may relate to quality of care, treatment, and service issues.

HR.4.50 Clinical privileges and appointments/reappointments are reviewed and revised at least every two years.

HR.4.60 Through HR.5.40 Not applicable

Management of Information

IM.1.10 The organization plans and designs information management processes to meet internal and external information needs.

IM.2.10 Information privacy and confidentiality are maintained.

IM.2.20 Not applicable

IM.2.30 Not applicable

IM.3.10 The organization has processes in place to effectively manage information, including the capturing, reporting, processing, storing, retrieving, disseminating, and displaying of clinical/service and nonclinical data and information.

IM.4.10 The information management system provides information for use in decision making.

IM.5.10 Knowledge-based information resources are readily available, current, and authoritative.

IM.6.10 Through IM.6.40 Not applicable

IM.6.50 Designated qualified personnel accept and transcribe verbal orders from authorized individuals.

IM.6.60 Through IM.6.120 Not applicable

IM.6.130 Clinical record documentation includes the provision of education and its effectiveness.

IM.6.140 Through IM.6.280 Not applicable

Standards, Rationales, Elements of Performance, and Scoring

Ethics, Rights, and Responsibilities

Standard RI.1.10

Not applicable

Standard RI.1.20 Through RI.2.80

Not applicable

Standard RI.2.90

Residents and, when appropriate, their families are informed about the outcomes of care, treatment, and services that have been provided, including unanticipated outcomes.

Elements of Performance for RI.2.90

C Ⓜ 1. At a minimum, the resident and when appropriate, his or her family, is informed about outcomes of care, treatment, and services that have been provided that the resident (or family) must be knowledgeable about to participate in current and future decisions affecting the resident's care, treatment, and services.

C Ⓜ 2. At a minimum, the resident and when appropriate, his or her family, is informed about unanticipated outcomes of care, treatment, and services that relate to sentinel events considered reviewable* by the Joint Commission.

C Ⓜ 3. The responsible licensed independent practitioner or his or her designee informs the resident (and when appropriate, his or her family) about those unanticipated outcomes of care, treatment, and services related to sentinel events, when the resident is not already aware of the occurrence, or further discussion is needed (*see* EP 2 above).†

Standard RI.2.100 Through RI.2.150

Not applicable

---

* *See* the "Sentinel Events" chapter of this book for a definition of reviewable sentinel events.

† In settings where there is no licensed independent practitioner, the staff member responsible for the care of the resident is responsible for sharing information about such outcomes.

Standard RI.2.160

Residents have the right to pain management.

Rationale for RI.2.160

Residents may experience pain. Unrelieved pain has adverse physical and psychological effects. The organization respects and supports the right of residents to pain management. In accordance with the organization's mission, this may occur through referral.

Element of Performance for RI.2.160

A 1. The organization plans, supports, and coordinates activities and resources to ensure that pain is recognized and addressed appropriately and in accordance with the care, treatment, and services provided including the following:
- Assessing for pain
- Educating all relevant providers about assessing and managing pain
- Educating residents and families, when appropriate, about their roles in managing pain and the potential limitations and side effects of pain treatments ⚠3

Standard RI.2.170 Through RI.3.10

Not applicable

Provision of Care, Treatment, and Services

Standard PC.1.10 Through PC.4.120

Not applicable

Standard PC.5.10

The organization provides care, treatment, and services for each resident according to the plan for care, treatment, and services.

Elements of Performance for PC.5.10

1. Not applicable
2. Not applicable
3. Not applicable
4. Use at least two resident identifiers (neither to be the resident's room number) whenever administering medications or blood products; taking blood samples and other specimens for clinical testing, or providing any other treatments or procedures.

Note: *The preceding requirement is not scored here. It is scored at NPSG.01.01.01.*

Standard PC.5.20 Through PC.5.70

Not applicable

Standard PC.6.10

The resident receives education and training specific to the resident's needs and as appropriate to the care, treatment, and services provided.

Rationale for PC.6.10

Residents must be given sufficient information to make decisions and to take responsibility for self-management activities related to their needs. Residents and, as appropriate, their families are educated to improve individual outcomes by promoting healthy behavior and appropriately involving residents in their care, treatment, and service decisions.

Elements of Performance for PC.6.10

A 1. Education provided is appropriate to the resident's needs.

C Ⓜ 2. The assessment of learning needs addresses cultural and religious beliefs, emotional barriers, desire and motivation to learn, physical or cognitive limitations, and barriers to communication as appropriate.

A 3. As appropriate to the resident's condition and assessed needs and the organization's scope of services, the resident is educated about the following:

- The plan for care, treatment, and services
- His or her condition or illness and preventive interventions
- Basic health practices and safety
- The safe and effective use of medications
- Nutrition interventions, modified diets, or oral health
- Safe and effective use of medical equipment or supplies when provided by the organization
- Understanding pain, the risk for pain, the importance of effective pain management, the pain assessment process, and methods for pain management
- Habilitation or rehabilitation techniques to help them reach the maximum independence possible
- Environmental and physical plant safety issues, such as fire safety, evacuation, storage of chemical agents, and so on
- Use of nonmedical equipment, including, but not limited to, operating call lights, beds, and personal appliances

Standard PC.6.20 Through PC.8.70

Not applicable

Standard PC.9.10

Blood and blood components are administered safely, as appropriate to the setting.

Element of Performance for PC.9.10

1. Through 9. Not applicable

A 10. If the organization provides for the maintenance and transfusion of blood or blood components, it meets all applicable law and regulation. ⚠3

Standard PC.9.20 Through PC.15.50

Not applicable

Standard PC.16.10

The director named on the CLIA certificate establishes policies and procedures that define the context in which waived test results are used in resident care, treatment, and services.

Elements of Performance for PC.16.10

A 1. The director named on the CLIA certificate determines the context in which waived tests are used.

C Ⓜ 2. Clinical use of results is consistent with the organization's policies and the manufacturer's recommendations for waived tests. ⚠3

A 3. Quantitative test result reports in the clinical record are accompanied by reference ranges specific to the test method used and population served.

Note: *Semiquantitative results, such as urine macroscopic and urine dipsticks, are not required to comply with this EP.*

A 4. For qualitative and quantitative tests, criteria for confirmatory testing is specified in the written procedures.

A 5. These written procedures are based on clinical usage and limitations of the test methodology.

C Ⓜ 6. The criteria for confirmatory testing is followed as specified in the written procedures. ⚠3

Standard PC.16.20

The director named on the CLIA certificate identifies the staff responsible for performing and supervising waived testing.

Elements of Performance for PC.16.20

A 1. The identity of staff members who perform testing is documented.

A 2. The identity staff members who direct or supervise testing is documented.

Note: *These individuals may be employees of the organization, contracted staff, or employees of a contracted service.*

Standard PC.16.30

Staff receive specific training and orientation for the tests they perform, and demonstrate satisfactory levels of competence.

Rationale for PC.16.30

For waived tests to be performed properly, the staff performing them must be qualified to do so. Staff members who perform waived testing have specific training for each test performed. This training can be acquired through organization or other training programs, such as those provided by another health care organization or manufacturer.

Elements of Performance for PC.16.30

A 1. Staff members who perform testing have been oriented according to the organization's specific services.

A 2. Staff members who perform testing have been trained for each test he or she is authorized to perform.

A 3. Staff members who perform testing that requires the use of an instrument have been trained on the use and maintenance of that instrument.

A 4. Competence is assessed according to organization policy at defined intervals, but at least at the time of orientation and annually thereafter.

A 5. Current competency is assessed using at least two of the following methods per person per test:
- Performing a test on a blind specimen*
- Having the supervisor or qualified delegate periodically observe routine work
- Monitoring each user's quality control performance
- Having written testing that is specific to the method assessed ⚠3

A 6. The director named on the CLIA certificate or qualified designee evaluates and documents evidence of orientation, training, and competency.

Note: *Staff who perform instrument-based testing, including (but not limited to) physicians, licensed independent practitioners, contracted staff, and RNs, participate in training and competence demonstrations.*

Standard PC.16.40

Policies and procedures governing specific testing-related processes are current, approved, and readily available.

* **Blind specimen** A sample with known value tested by personnel who do not know the expected result.

Rationale for PC.16.40

Current and up-to-date policies and procedures are an important reference tool in managing laboratory testing activities. Testing policies and procedures include requirements that are in compliance with the manufacturer's recommendations regarding all the following, as applicable:

- Specimen type (e.g., a method for whole blood is not used for spinal fluid)
- Storage considerations for test components (e.g., compliance with directions such as store away from direct light, temperature requirements, open container expiration dates, and so forth)
- Instrument maintenance and function checks such as calibration
- Quality control frequency and type
- Result follow-up recommendations (e.g., a recommendation to repeat the test when the results are higher or lower than the reportable range of the test)*
- Tests approved by the FDA for home use only are not used for professional purposes (e.g., glucose meters cleared for home use only are not used in a hospital setting by nursing staff except as resident education)

Elements of Performance for PC.16.40

A 1. The director named on the CLIA certificate or a qualified designee approves policies and procedures at the following times:
- Before initial use of the test for patient testing
- Periodically thereafter, defined by the director but at least once every three years
- When there are changes in procedures†

A 2. Written policies and procedures address the following items:
- Specimen type, collection, identification, and required labeling
- Specimen preservation, as appropriate
- Instrument maintenance and function checks, such as calibration
- Storage conditions for test components

Note: *No reagent is used after its expiration date.*
- Quality control (including frequency and type) and remedial action
- Result reporting

Note: *Individual patient results are not reported unless the quality control is acceptable.*
- Equipment performance evaluation
- Test performance

A 3. If manufacturers' manuals or package inserts are used as the policies or procedures for each test, they must be enhanced to include specific operational policies (e.g., detailed quality control protocols and any other institution-specific procedures regarding the test or instrument).

---

* **Reportable range** The span of test result values over which the laboratory can verify the accuracy of the instrument or test system measurement response.

† **Changes in procedures** Manufacturer updates to package inserts can include procedural changes or a different manufacturer is used.

A 4. Current and complete policies and procedures are readily available to the person performing the test.

A 5. Written policies, procedures, and manufacturer's instructions are followed. ⚠3

Standard PC.16.50

Quality control checks are conducted on each procedure.

Elements of Performance for PC.16.50

A 1. The director named on the CLIA certificate establishes a written quality control plan that specifies how procedures will be controlled for quality, establishes timetables, and explains the rationale for choice of procedures and timetables.

A 2. The documented quality control rationale is based on the following:
- How the test is used
- Reagent stability
- Manufacturers' recommendations
- The organization's experience with the test
- Currently accepted guidelines

A 3. Quality control procedures are performed at least as frequently as recommended by the manufacturer or defined by the organization's policies. ⚠3

Note: *If frequency of quality control is not defined by the manufacturer, the organization defines frequency of quality control.*

C Ⓜ 4. For instrument-based waived testing, quality control requirements include two levels of control, if commercially available. ⚠3

C Ⓜ 5. For instrument-based waived testing, quality control procedures are performed at least once each day on each instrument used that day for resident testing. ⚠3

Standard PC.16.60

Quality control and test result records are maintained.

Elements of Performance for PC.16.60

C Ⓜ 1. Quality control results are documented, including internal and external (liquid and electronic).

Note: *Quality control results may be located in the clinical record.*

C Ⓜ 2. Test results are documented in the clinical record.

A 3. Individual test results are associated with quality control and instrument records.

Note: *A formal log is not required, but a functional audit trail is maintained that allows retrieval of individual test results and their association with quality control and instrument records.*

A 4. Quality control and test result records are retained for at least two years.

Standard PC.17.10

Not applicable

Standard PC.17.20

Not applicable

Standard PC.17.30

Not applicable

Medication* Management

Standard MM.1.10

Not applicable

Standard MM.2.10

Not applicable

Standard MM.2.20

Medications are properly and safely stored.

Rationale for MM.2.20

Appropriate medication storage increases patient safety. Medication storage is designed to assist in maintaining medication integrity, promote the availability of medications when needed, minimize the risk of medication diversion, and reduce potential dispensing errors.

---

* For the purpose of these standards, *medication* includes prescription medications, sample medications, herbal remedies, vitamins, nutraceuticals, over-the-counter drugs, vaccines, diagnostic and contrast agents used on or administered to persons to diagnose, treat, or prevent disease or other abnormal conditions; radioactive medications; respiratory therapy treatments; parenteral nutrition; blood derivatives; intravenous solutions (plain, with electrolytes, and/or drugs); and any product designated by the Food and Drug Administration (FDA) as a drug. The definition of *medication* does not include enteral nutrition solutions (which are considered food products), oxygen, and other medical gases.

Note: *The following elements of performance also apply to emergency medications.*

Elements of Performance for MM.2.20

1. Through 7. Not applicable

8. Identify and, at a minimum, annually review a list of look-alike/sound-alike drugs used: in the organization, and take action to prevent errors involving the interchange of these drugs.

   Note: *The preceding requirement is not scored here. It is scored at NPSG.03.03.01.*

9. Not applicable

A 10. Standardize and limit the number of drug concentrations available in the organization.

A Ⓜ 11. Concentrated electrolytes are removed from care units or areas (unless resident safety is at risk if the concentrated electrolyte is not immediately available on a specific care unit or area; in such situations, specific precautions are taken to prevent inadvertent administration). ⚠3

MM.2.30 Through MM.8.10

Not applicable

Surveillance, Prevention and Control of Infection

IC.1.10 Through IC.9.10

Not applicable

Improving Organization Performance

Standard PI.1.10

The organization collects data to monitor its performance.

Rationale for PI.1.10

Data help determine performance improvement priorities. The data collected for high-priority and required areas are used to monitor the stability of existing processes, identify opportunities for improvement, identify changes that lead to improvement, or sustain improvement. Data collection helps identify specific areas that require further study. These areas are determined by considering the information provided by the data about process stability, risks, and sentinel events, and priorities set by the leaders. Data may come from internal sources such as staff or external sources such as patients, referral sources, and so on. In addition, the organization identifies those areas needing improvement and identifies desired changes. Performance measures are used to determine whether the changes result in desired outcomes. The organization identifies the frequency and detail of data collection.

Note: *The organization also collects data on the following areas that will be scored in their respective chapters:*

- *Evaluation and improvement of conditions in the environment* (see *the "Management of the Environment of Care" chapter)*
- *Staffing effectiveness* (see *the "Management of Human Resources" chapter)*

Note: *For long term care organizations that serve residents with dementia, the organization may measure performance in the following areas: psychotropic drugs, incidents, acute behavioral events, family involvement, do-not-resuscitate orders, appropriate use of services, transfers, programs that meet resident needs, infection control, environmental adaptations, and safety.*

Elements of Performance for PI.1.10

A 1. The organization collects data for priorities identified by leaders (*see* Standard LD.4.50).

A 2. The organization considers collecting data in the following areas:
- Staff opinions and needs
- Staff perceptions of risks to individuals and suggestions for improving resident safety
- Staff willingness to report unanticipated adverse events

A 3. The organization collects data on the perceptions of care, treatment, and services* of residents including the following:
- Their specific needs and expectations
- How well the organization meets these needs and expectations
- How the organization can improve resident safety
- The effectiveness of pain management, when applicable

The organization collects data that measure the performance of each of the following potentially high-risk processes, when provided (EPs 4–6, 8):

A 4. Medication management

A 5. Blood and blood product use

A 6. Restraint use

7. Not applicable

A 8. Behavior management and treatment

9. Through 12. Not applicable

---

* The Joint Commission is moving from the phrase *satisfaction with care, treatment, and services* toward the more inclusive phrase *perception of care, treatment, and services* to better measure the performance of organizations meeting the needs, expectations, and concerns of residents. By using this term, the organization will be prompted to assess not only residents' and/or families' satisfaction with care, treatment, and services, but also whether the organization meets their needs and expectations.

Relevant information developed from the following activities (EPs 13–17) is integrated into performance improvement initiatives. This occurs in a way consistent with any organization policies or procedures intended to preserve any confidentiality or privilege of information established by applicable law.

A 13. Risk management

A 14. Utilization management

A 15. Quality control

A 16. Infection control surveillance and reporting

A 17. Research, as applicable

Standard PI.1.20

Not applicable

Standard PI.2.10

Data are systematically aggregated and analyzed.

Rationale for PI.2.10

Aggregating and analyzing data means transforming data into information. Aggregating data at points in time enables the organization to judge a particular process's stability or a particular outcome's predictability in relation to performance expectations. Accumulated data are analyzed in such a way that current performance levels, patterns, or trends can be identified.

Elements of Performance for PI.2.10

A 1. Collected data are aggregated and analyzed.

A 2. Data are aggregated at the frequency appropriate to the activity or process being studied.

A 3. Statistical tools and techniques are used to analyze and display data.

4. Data are analyzed and compared internally over time and externally* with other sources of information when available.

5. Comparative data are used to determine if there is excessive variability or unacceptable levels of performance, when available.

Standard PI.2.20

Undesirable patterns or trends in performance are analyzed.

---

* External sources of information include recent scientific, clinical, and management literature, including sentinel event alerts; well-formulated practice guidelines or parameters; performance measures; reference databases; other organizations with similar processes, and standards that are periodically reviewed and revised.

Elements of Performance for PI.2.20

A 1. Analysis is performed when data comparisons indicate that levels of performance, patterns, or trends vary substantially from those expected.

A 2. Analysis occurs for those topics chosen by leaders as performance improvement priorities.

A 3. Analysis is performed when undesirable variation occurs which changes priorities.

An analysis is performed for the following (EPs 4–6, 9–10):

A 4. All confirmed transfusion reactions, if applicable to the organization

A 5. All serious adverse drug events, if applicable and as defined by the organization

A 6. All significant medication errors, if applicable and as defined by the organization

7. Not applicable

8. Not applicable

A 9. Hazardous conditions

A 10. Staffing effectiveness issues

Standard PI.2.30

Not applicable

Standard PI.3.10

Information from data analysis is used to make changes that improve performance and resident safety and reduce the risk of sentinel events.

Elements of Performance for PI.3.10

A 1. The organization uses the information from data analysis to identify and implement changes that will improve the quality of care, treatment, and services.

A 2. The organization identifies and implements changes that will reduce the risk of sentinel events.

A 3. The organization uses the information from data analysis to identify changes that will improve resident safety.

A 4. Changes made to improve processes or outcomes are evaluated to ensure that they achieve the expected results.

A 5. Appropriate actions are undertaken when planned improvements are not achieved or sustained.

Standard PI.3.20

Not applicable

Leadership

Standards, Rationales, Elements of Performance, and Scoring

Introduction to Leadership Structure, Standards LD.01.01.01 through LD.01.07.01

Each organization, regardless of its complexity, has a structured leadership. Many leadership responsibilities directly affect the provision of care, treatment, or services, as well as the day-to-day operations of the organization. In some cases, these responsibilities will be shared among leaders, and, in other cases, a particular leader has primary responsibility. Individual leaders may have several different roles. Regardless of the organization's structure, it is important that leaders carry out all their responsibilities.

A variety of individuals may work in the organization, including licensed independent practitioners, staff, volunteers, students, and independent contractors. These standards describe the overall responsibility of the governance for the safety and quality of care, treatment, or services provided by all of these individuals.

How well the leaders work together is key to effective organization performance, and the standards emphasize this. Leaders with different responsibilities—governance, management, and the clinical staff—bring different skills, experiences, and perspectives to the organization. Working together means that leaders have the opportunity to participate in discussions and have their opinions heard. Depending upon the topic and the organization, individuals may participate in decision making, and the governing body may delegate decision making to certain leaders. Final decisions, however, are always the ultimate responsibility of governance; this key principle is assumed in any standard that describes how leaders work together.

Standard LD.01.03.01

Governance is ultimately accountable for the safety and quality of care, treatment, or services.

Rationale for LD.01.03.01

Governance's ultimate responsibility for safety and quality derives from its legal responsibility and operational authority for organization performance. In this context, governance provides for internal structures and resources, including staff, that support safety and quality.

Elements of Performance for LD.01.03.01

A 1. Governance defines in writing its responsibilities.

A 2. Governance provides for organization management and planning.

A 3. Governance approves the organization's written scope of services.

A 4. Governance selects the administrator.

A 5. Governance provides for the resources needed to maintain safe, quality care, treatment, or services. (3)

A 6. Governance works with other leaders to annually evaluate the organization's performance in relation to its mission, vision, and goals.

A 11. If the organization has an organized medical staff, the governance approves its bylaws, rules, and regulations.

Introduction to Leadership Relationships, Standards LD.02.01.01 through LD.02.03.01

How well leaders work together and manage conflict affects an organization's performance. In fulfilling its role, the governance involves senior managers and leaders of the clinical staff in governance and management functions.

Good relationships thrive when leaders work together to develop the mission, vision, and goals of the organization; encourage honest and open communication; and address conflicts of interest.

Standard LD.02.01.01

The mission, vision, and goals of the organization support the safety and quality of care, treatment, or services.

Rationale for LD.02.01.01

The primary responsibility of leaders is to provide for the safety and quality of care, treatment or services. The purpose of the organization's mission, vision, and goals is to define how the organization will achieve safety and quality. The leaders are more likely to be aligned with the mission, vision and goals when they create them together. The common purpose of the organization is most likely achieved when it is understood by all who work in or are served by the organization.

Element of Performance for LD.02.01.01

A 3. Leaders communicate the mission, vision, and goals to staff and the population the organization serves.

Introduction to Organization Culture and System Performance, Standards LD.03.01.01 through LD.03.06.01

An organization's culture reflects the beliefs, attitudes, and priorities of its members, and it influences the effectiveness of performance. Although there may be a dominant culture, in many larger organizations diverse cultures exist that may or may not share the same values. In fact, diverse cultures can exist even in smaller organizations. Organization performance can be effective in either case. Successful organizations will work to develop a culture of safety and quality.

In a culture of safety and quality, all individuals are focused on maintaining excellence in performance. They accept the safety and quality of resident care, treatment, or services as personal responsibilities and work together to minimize any harm that might result from unsafe or poor quality of care, treatment, or services. Leaders create this culture by demonstrating their commitment to safety and quality and by taking actions to achieve the desired state. In a culture of this kind, one finds teamwork, open discussions of concerns about safety and quality, and the encouragement of and reward for internal and external reporting of safety and quality issues. The focus of attention is on the performance of systems and processes instead of the individual, although reckless behavior and a blatant disregard for safety are not tolerated. Organizations are committed to ongoing learning and have the flexibility to accommodate changes in technology, science, and the environment.

The leaders provide for the effective functioning of the organization, with a focus on safety and quality. Leaders plan, support, and implement key systems critical to this effort. The Joint Commission has identified five key systems that influence the effective performance of an organization. They are:

- Using data
- Planning
- Communicating
- Changing performance
- Staffing

Leadership provides the foundation for effective performance. The five key systems serve as pillars that are based on the foundation set by leadership and in turn support the many organization-wide processes (such as medication management) that are important to individual care, treatment, or services. Culture permeates the entire structure.

The five key systems are interrelated and need to function well together. The integration of these systems throughout the organization will facilitate the effective performance of the organization as a whole. Leaders develop a vision and goals for the performance of these systems and evaluate their performance. Leaders use results to develop strategies for future improvements.

Performance of many aspects of these systems may be directly observable. But in many cases, organizations demonstrate compliance through performance in standards located in other sections of this manual. These leadership standards are cited when patterns of performance suggest organization-wide issues.

The effective performance of these systems results in a culture in which safety and quality are priorities. The organization demonstrates this through a proactive, nonpunitive culture that is monitored and sustained by related reporting systems and improvement initiatives.

Many of the concepts in the following section have long existed in the standards.

Standard LD.03.01.01

Leaders create and maintain a culture of safety and quality throughout the organization.

Rationale for LD.03.01.01

Safety and quality thrive in an environment that supports teamwork and respect for other people, regardless of their position in the organization. Leaders demonstrate their commitment to quality and set expectations for those who work in the organization. Leaders evaluate the culture on a regular basis, using a variety of methods, such as formal surveys, focus groups, staff interviews, and data analysis.

Leaders encourage teamwork and create structures, processes, and programs that allow this positive culture to flourish. Disruptive behavior that intimidates others and affects morale or staff turnover can be harmful to resident care. Leaders must address disruptive behavior of individuals working at all levels of the organization, including management, clinical and administrative staff, licensed independent practitioners, and governing body members.

Elements of Performance for LD.03.01.01

A 1. Leaders regularly evaluate the culture of safety and quality.

A 2. Leaders prioritize and implement changes identified by the evaluation.

A 3. Leaders provide opportunities for all individuals who work in the organization to participate in safety and quality initiatives.

A 4. The organization has a code of conduct that defines acceptable, disruptive, and inappropriate behaviors.

A 5. Leaders create and implement a process for managing disruptive and inappropriate behaviors. ⚠3

A 6. Leaders provide education that focuses on safety and quality for all individuals. (See also LD.04.04.05, EP 6)

A 7. Leaders establish a team approach among all staff at all levels.

A 8. All individuals who work in the organization, including staff and licensed independent practitioners, are able to openly discuss issues of safety and quality.

A 9. Literature and advisories relevant to resident safety are available to all individuals who work in the organization.

A 10. Leaders define how members of the population(s) served can help identify and manage issues of safety and quality within the organization.

Standard LD.03.02.01

The organization uses data and information to guide decisions and to understand variation in the performance of processes supporting safety and quality.

Rationale for LD.03.02.01

Data help organizations make the right decisions. When decisions are supported by data, organizations are more likely to move in directions that help them achieve their goals. Successful organizations measure and analyze their performance. When data are analyzed and turned into information, this process helps organizations see patterns and trends and understand the reasons for their performance. Many types of data are used to evaluate performance, including data on outcomes of care, performance on safety and quality initiatives, resident satisfaction, process variation, and staff perceptions.

Elements of Performance for LD.03.02.01

A 1. Leaders set expectations for using data and information to improve the safety and quality of care, treatment, or services.

A 2. Leaders are able to describe how data and information are used to create a culture of safety and quality.

A 3. The organization uses processes to support systematic data and information use.

A 4. Leaders provide the resources needed for data and information use, including staff, equipment, and information systems.

A 5. The organization uses data and information in decision making that supports the safety and quality of care, treatment, or services.

A 6. The organization uses data and information to identify and respond to internal and external changes in the environment.

A 7. Leaders evaluate how effectively data and information are used throughout the organization.

Standard LD.03.03.01

Leaders use organizationwide planning to establish structures and processes that focus on safety and quality.

Rationale for LD.03.03.01

Planning is essential to the following:

- The achievement of short- and long-term goals.
- Meeting the challenge of external changes

- The design of services and work processes
- The creation of communication channels
- The improvement of performance
- The introduction of innovation

Planning includes contributions from the populations served, from those who work for the organization, and from other interested groups or individuals.

Elements of Performance for LD.03.03.01

A 1. Planning activities focus on improving resident safety and health care quality.

A 2. Leaders can describe how planning supports a culture of safety and quality.

A 3. Planning is systematic, and it involves designated individuals and information sources.

A 4. Leaders provide the resources needed to support the safety and quality of care, treatment, or services. (3)

A 5. Safety and quality planning is organizationwide.

A 6. Planning activities adapt to changes in the environment.

A 7. Leaders evaluate the effectiveness of planning activities.

Standard LD.03.04.01

The organization communicates information related to safety and quality to those who need it, including staff, residents, families, and external interested parties.

Rationale for LD.03.04.01

Effective communication is essential among individuals and groups within the organization and between the organization and external parties. Poor communication often contributes to adverse events and can compromise safety and quality of care, treatment or services. Effective communication is timely, accurate, and usable by the audience.

Elements of Performance for LD.03.04.01

A 1. Communication processes foster the safety of the resident and the quality of care.

A 2. Leaders are able to describe how communication supports a culture of safety and quality.

A 3. Communication is designed to meet the needs of internal and external users.

A 4. Leaders provide the resources required for communication, based on the needs of resident, staff, and administration.

A 5. Communication supports safety and quality throughout the organization. (*See also* LD.04.04.05, EPs 6 and 12)

A 6. When changes in the environment occur, the organization communicates those changes effectively.

A 7. Leaders evaluate the effectiveness of communication methods.

Standard LD.03.05.01

Leaders implement changes in existing processes to improve the performance of the organization.

Rationale for LD.03.05.01

Change is inevitable, and agile organizations are able to manage change and rapidly execute new plans. The ability of leaders to manage change is necessary for performance improvement, for successful innovation, and to meet environmental challenges. The organization integrates change into all relevant processes so that its effectiveness can be sustained, assessed, and measured.

Elements of Performance for LD.03.05.01

A 1. Structures for managing change and performance improvements exist that foster the safety of the resident and the quality of care, treatment, or services.

A 2. Leaders are able to describe how the organization's approach to performance improvement and its capacity for change support a culture of safety and quality.

A 3. The organization has a systematic approach to change and performance improvement.

A 4. Leaders provide the resources required for performance improvement and change management, including sufficient staff, access to information, and training.

A 5. The management of change and performance improvement supports both safety and quality throughout the organization.

A 6. The organization's internal structures can adapt to changes in the environment.

A 7. Leaders evaluate the effectiveness of processes for the management of change and performance improvement.

Standard LD.03.06.01

Those who work in the organization are focused on improving safety and quality.

Rationale for LD.03.06.01

The safety and quality of care, treatment, or services are highly dependent on the people who work in the organization. The mission, scope, and complexity of services define the design of work processes and the skills and number of individuals needed. In a successful organization, work processes and the environment make safety and quality paramount. This standard, therefore, applies to all those who work in or for the organization, including staff and licensed independent practitioners.

Elements of Performance for LD.03.06.01

A 1. Leaders design work processes to focus individuals on safety and quality issues.

A 2. Leaders are able to describe how those who work in the organization support a culture of safety and quality.

A 3. Leaders provide for a sufficient number and mix of individuals to support safe, quality care, treatment, or services. ⚠3

A 4. Those who work in the organization are competent to complete their assigned responsibilities. ⚠3

A 5. Those who work in the organization adapt to changes in the environment.

A 6. Leaders evaluate the effectiveness of those who work in the organization to promote safety and quality.

Introduction to Leadership Operations, Standards LD.04.01.01 through LD.04.04.05

Although some leaders may not be involved in the day-to-day, hands-on operations of the organization, their decisions and work affect, either directly or indirectly, every aspect of operations. They are the driving force behind the culture of the organization. Leaders establish the ethical framework in which the organization operates, create policies and procedures, and secure resources and services that support resident safety and quality care, treatment, or services. Policies, procedures, resources, and services are all influenced by the culture of the organization, and, in turn, they influence the culture.

Standard LD.04.01.01

The organization complies with law and regulation.

Elements of Performance for LD.04.01.01

A 1. The organization is licensed, certified, or has a permit, in accordance with law and regulation, to provide the care, treatment, or services for which the organization is seeking accreditation from The Joint Commission. ▲2

Note 1: *Applicable law and regulation include, but are not limited to, individual and facility licensure, certification, Food and Drug Administration regulations, Drug Enforcement Agency regulations, Center for Medicare and Medicaid Services regulations, Occupational Safety and Health Administration regulations, Department of Transportation regulations, Health Insurance Portability and Accountability Act, and other local, state, and federal laws and regulations.*

Note 2: *Each service location that performs laboratory testing (waived or non waived) must have a Clinical Laboratory Improvement Amendments of 1988 (CLIA '88) certificate, as specified by the federal CLIA regulations (42 CFR 493.55 and 493.3) and applicable state law.*

A 2. The organization provides care, treatment, or services in accordance with licensure requirements, laws, and rules and regulations. (3)

A 3. Leaders act on or comply with reports or recommendations from external authorized agencies, such as accreditation, certification, or regulatory bodies.

Standard LD.04.01.07

The organization has policies and procedures that guide and support resident care, treatment, or services.

Elements of Performance for LD.04.01.07

A 1. Leaders review and approve policies and procedures that guide and support resident care, treatment, or services.

A 2. The organization manages the implementation of policies and procedures.

Standard LD.04.02.03

Ethical principles guide the organization's business practices.

Elements of Performance for LD.04.02.03

A 1. The organization has a process that allows staff, residents, and families to address ethical issues or issues prone to conflict.

A 2. The organization uses its process to address ethical issues or issues prone to conflict.

A 3. The organization follows ethical practices for marketing and billing.

A 4. Marketing materials accurately represent the organization and address the care, treatment, or services that the organization provides either directly or by contractual arrangement.

---

* For more information on how to obtain a CLIA certificate, *see* http://www.cms.hhs.gov/CLIA/downloads/HowObtainCLIACertificate.pdf.

A 5. Care, treatment, or services are provided based on resident needs, regardless of compensation or financial risk sharing with those who work in the organization, including staff and licensed independent practitioners.

A 6. When leaders excuse staff members from a job responsibility, care, treatment, or services are not affected in a negative way.

A 7. Residents receive information about charges for which they will be responsible.

A 8. Residents are informed whenever services, charges, or coverage change.

Standard LD.04.02.05

When internal or external review results in the denial of care, treatment, or services or payment, the organization makes decisions regarding the ongoing provision of care, treatment, or services and discharge or transfer, based on the assessed needs of the resident.

Rationale for LD.04.02.05

The organization is professionally and ethically responsible for providing care, treatment, or services within its capability and law and regulation. At times, such care, treatment, or services are denied because of payment limitations. In these situations, the decision to continue providing care, treatment, or services or to discharge the resident is based solely on the resident's identified needs.

Element of Performance for LD.04.02.05

A 2. The safety and quality of care, treatment, or services do not depend on the resident's ability to pay.

Introduction to Oversight of Care, Treatment, or Services Provided through Contractual Agreement, Standard LD.04.03.09

The same level of care should be delivered to residents, regardless of whether services are provided directly by the organization or through contractual agreement. Leaders provide oversight to make sure that care, treatment, or services provided directly are safe and effective. Likewise, leaders must also oversee contracted services to make sure that they are provided safely and effectively. Standard LD.04.03.09 outlines the requirements for leadership oversight of care, treatment, or services provided through contractual agreement.

The only contractual agreements subject to the requirements in Standard LD.04.03.09 are those for the provision of care, treatment, or services provided to the organization's residents. This standard does not apply to contracted services that are not directly related to resident care. In addition, contracts for consultation or referrals are not subject to the requirements in LD.04.03.09. However, regardless of whether a contract is subject to this standard, the actual performance of any contracted service is evaluated at the other standards in this manual appropriate to the nature of the contracted service.

Monitoring Contracted Services

The expectations that leaders set for the performance of contracted services should reflect basic principles of risk reduction, safety, staff competence, and performance improvement. Although leaders have the same responsibility for oversight of contracted services outside the organization's expertise as they do for contracted services within the organization's expertise, it is more difficult to determine how to monitor such services. In these cases, information from relevant professional organizations can provide guidance for setting expectations.

The EPs do not prescribe the methods for evaluating contracted services; leaders are expected to select the best methods for their organization to oversee the quality and safety of services provided through contractual agreement. Some examples of sources of information that may be used for evaluating contracted services include the following:

- Review of information about the contractor's Joint Commission accreditation or certification status
- Direct observation of the provision of care
- Audit of documentation, including medical records
- Review of incident reports
- Review of periodic reports submitted by the individual or organization providing services under contractual agreement
- Collection of data that address the efficacy of the contracted service
- Review of performance reports based on indicators required in the contractual agreement
- Input from staff and residents
- Review of resident satisfaction studies
- Review of results of risk management activities

In the event that contracted services do not meet expectations, leaders take steps to improve care, treatment, or services. In some cases it may be best to work with the contractor to make improvements, whereas in other cases it may be best to renegotiate or terminate the contractual relationship. When the leaders anticipate the renegotiation or termination of a contractual agreement, planning needs to occur so that the continuity of care, treatment, or services is not disrupted.

Credentialing and Privileging

In most cases, each licensed independent practitioner providing services through a contractual agreement must be credentialed and privileged by the organization using their services, following the process described in the "Management of Human Resources" chapter. However, there is one special circumstance when this is not required:

- Off-site services provided by a Joint Commission–accredited contractor.

Standard LD.04.03.09

Care, treatment, or services provided through contractual agreement are provided safely and effectively.

Elements of Performance for LD.04.03.09

A 1. Clinical leaders have an opportunity to provide advice about the sources of clinical services to be provided through contractual agreements.

A 2. The organization describes in writing the nature and scope of services provided through contractual agreements.

A 3. Designated leaders approve contractual agreements.

A 4. Leaders monitor contracted services by establishing expectations for the performance of the contracted services.

Note: *When the organization contracts with another accredited organization for resident care, treatment, or services to be provided off site, it can do the following:*
- *Verify that all licensed independent practitioners who will be providing resident care, treatment, or services have appropriate privileges by obtaining, for example, a copy of the list of privileges.*
- *Specify in the written agreement that the contracted organization will ensure that all contracted services provided by licensed independent practitioners will be within the scope of their privileges.*

A 5. Leaders monitor contracted services by communicating the expectations in writing to the provider of the contracted services.

Note: *A written description of the expectations can be provided either as part of the written agreement or in addition to it.*

A 6. Leaders monitor contracted services by evaluating these services in relation to the organization's expectations.

A 7. The leaders take steps to improve contracted services that do not meet expectations.

Note: *Examples of improvement efforts to consider include the following:*
- *Increase monitoring of the contracted services*
- *Provide consultation or training to the contractor*
- *Renegotiate the contract terms*
- *Apply defined penalties*
- *Terminate the contract*

A 8. When contractual agreements are renegotiated or terminated, the organization maintains the continuity of resident care. ⚠3

A 10. Reference and contract laboratory services meet the federal regulations for clinical laboratories and maintain evidence of the same.

Standard LD.04.04.01

Leaders establish priorities for performance improvement. (*See also* the "Improving Organization Performance" chapter)

Elements of Performance for LD.04.04.01

A 1. Leaders set priorities for performance improvement activities and resident health outcomes.

A 2. Leaders give priority to high-volume, high-risk, or problem-prone processes for performance improvement activities.

A 3. Leaders reprioritize performance improvement activities in response to changes in the internal or external environment.

A 4. Performance improvement occurs organization-wide.

Standard LD.04.04.03

New or modified services or processes are well-designed.

Elements of Performance for LD.04.04.03

A 1. The organization's design of new or modified services or processes incorporates: The needs of residents, staff, and others.

A 2. The organization's design of new or modified services or processes incorporates: The results of performance improvement activities.

A 3. The organization's design of new or modified services or processes incorporates: Information about potential risks to residents.

A 4. The organization's design of new or modified services or processes incorporates: Evidence-based information in the decision-making process.

Note: *For example, evidence-based information could include practice guidelines, successful practices, information from current literature, and clinical standards.*

A 5. The organization's design of new or modified services or processes incorporates: Information about sentinel events.

A 6. The organization tests and analyzes its design of new or modified services or processes to determine whether the proposed design or modification is an improvement.

A 7. The leaders involve staff and residents in the design of new or modified services or processes.

Introduction to Standard LD.04.04.05

This standard describes a safety program that integrates safety priorities into all processes, functions, and services within the organization, including resident care, support, and contract services. It addresses the responsibility of leaders to establish an organization-wide safety program; to proactively explore potential system failures; to analyze and take action on problems that have occurred; and to encourage the reporting of adverse events and near misses, both internally and externally. The organization's culture of safety and quality supports the safety program. (*See also* LD.03.01.01)

This standard does not require the creation of a new structure or office in the organization. It only emphasizes the need to integrate resident-safety activities, both existing and newly created, with the organization's leadership, which is ultimately responsible for this integration.

Standard LD.04.04.05

The organization has an organizationwide, integrated resident safety program.

Elements of Performance for LD.04.04.05

A 1. The organization implements an organizationwide resident safety program.

A 2. One or more qualified individuals or an interdisciplinary group manages the safety program.

A 3. The scope of the safety program includes the full range of safety issues, from potential or no-harm errors (sometimes referred to as near misses, close calls, or good catches) to hazardous conditions and sentinel events.

A 4. All departments, programs, and services within the organization participate in the safety program.

A 5. As part of the safety program, the organization creates procedures for responding to system or process failures.

Note: *Responses might include continuing to provide care, treatment, or services to those affected, containing the risk to others, and preserving factual information for subsequent analysis.*

A 6. The organization provides and encourages the use of systems for blame-free internal reporting of a system or process failure or the results of a proactive risk assessment. (*See also* LD.03.01.01, EP 8; LD.03.04.01, EP 5)

A 7. The organization defines *sentinel event* and communicates this definition throughout the organization.

Note: *At a minimum, the organization's definition includes those events subject to review in the "Sentinel Events" (SE) chapter of this book. The definition may include any process variation that does not affect the outcome or result in an adverse event, but for which a recurrence carries significant chance of a serious adverse outcome or result in an adverse event, often referred to as a* near miss.

A 8. The organization conducts thorough and credible root cause analyses in response to sentinel events, as described in the "Sentinel Events" (SE) section of this book. △3

A 9. The organization makes support systems available for staff who have been involved in an adverse or sentinel event.

Note: *Support systems recognize that conscientious health care workers who are involved in sentinel events are themselves victims of the event and require support. Support systems provide staff with additional help and support as well as additional resources through the human resources function or an employee assistance program. Support systems also focus on the process rather than blaming the involved individuals.*

A 10. At least every 12 months, the organization selects one high-risk process and conducts a proactive risk assessment.

Note: *See the Introduction to this standard for suggested components of a proactive risk assessment.*

A 11. To improve safety, the organization analyzes and uses information about system or process failures and the results of proactive risk assessments.

A 12. The organization disseminates lessons learned from root cause analyses, system or process failures, and the results of proactive risk assessments to all staff who provide services for the specific situation. (*See also* LD.03.04.01, EP 5)

A 13. At least once a year, the organization provides governance with written reports on the following:
- All system or process failures
- The number and type of sentinel events
- Whether the organization and the families were informed of the event
- All actions taken to improve safety, both proactively and in response to actual occurrences

A 14. The organization encourages external reporting of significant adverse events, including voluntary reporting programs in addition to mandatory programs.

Note: *Examples of voluntary programs include The Joint Commission's Sentinel Event Database and the Food and Drug Administration's (FDA) MedWatch. Mandatory programs are often state initiated.*

Management of the Environment of Care

Standard EC.1.10

The organization manages safety risks.

Rationale for EC.1.10

Each organization has inherent safety risks associated with providing services for residents, the performance of daily activities by staff, and the physical environment in which services occur. It is important that each organization identifies these risks and plans and implements processes to minimize the likelihood of those risks causing incidents.

Elements of Performance for EC.1.10

A 1. The organization develops and maintains a written management plan describing the processes it implements to effectively manage the environmental safety of residents, staff, and other people coming to the organization's facilities.

A 2. The organization identifies a person(s), as designated by leadership, to coordinate the development, implementation, and monitoring of the safety-management activities.

A 3. The organization identifies a person(s) to intervene whenever conditions immediately threaten life or health, or threaten damage to equipment or buildings.

A 4. The organization conducts comprehensive, proactive risk assessments that evaluate the potential adverse impact of buildings, grounds, equipment, occupants, and internal physical systems on the safety and health of residents, staff, and other people coming to the organization's facilities.

C Ⓜ 5. The organization uses the risks identified to select and implement procedures and controls to achieve the lowest potential for adverse impact on the safety and health of residents, staff, and other people coming to the organization's facilities.

C Ⓜ 6. The organization establishes safety policies and procedures that are practiced and reviewed as frequently as necessary, but at least every three years.

7. Not applicable

A 8. The organization ensures that a process exists for responding to product-safety recalls by appropriate organization staff.

A 9. The organization ensures that all grounds and equipment are maintained appropriately.

Standard EC.1.20

The organization maintains a safe environment.

Rationale for EC.1.20

It is essential that the organization conduct periodic environmental tours to determine if its current processes for managing resident, public, and staff safety risks are being practiced correctly and are effective. These tours can also be used to assess staff knowledge and behaviors, identify new or altered risks in areas where construction or changes in services have occurred, and identify opportunities to improve the environment.

Elements of Performance for EC.1.20

A 1. The organization conducts environmental tours to identify environmental deficiencies, hazards, and unsafe practices.

C Ⓜ 2. The organization conducts environmental tours at least every six months in all areas where residents are served.

C Ⓜ 3. The organization conducts environmental tours at least annually in areas where residents are not served.

Standard EC.1.25

Not applicable

Standard EC.1.27

Not applicable

Standard EC.1.30

The organization develops and implements a policy to prohibit smoking except in specified circumstances.

Rationale for EC.1.30

This standard is intended to reduce the following risks:

- To people who smoke, including possible adverse effects on care, treatment, and services
- Of passive smoking for others
- Of fire

The standard prohibits smoking in all areas of all building(s) under the organization's control, except for residents in circumstances specified in the following EPs.

Elements of Performance for EC.1.30

A 1. The organization develops a policy regarding smoking in all areas of all building(s) under the organization's control.

A 2. The organization's policy prohibits smoking in all areas of all building(s) under the organization's control (no medical exceptions allowed) for all children or youth residents.

A 3. The organization's policy may permit residents to smoke in the organization's buildings when a resident meets criteria developed and approved by the organization's leaders.

C Ⓜ 4. When residents are permitted to smoke in the organization's buildings, they smoke only under the following circumstance(s):
- In designated locations environmentally separate from care, treatment, and service areas*
- After the organization has taken measures to minimize fire risks ⚠3

C Ⓜ 5. Residents who do smoke in the organization's buildings are provided education, including information about options for smoking cessation.

A 6. The organization identifies and implements a process(es) for monitoring compliance with the policy.

A 7. The organization develops strategies to eliminate the incidence of policy violations when identified.

Standard EC.2.10

Not applicable

Standard EC.3.10

The organization manages its hazardous materials (HAZMAT) and waste† risks.

Rationale for EC.3.10

Organizations must identify materials they use that need special handling and implement processes to minimize the risks of their unsafe use and improper disposal.

Elements of Performance for EC.3.10

A 1. The organization develops and maintains a written management plan describing the processes it implements to effectively manage hazardous materials and wastes.

A 2. The organization creates and maintains an inventory that identifies HAZMAT and waste used, stored, or generated using criteria consistent with applicable law and regulation (for example, the Environmental Protection Agency [EPA] and the Occupational Safety and Health Administration [OSHA]).

---

* **Note:** *This does not require that a designated smoking area be a specific distance from care, treatment, and service areas. A physically separate, well-ventilated room (a designated area for authorized smoking by residents that is exhausted to the outside) is acceptable.*

† **HAZMAT and waste** Materials whose handling, use, and storage are guided or regulated by local, state, or federal regulation. Examples include OSHA's Regulations for Bloodborne Pathogens (regarding blood, other infectious materials, contaminated items that could release blood or other infectious materials, or contaminated sharps), the Nuclear Regulatory Commission's regulations for handling and disposal of radioactive waste, management of hazardous vapors (such as glutaraldehyde, ethylene oxide, and nitrous oxide), chemicals regulated by the EPA, Department of Transportation requirements, and hazardous energy sources (for example, ionizing or nonionizing radiation, lasers, microwaves, and ultrasound).

The organization establishes and implements processes for selecting, handling, storing, transporting, using, and disposing of hazardous materials and waste from receipt or generation through use and/or final disposal, including managing the following:

C Ⓜ 3. Chemicals

A 4. Chemotherapeutic materials ⚠3

A 5. Radioactive materials ⚠3

C Ⓜ 6. Infectious and regulated medical wastes, including sharps ⚠3

A 7. The organization provides adequate and appropriate space and equipment for safely handling and storing HAZMAT and waste.

8. Not applicable

A 9. The organization identifies and implements emergency procedures that include the specific precautions, procedures, and protective equipment used during HAZMAT and waste spills or exposures. ⚠3

A 10. The organization maintains documentation, including required permits, licenses, and adherence to other regulations.

C Ⓜ 11. The organization maintains required manifests for handling HAZMAT and waste.

C Ⓜ 12. The organization properly labels HAZMAT and waste.

A 13. The organization effectively separates HAZMAT and waste storage and processing areas from other areas of the facility.

Standard EC.4.10

Not applicable

Emergency Management

Introduction

Catastrophic emergencies are a threat to any health care organization, regardless of size, scope, or location. A single emergency* can temporarily affect demand for services; however, multiple emergencies that occur concurrently or sequentially can adversely impact patient safety and the organization's ability to provide care, treatment, and services for an extended length of time. This is especially true in situations

* **Emergency** A natural or manmade event that significantly disrupts the environment of care (for example, damage to the organization's building[s] and grounds due to severe winds, storms, or earthquakes); that significantly disrupts care, treatment and services (for example, loss of utilities such as power, water, or telephones due to floods, civil disturbances, accidents, or emergencies within the organization or in its community); or that results in sudden, significantly changed, or increased demands for the organization's services (for example, bioterrorist attack, building collapse, plane crash in the organization's community). Some emergencies are called *disasters* or *potential injury creating events (PICEs)*.

where the community cannot adequately support the organization. Power failures, water and fuel shortages, flooding, and communication breakdowns are just a few of the hazards that can disrupt patient care, and pose risks to staff and the organization.

No organization can predict the nature of a future emergency, nor can it predict the date of its arrival. However, organizations can plan for managing six critical areas of emergency response in order to assess their needs and prepare staff to respond to events most likely to occur regardless of the cause(s) of an emergency situation. The six critical areas of emergency management are as follows:

1. **Communication (*see* EC.4.13).** In the event that community infrastructure is damaged and/or an organization's power or facilities experience debilitation, communication pathways, whether dependent on fiber optic cables, electricity, satellite, or other conduits, are likely to fail. Organizations must develop a plan to maintain communication pathways both within the organization and to critical community resources.
2. **Resources and assets (*see* EC.4.14).** A solid understanding of the scope and availability of an organization's resources and assets is as important, and perhaps more important, during an emergency than during times of normal operation. Materials and supplies, vendor and community services, as well as state and federal programs, are some of the essential resources that organizations must know how to access in times of crisis in order to ensure patient safety and sustain care, treatment, and services.
3. **Safety and security (*see* EC.4.15).** The safety and security of residents is the prime responsibility of the organization during an emergency. As emergency situations develop and parameters of operability shift, organizations must provide a safe and secure environment for their residents and staff.
4. **Staff responsibilities (*see* EC.4.16).** During an emergency, the probability that staff responsibilities will change is high. As new risks develop along with changing conditions, staff will need to adapt their roles to meet new demands on their ability to care for patients. If staff cannot anticipate how they may be called to perform during an emergency, the likelihood that the organization will not sustain itself during an emergency increases.
5. **Utilities management (*see* EC.4.17).** An organization is dependent on the uninterrupted function of its utilities during an emergency. The supply of key utilities, such as power or potable water, ventilation, and fuel must not be disrupted or adverse events may occur as a result.
6. **Patient clinical and support activities (*see* EC.4.18).** The clinical needs of patients during an emergency are of prime importance. The organization must have clear, reasonable plans in place to address the needs of patients during extreme conditions when the organization's infrastructure and resources are taxed.

When organizations have a sound understanding of their response to these six critical areas of emergency management, they have developed an "all hazards" approach that supports a level of preparedness sufficient to address a range of emergencies, regardless of the cause. Organizations should also identify potential hazards, threats, and adverse events, and assess their impact on the care, treatment, and services they must sustain during an emergency. This assessment is known as a Hazard Vulnerability Analysis* (HVA) and is designed to assist organizations in gaining a realistic understanding of their vulnerabilities, and to help focus their resources and planning efforts. Finally, organizations should use the information from their assessments to develop Emergency Operations Plans (EOPs), which should be tested regularly, and use the lessons learned to improve.

Organizations should note that additional standards in other chapters are integral to organization-wide emergency preparedness, including processes for the following:
- Maintaining continuity of information (Management of Information chapter)
- Responding to an influx, or the risk of influx, of infectious patients (Surveillance, Prevention, and Control of Infection chapter)
- Granting disaster privileges (Management of Human Resources chapter)
- Assigning disaster responsibilities (Management of Human Resources chapter)

Standard EC.4.11

The organization plans for managing the consequences of emergencies.

Rationale for EC.4.11

An emergency in a health care organization or in its community can suddenly and significantly affect demand for its services or its ability to provide those services. Therefore, it is important that organizations define a comprehensive approach to identifying risks and mobilizing an effective response within the organization as well as in collaboration and coordination with essential response partners in the community.

Elements of Performance for EC.4.11

A 1. The organization's leaders including the administrator, the medical director, the nursing leader, and other clinical leaders actively participate in emergency management planning.

A 2. The organization conducts a Hazard Vulnerability Analysis (HVA) to identify events that could affect demand for its services or its ability to provide those services, the likelihood of those events occurring, and the consequences of those events.

Note: *The HVA is evaluated at least annually as part of EP 11.*

A 3. The organization prioritizes those hazards, threats and events identified in its HVA.

A 4. When developing its EOP (*see* EC.4.12), the organization communicates its needs and vulnerabilities to community emergency response agencies and identifies the capabilities of its community in meeting their needs.

* **Hazard vulnerability analysis** The identification of potential emergencies and the direct and indirect effects these emergencies may have on the organization's operations and the demand for its services.

A 5. For each emergency identified in its HVA, the organization defines mitigation activities designed to reduce the risk of and potential damage due to an emergency.

A 6. For each emergency identified in its HVA, the organization defines preparedness activities that will organize and mobilize essential resources.

A 7. For each emergency identified in its HVA, the organization defines response strategies and actions to be activated during the emergency.

A 8. For each emergency identified in its HVA, the organization defines recovery strategies and actions designed to help restore the systems that are critical to resuming normal care, treatment, and services.

A 9. The organization keeps a documented inventory of the assets and resources it has on site, that would be needed during an emergency (at a minimum, personal protective equipment, water, fuel, staffing, medical, and pharmaceuticals resources and assets).

Note: *The inventory is evaluated at least annually as part of EP 11.*

A 10. The organization establishes methods for monitoring quantities of assets and resources during an emergency.

A 11. The objectives, scope, performance, and effectiveness of the organization's emergency management planning efforts are evaluated at least annually.

Standard EC.4.12

The organization develops and maintains an Emergency Operations Plan.

Rationale for EC.4.12

A successful response relies upon planning around the management of six critical areas: communications; resources and assets; safety and security; staffing; utilities; and clinical activities. It is important for organizations to develop a comprehensive Emergency Operations Plan (EOP) as documentation to help guide the organization in its emergency response and recovery efforts. While the EOP can be formatted in a variety of ways, it must address these six critical areas to serve as a blueprint for managing care and safety during an emergency.

Some emergencies can escalate unexpectedly and strain the organization and the entire community. An organization cannot mitigate risks, plan thoroughly, and sustain an effective response and recovery without preparing its staff and collaborating with the community, suppliers and external response partners as well. Such an approach will aid the organization in developing a scalable response capability and in defining the timing and criteria for decisions that involve sheltering in place, resident transfer, facility closings, or evacuation.

Elements of Performance for EC.4.12

A 1. The organization develops and maintains a written EOP that describes an "all-hazards" command structure for coordinating six critical areas (*see* EC.4.13 through EC.4.18) within the organization during an emergency.

A 2. The EOP establishes an incident command structure.

A 3. The EOP identifies to whom staff report in the organization's incident command structure.

A 4. The EOP describes processes for initiating and terminating the response and recovery phases, including who has the authority to activate the phases.

A 5. The EOP describes processes for initiating and terminating the response and recovery phases, including how the phases are to be activated.

A 6. The EOP identifies the organization's capabilities and establishes response efforts when the organization cannot be supported by the local community for at least 96 hours in the six critical areas.

Note: *Acceptable response efforts could include the following:*
- *Conservation of resources*
- *Curtailment of services*
- *Supplementing of resources from outside the local community*
- *Staged evacuation*
- *Total evacuation*

A 7. The EOP identifies alternative sites for care, treatment or service that meet the needs of its residents during emergencies.

Standard EC.4.13

The organization establishes emergency communications strategies.

Rationale for EC.4.13

The organization maintains reliable surveillance and communications capability to detect emergencies and communicate response efforts to organization response personnel, residents and their families, and external agencies. The organization plans for back-up communications processes and technologies (e.g., cell phones, land lines, bulletin boards, fax machines, satellite phones, ham radio, text messages) if primary communications systems fail. It is important that responders and incident managers use common terminology; there simply is little or no room for misunderstanding in an emergency situation.

Elements of Performance for EC.4.13

A 1. The organization plans for notifying staff when emergency response measures are initiated.

A 2. The organization plans for ongoing communication of information and instructions to its staff once emergency response measures are initiated.

A 3. The organization defines processes for notifying external authorities when emergency response measures are initiated.

A 4. The organization plans for communicating with external authorities once emergency response measures are initiated.

A 5. The organization plans for communicating with residents and their families during emergencies, including notification when residents are relocated to alternative care sites.

A 6. The organization defines the circumstances and plans for communicating with the community and/or the media during emergencies.

A 7. The organization plans for communicating with purveyors of essential supplies, services, and equipment once emergency measures are initiated.

The organization plans for communicating in a timely manner with other health care organizations that together provide services to a contiguous geographic area (for example, among health care organizations serving a town or borough) regarding the following (EPs 8–11):

A 8. Essential elements of their command structures and control centers for emergency response

A 9. Names and roles of individuals in their command structures and command center telephone numbers

A 10. Resources and assets that potentially could be shared in an emergency response

A 11. Names of residents and deceased individuals brought to their organizations in accordance with applicable law and regulation, when requested

A 12. The organization defines the circumstances and plans for communicating information about residents to third parties (such as other health care organizations, the state health department, police, FBI, etc.).

A 13. The organization plans for communicating with identified alternative care sites.

A 14. The organization establishes back-up communication systems and technologies for the activities identified above.

Standard EC.4.14

The organization establishes strategies for managing resources and assets during emergencies.

Rationale for EC.4.14

During emergencies, health care organizations that continue to provide care, treatment, and services to their residents must sustain essential resources, materials, and facilities. The EOP should identify how resources and assets will be solicited and acquired from a range of possible sources, such as vendors, neighboring health care providers, other community organizations, state affiliates, or a regional parent company. To address emergencies of long duration or broad geographic scope, the organization's plan must proactively identify, locate, acquire, distribute and account for critical resources and supplies. The plan should also recognize the risk that some assets may not be available from planned sources and that contingency plans will be necessary for critical supplies. This situation may occur when multiple organizations are vying for a limited supply from the same vendor.

The infrastructure for supplying and supporting the health care organization is complex, and the HVA will help identify risks to this infrastructure that can be mitigated. Planning must address managing and maintaining the facility, but also must consider evacuation of the entire facility when the environment is no longer deemed safe.

Elements of Performance for EC.4.14

The organization plans for the following (EPs 1–11):

A 1. Obtaining supplies that will be required at the onset of emergency response (medical, pharmaceutical and non-medical)

A 2. Replenishing medical supplies and equipment that will be required throughout response and recovery, including personal protective equipment where required

A 3. Replenishing pharmaceutical supplies that will be required throughout response and recovery, including access to and distribution of caches (stockpiled by the organization or its affiliates, local, state or federal sources) to which the organization has access

A 4. Replenishing non-medical supplies that will be required throughout response and recovery (for example, food, linens, water, fuel for generators and transportation vehicles, etc.)

A 5. Managing staff support activities (for example, housing, transportation, incident stress debriefing, etc.)

A 6. Managing staff family support needs (for example, child care, elder care, communication, etc.)

A 7. Potential sharing of resources and assets (e.g., personnel, beds, transportation, linens, fuel, PPE, medical equipment and supplies, etc.) with other health care organizations within the community that could potentially be shared in an emergency response

A 8. Potential sharing of resources and assets with health care organizations outside of the community in the event of a regional or prolonged disaster

A 9. Evacuating (both horizontally and, when required by circumstances, vertically) when the environment cannot support care, treatment, and services

A 10. Transporting residents, their medications and equipment, and staff to an alternative care site or sites when the environment cannot support care, treatment, and services

A 11. Transporting pertinent information, including essential clinical and medication-related information, for residents to an alternative care site or sites when the environment cannot support care, treatment, and services

Standard EC.4.15

The organization establishes strategies for managing safety and security during emergencies.

Rationale for EC.4.15

Controlling the movement of individuals into, throughout, and out of the organization during an emergency is essential to the safety of residents and staff, and to the security of critical supplies, equipment, and utilities. The organization determines the type of access and movement to be allowed by staff, residents, visitors, emergency volunteers, vendors, maintenance and repair workers, utility suppliers, and other individuals when emergency measures are initiated. Factors influencing access and movement vary depending upon the type of emergency and local conditions (i.e., the decision by the organization to shelter staff families, the allowance for or prohibition against firearms, mutual aid agreements with nearby facilities or vendors, etc.).

During an emergency, the campus or immediate environment around the organization may be under the authority of the local police or sheriff serving the larger community. Access to and from the organization on local roads and interstates could be subject to local, state or even federal control. As an incident evolves, this responsibility and authority may shift from one agency to another. For this reason, it is important that the EOP includes reference to any existing community command structure to provide for ongoing communication and coordination with this structure. In the absence of such a command structure, the organization maintains direct contact with the agencies charged with community security.

Elements of Performance for EC.4.15

A 1. The organization establishes internal security and safety operations that will be required once emergency measures are initiated.

A 2. The organization identifies the roles of community security agencies (police, sheriff, national guard, etc.) and defines how the organization will coordinate security activities with these agencies.

A 3. The organization identifies a process that will be required for managing hazardous materials and waste once emergency measures are initiated.

4. Not applicable

A 5. The organization identifies residents who might be susceptible to wandering once emergency measures are initiated. ⚠3

The organization establishes processes for the following (EPs 6–8):

A 6. Controlling entrance into and out of the health care facility during emergencies

A 7. Controlling the movement of individuals within the health care facility during emergencies

A 8. Controlling traffic accessing the health care facility during emergencies

Standard EC.4.16

The organization defines and manages staff roles and responsibilities.

Rationale for EC.4.16

To provide safe and effective resident care during an emergency, staff roles are well defined; staff are oriented and trained in their assigned responsibilities; and staff maintains their competencies over time. Staff roles in emergencies are determined largely by the priority emergencies defined in the Hazard Vulnerability Analysis, and the reporting relationships in the command and control operations of the organization. As such, staff must stand ready to adjust to changes in resident volume or acuity, work procedures or conditions, and response partners within and outside the organization. (**Note:** *Standards in the Management of Human Resources chapter define the processes for accepting volunteer practitioners during emergencies.*) Staff roles and responsibilities may be documented in the EOP using a variety of formats: job action sheets, checklists, flow charts, etc.

Elements of Performance for EC.4.16

A 1. Staff roles and responsibilities are defined in the EOP for all critical areas (communication, resources and assets, safety and security, utilities, and clinical activities).

A 2. Staff are trained for their assigned roles during emergencies.

A 3. The organization communicates to licensed independent practitioners their roles in emergency response and to whom they report during an emergency.

A 4. The organization establishes a process for identifying care providers and other personnel (such as identification cards, wrist bands, vests, hats, badges, computer print-outs, etc.) assigned to particular areas during emergencies.

Standard EC.4.17

The organization establishes strategies for managing utilities during emergencies.

Rationale for EC.4.17

Different types of emergencies can have the same detrimental impact on an organization's utility systems. For example, brush fires, ice storms, and industrial accidents can all result in a loss of utilities required for care, treatment, services, related transport and building operations. Organizations, therefore, must have alternative means of providing for essential utilities, whether through negotiated relationships with the primary suppliers; Memoranda of Understanding (MOUs) with other organizations in the community; alternative equipment at the organization; or provision through a parent entity, etc. Organizations should determine how long they expect to remain open to care for residents, and plan for their utilities accordingly. Because some emergencies may be regional in scope or of long duration, organizations should not rely solely on single source providers in the community. Where possible, organizations should identify other suppliers outside of the local community in case the communities' infrastructure is severely compromised and unable to support the organization.

Elements of Performance for EC.4.17

The organization identifies an alternative means of providing for the following utilities in the event that their supply is compromised or disrupted (EPs 1–5):

A 1. Electricity

A 2. Water needed for consumption and essential care activities

A 3. Water needed for equipment and sanitary purposes

A 4. Fuel required for building operations or essential transport activities

A 5. Other essential utility needs (for example, ventilation, medical gas/vacuum systems, etc.)

Standard EC.4.18

The organization establishes strategies for managing resident clinical and support activities during emergencies.

Rationale for EC.4.18

The fundamental goal of emergency management planning is to protect life and prevent disability. The manner in which care, treatment, and services are provided may vary by type of emergency. However, certain clinical activities are so fundamental to safe and effective care that the organization should determine how it will re-schedule or manage resident clinical needs even under the most dynamic situations or in the most austere care environments.

The emergency triage process will typically result in residents being quickly treated and discharged, admitted for a longer stay, or transferred to a more appropriate source of care. It is especially important to identify and triage residents whose clinical needs are outside of the usual scope of service of the organization. A catastrophic emergency may result in the decision to keep all residents on the premises in the interest of safety or, conversely, in the decision to evacuate all residents because the facility is no longer safe. Planning for clinical services must address these situations accordingly.

Elements of Performance for EC.4.18

The organization plans to manage the following during emergencies (EPs 1–5):

A 1. The clinical activities required as part of resident scheduling, triage, assessment, treatment, admission, transfer, discharge, and evacuation

A 2. Clinical services for vulnerable populations served by the organization, including residents who are pediatric, geriatric, disabled, or have serious chronic conditions or addictions

A 3. Personal hygiene and sanitation needs of its residents

A 4. The mental health service needs of its residents

A 5. Mortuary services

A 6. The organization plans for documenting and tracking residents' clinical information

Standard EC.4.20 Through EC.5.50

Not applicable

Standard EC.6.10

The organization manages medical equipment risks.

Rationale for EC.6.10

Medical equipment is a significant contributor to the quality of care. It is used in treatment, diagnostic activities, and monitoring of the residents. It is essential that the equipment is appropriate for the intended use; that staff, including licensed independent practitioners, be trained to use the equipment safely and effectively; and it is essential that equipment is maintained appropriately by qualified individuals.

Elements of Performance for EC.6.10

A 1. The organization develops and maintains a written management plan describing the processes it implements to manage the effective, safe, and reliable operation of medical equipment.

A 2. The organization identifies and implements a process(es) for selecting and acquiring medical equipment.*

A 3. The organization establishes and uses risk criteria† for identifying, evaluating, and creating an inventory of equipment to be included in the medical equipment management plan before the equipment is used. These criteria address the following:

- Equipment function (diagnosis, care, treatment, life support, and monitoring)
- Physical risks associated with use
- Equipment incident history

* **Note:** *The acquisition process includes initially evaluating the condition and function of the equipment when received and evaluating the training of users before use on residents.*

† **Note:** *The organization may choose not to use risk criteria to limit the types of equipment to be included in the medical equipment management plan, rather include all medical equipment.*

A 4. The organization identifies appropriate inspection and maintenance strategies for all equipment in the inventory for achieving effective, safe, and reliable operation of all equipment in the inventory.*

A 5. The organization defines intervals for inspecting, testing, and maintaining appropriate equipment in the inventory (that is, those pieces of equipment in the inventory benefiting from scheduled activities to minimize the clinical and physical risks) that are based upon criteria such as manufacturers' recommendations, risk levels, and current organization experience.

A 6. The organization identifies and implements processes for monitoring and acting on equipment hazard notices and recalls.

A 7. The organization identifies and implements processes for monitoring and reporting incidents in which a medical device is suspected or attributed to the death, serious injury, or serious illness of any individual, as required by the Safe Medical Devices Act of 1990.

A 8. The organization identifies and implements processes for emergency procedures that address the following:
- What to do in the event of equipment disruption or failure
- When and how to perform emergency clinical interventions when medical equipment fails
- Availability of backup equipment
- How to obtain repair services

Standard EC.6.20

Medical equipment is maintained, tested, and inspected.

Elements of Performance for EC.6.20

C Ⓜ 1. The organization documents a current, accurate, and separate inventory of all equipment identified in the medical equipment management plan, regardless of ownership.

A 2. The organization documents performance and safety testing of all equipment identified in the medical equipment management program before initial use.

A 3. The organization documents inspection and maintenance of equipment used for life support† that is consistent with maintenance strategies to minimize clinical and physical risks identified in the equipment management plan (*see* Standard EC.6.10). ⚠3

* **Note:** *Organizations may use different strategies for different items as appropriate. For example, strategies such as predictive maintenance, interval-based inspections, corrective maintenance, or metered maintenance may be selected to ensure reliable performance.*

† **Life support equipment** Those devices intended to sustain life and whose failure to perform their primary function, when used according to manufacturer's instructions and clinical protocol, is expected to result in imminent death in the absence of immediate intervention (examples include ventilators, anesthesia machines, and heart-lung bypass machines).

C Ⓜ 4. The organization documents inspection and maintenance of non–life support equipment in the inventory that is consistent with maintenance strategies to minimize clinical and physical risks identified in the equipment management plan (*see* Standard EC.6.10).

5. Not applicable

A Ⓜ 6. The organization documents chemical and biological testing of water used in renal dialysis and other applicable tests based upon regulations, manufacturers' recommendations, and organization experience. ⚠3

Standard EC.6.30 Through EC.6.130

Not applicable

Standard EC.7.10

The organization manages its utility risks.

Rationale for EC.7.10

Utility systems* are essential to the proper operation of the environment of care and significantly contribute to effective, safe, and reliable provision of care to residents in health care organizations. It is important that health care organizations establish and maintain a utility systems management program to promote a safe, controlled, and comfortable environment that does the following:

- Ensures operational reliability of utility systems
- Reduces the potential for organization-acquired illness to be transmitted through the utility systems
- Assesses the reliability and minimizes potential risks of utility system failures

Elements of Performance for EC.7.10

1. Through 6. Not applicable

A 7. The organization develops and maintains a written management plan describing the processes it implements to manage the effective, safe, and reliable operation of utility systems.

A 8. The organization designs and installs utility systems that meet the resident care and operational needs of the services in the organization's buildings.

A 9. The organization establishes risk criteria† for identifying, evaluating, and creating an inventory of operating components of systems before the equipment is used.

---

* **Utility systems** May include electrical distribution; emergency power; vertical and horizontal transport; heating, ventilating, and air conditioning; plumbing, boiler, and steam; piped gases; vacuum systems; or communication systems, including data-exchange systems.

† **Note:** *The organization may choose not to use risk criteria to limit the types of utility systems to be included in the utility management plan, but rather include all utility systems.*

These criteria address the following:
- Life support
- Infection control
- Support of the environment
- Equipment support
- Communication

A 10. The organization develops appropriate strategies for all utility systems equipment in the inventory for ensuring effective, safe, and reliable operation of all equipment in the inventory.*

A 11. The organization defines intervals for inspecting, testing, and maintaining appropriate utility systems equipment in the inventory (that is, those pieces of equipment in the inventory benefiting from scheduled activities to minimize the clinical and physical risks) that are based upon criteria such as manufacturers' recommendations, risk levels, and current organization experience.

A 12. The organization identifies and implements emergency procedures for responding to utility system disruptions or failures that address the following:
- What to do if utility systems malfunction
- Identification of an alternative source of organization-defined essential utilities
- Shutting off the malfunctioning systems and notifying staff in affected areas
- How and when to perform emergency clinical interventions when utility systems fail
- Obtaining repair services ⚠3

A 13. The organization maps the distribution of utility systems. ⚠3

C Ⓜ 14. The organization labels controls for a partial or complete emergency shutdown. ⚠3

A 15. The organization identifies and implements processes to minimize pathogenic biological agents in cooling towers, domestic hot/cold water systems, and other aerosolizing water systems. ⚠3

A 16. The organization designs, installs, and maintains ventilation equipment to provide appropriate pressure relationships, air-exchange rates, and filtration efficiencies for ventilation systems serving areas specially designed† to

---

* **Note:** *Organizations may use different strategies as appropriate. For example, strategies such as predictive maintenance, interval-based inspections, corrective maintenance, or metered maintenance may be selected to ensure reliable performance.*

† **Areas specially designed** Include spaces such as rooms for residents diagnosed or suspected of having airborne communicable diseases (for example, pulmonary or laryngeal tuberculosis), residents in protective-isolation rooms (for example, those receiving bone marrow transplants), laboratories, pharmacies, and sterile supply rooms.

control airborne contaminants (such as biological agents, gases, fumes, and dust). ⚠3

Standard EC.7.20

Not applicable

Standard EC.7.30

The organization maintains, tests, and inspects its utility systems.

Note: *Organizations that offer care, treatment, and services in leased facilities need to communicate maintenance expectations for building equipment not under their control to their landlord through contractual language, lease agreements, memos, and so forth. These organizations are not required to possess maintenance documentation, but must only have access to such documentation as needed and during survey. It is also important that the landlord communicate to the organization any building equipment problems identified that could negatively affect the safety or health of residents, staff, and other people coming to the organization, as well as the landlord's plan to resolve such issues.*

Elements of Performance for EC.7.30

C Ⓜ 1. The organization maintains documentation of a current, accurate, and separate inventory of utility components identified in the utility management plan.

A Ⓜ 2. The organization maintains documentation of performance and safety testing of each critical component identified in the plan before initial use.

A Ⓜ 3. The organization maintains documentation of maintenance of critical components of life support utility systems/equipment consistent with maintenance strategies identified in the utility management plan (*see* standard EC.7.10).

A Ⓜ 4. The organization maintains documentation of maintenance of critical components of infection control utility systems/equipment for high-risk residents consistent with maintenance strategies identified in the utility management plan (*see* standard EC.7.10).

C Ⓜ 5. The organization maintains documentation of maintenance of critical components of non–life support utility systems/equipment in the inventory consistent with maintenance strategies identified in the utility management plan (*see* standard EC.7.10).

Standard EC.7.40

Not applicable

Standard EC.7.50

The organization maintains, tests, and inspects its medical gas and vacuum systems.

Note: *This standard does not require organizations to have the medical gas and vacuum systems discussed in the following EPs. However, if an organization has these types of systems, then the following maintenance, testing, and inspection requirements apply.*

Elements of Performance for EC.7.50

A 1. The organization inspects, tests, and maintains critical components of piped medical gas systems including master signal panels, area alarms, automatic pressure switches, shutoff valves, flexible connectors, and outlets. ⚠3

A 2. The organization tests piped medical gas and vacuum systems when the systems are installed, modified, or repaired including cross-connection testing, piping purity testing, and pressure testing. ⚠3

A 3. The organization maintains the main supply valve and area shut-off valves of piped medical gas and vacuum systems to be accessible and clearly labeled. ⚠3

Standard EC.8.10

Not applicable

Standard EC.8.20

Not applicable

Standard EC.8.30

Not applicable

Standard EC.9.10

The organization monitors conditions in the environment.

Elements of Performance for EC.9.10

A 1. The organization establishes and implements process(es) for reporting and investigating the following:*
- Injuries to residents or others coming to the organization's facilities as well as incidents of property damage
- Occupational illnesses and injuries to staff
- Security incidents involving residents, staff, or others coming to the organization's facilities or property

---

* Organizations have the flexibility to develop a single reporting method that addresses one or more of the items listed.

- Hazardous materials and waste spills, exposures, and other related incidents
- Fire-safety management problems, deficiencies, and failures
- Equipment-management problems, failures, and user errors
- Utility systems management problems, failures, or user errors

A 2. The organization's leaders assign a person(s) (hereafter referred to as the "assigned person[s]") to monitor and respond to conditions in the organization's environment. The assigned individual performs the following tasks:
- Coordinates the ongoing, organizationwide collection of information about deficiencies and opportunities for improvement in the environment of care
- Coordinates the ongoing collection and dissemination of other sources of information, such as published hazard notices or recall reports
- Coordinates the preparation of summaries of deficiencies, problems, failures, and user errors related to managing the environment of care*
- Coordinates the preparation of summaries on findings, recommendations, actions taken, and results of performance improvement (PI) activities
- Participates in hazard surveillance and incident reporting
- Participates in developing safety policies and procedures

A 3. The organization establishes and implements a process(es) for ongoing monitoring of performance regarding actual or potential risk(s) in each of the environment of care management plans.†

A 4. Each of the environment of care management plans are evaluated at least annually.

A 5. The objectives, scope, performance, and effectiveness of each of the environment of care management plans are evaluated at least annually.

6. Through 9. Not applicable

A 10. Environmental safety monitoring and response activities are communicated to the resident safety program required in the "Leadership" chapter of this book.

Standard EC.9.20

The organization analyzes identified environment issues and develops recommendations for resolving them.

---

* **Note:** *Incidents involving residents may be reported to appropriate staff such as staff in quality assessment, improvement, or other functions. However, at least a summary of incidents is shared with the person designated to coordinate safety management activities (see standard EC.1.10). Review of incident reports often requires that various legal processes be followed to preserve confidentiality. Opportunities to improve care, treatment, and services or to prevent future similar incidents are not lost as a result of the legal process followed.*

† The environment of care plans are for managing safety, security, hazardous materials and waste, emergency management, fire safety, medical equipment, and utilities.

Elements of Performance for EC.9.20

A 1. The organization establishes an ongoing process for resolving environment of care issues that involves representatives from clinical, administrative, and support services.

C Ⓜ 2. A multidisciplinary improvement team meets at least bimonthly to address environment of care issues.*

A 3. The organization analyzes environment of care issues in a timely manner.

A 4. Recommendations are developed and approved as appropriate.

A 5. Appropriate staff establishes measurement guidelines.

A 6. Environment of care issues are communicated to the organization's leaders and person(s) responsible for PI activities.

7. Not applicable

A 8. A recommendation for one or more PI activities is communicated at least annually to the organization's leaders based on the ongoing performance monitoring of the environment of care management plans.

A 9. Recommendations for resolving environmental safety issues are communicated, when appropriate, to those responsible for managing the resident safety program required in the "Leadership" chapter of this book.

Standard EC.9.30

The organization improves the environment.

Elements of Performance for EC.9.30

A 1. Appropriate staff participates in implementing recommendations.

A 2. Appropriate staff monitors the effectiveness of the recommendation's implementation.

A 3. Monitoring results are reported through appropriate channels, including the organization's leaders.

A 4. Monitoring results are reported to the multidisciplinary improvement team responsible for resolving environment of care issues.

A 5. Results of monitoring are reported (when appropriate) to those responsible for managing the resident safety program required in the "Leadership" chapter of this book.

---

* **Note:** *Meetings held less frequently than bimonthly are acceptable when supported by current organization experience and the multidisciplinary improvement team's approval. Ongoing justification of meeting frequency depends on a satisfactory annual evaluation of performance as required by EC.9.10.*

Management of Human Resources

Standard HR.1.10

Not applicable

Standard HR.1.15

Not applicable

Standard HR.1.20

Staff qualifications are consistent with his or her job responsibilities.

Elements of Performance for HR.1.20

1. Through 7. Not applicable

A 8. All staff that provide resident care, treatment, and services possess a license, certification, or registration as required by law and regulation. ▲2

9. Not applicable

10. Not applicable

C Ⓜ 11. Prior to the provision of care, treatment or services, the qualifications and competence of a non-employee individual, brought into the organization by a licensed independent practitioner to provide care, treatment or services within the scope of the organization's services are assessed by the organization and determined to be commensurate with the qualifications and competence required if the individual were to be employed by the organization to perform the same or similar services. △3

Note: *When the service to be provided by the individual is not currently performed by anyone employed by the organization, it is leadership's responsibility to consult the appropriate professional organization guidelines with respect to expectations for credentials and competence.*

C Ⓜ 12. The organization reviews the qualifications, performance, and competence of each non-employee individual brought into the organization by a licensed independent practitioner to provide care, treatment, or services at the same frequency as individuals employed by the organization.

Standard HR.1.25

The organization may assign disaster responsibilities to volunteer practitioners.

Rationale for HR.1.25

When the disaster plan has been implemented (*see* standard EC.4.10 for a description of emergency management planning requirements) and the immediate needs of the residents cannot be met, the organization may implement a modified process for determining qualifications and competence of volunteer practitioners* (*see* EPs 5–8). The volunteer practitioners that are addressed by this standard only include those practitioners that are required by law and regulation to have a license, certification, or registration to practice their profession. The usual process to determine the qualifications and competence of these practitioners would not allow a volunteer practitioner to provide immediate care, treatment, and services in the event of a disaster (refer to the Glossary for definitions of disaster and emergency) due to the length of time it would take to complete the process. A similar modified process for the assignment of disaster privileges for volunteer licensed independent practitioners exists at standard HR.4.35.

While this standard allows for a method to streamline the process for determining qualifications and competence, safeguards must be in place to assure that the volunteer practitioners are competent to provide safe and adequate care, treatment, and services. Even in a disaster, the integrity of the following two parts of the usual process for determining qualifications and competence must be maintained:

1. Verification of licensure, certification, or registration required to practice a profession
2. Oversight of the care, treatment, and services provided

This option to assign disaster responsibilities to volunteer practitioners is made on a case-by-case basis in accordance with the needs of the organization and its residents, and on the qualifications of its volunteer practitioners.

There are a number of state and federal systems engaged in pre-event verification of qualifications that may facilitate the assigning of disaster responsibilities to volunteer practitioners at the time of a disaster. Examples of such systems include the Medical Reserve Corps (MRC[†]) and the Emergency System for Advance Registration of Volunteer Health Professionals (ESAR-VHP[‡]). It is expected that additional programs will emerge and evolve.

---

* Individuals who are qualified to practice a health care profession (for example, a nurse) and are engaged in the provision of care and services. Practitioners are often required to be licensed as defined by law.

[†] **MRC** Medical Reserve Corps units are comprised of locally based medical and public health volunteers who can assist their communities during emergencies, such as an influenza epidemic, a chemical spill, or an act of terrorism. The MRC Program was formed in 2002, in cooperation with the White House's USA Freedom Corps, as one of the charter programs of Citizen Corps. Pre-identifying, training, and organizing medical and public health professionals to strengthen their communities through volunteerism is at the core of the MRC concept. MRC volunteers offer their expertise throughout the year by supporting local public health initiatives, such as immunization and prevention activities. When an emergency community need occurs, MRC volunteers can work in coordination with existing local emergency response programs.

[‡] **ESAR-VHP** The Emergency System for Advance Registration of Volunteer Health Professionals (ESAR-VHP) program, created by the Health Resources and Services Administration (HRSA), allows for the advance registration and credentialing of health care professionals needed to augment a hospital or other medical facility to meet increased resident/victim care and increased surge capacity needs.

Elements of Performance for HR.1.25

A 1. Disaster responsibilities are assigned only when the following two conditions are present: the emergency management plan has been activated, and the organization is unable to meet immediate resident needs.

A 2. The organization identifies in writing the individual(s) responsible for assigning disaster responsibilities.

A 3. The organization describes in writing a mechanism (for example, direct observation, mentoring, and clinical record review) to oversee the professional performance of volunteer practitioners who are assigned disaster responsibilities.

A 4. The organization has a mechanism to identify volunteer practitioners that have been assigned disaster responsibilities.

A 5. For volunteer practitioners to be assigned disaster responsibilities, the organization obtains for each volunteer practitioner at a minimum, a valid government-issued photo identification issued by a state or federal agency (for example, driver's license or passport) and at least one of the following:
- A current health care organization (such as a long term care, ambulatory care, laboratory, or hospital) picture identification card that clearly identifies professional designation
- A current license, certification, or registration
- Primary source verification of licensure, certification, or registration (if required by law and regulation to practice a profession)
- Identification indicating that the individual is a member of a Disaster Medical Assistance Team (DMAT*), or MRC, ESAR-VHP, or other recognized state or federal organizations or groups
- Identification indicating that the individual has been granted authority to render resident care, treatment, and services in disaster circumstances (such authority having been granted by a federal, state, or municipal entity)
- Identification by current organization member(s) who possesses personal knowledge regarding the volunteer practitioner's qualifications

A 6. Primary source verification of licensure, certification, or registration (if required by law and regulation to practice a profession) begins as soon as the immediate situation is under control, and is completed within 72 hours from the time the volunteer practitioner presents to the organization.

Note: *In the extraordinary circumstance that primary source verification of licensure, certification, or registration* (if required by law and regulation to practice a profession) *cannot be completed in 72 hours (for example, no means of communication or a lack of resources), it is expected that it be done*

---

* **DMAT** A group of medical and support personnel designed to provide emergency medical care during a disaster or other unusual event. The DMAT is a component of the National Disaster Medical System (NDMS). The Department of Health and Human Services in partnership with other federal agencies such as Department of Defense, Department of Veterans Affairs, and the Federal Emergency Management Agency administer the program.

as soon as possible. In this extraordinary circumstance, there must be documentation of the following: why primary source verification could not be performed in the required time frame; evidence of a demonstrated ability to continue to provide adequate care, treatment, and services; and an attempt to rectify the situation as soon as possible. Primary source verification of licensure, certification, or registration (if required by law and regulation to practice a profession) would not be required if the volunteer practitioner has not provided care, treatment, and services under the disaster responsibilities.

A 7. The organization oversees the professional practice of volunteer practitioners.

A 8. The organization makes a decision (based on information obtained regarding the professional practice of the volunteer practitioner) within 72 hours related to the continuation of the disaster responsibilities initially assigned.

Standard HR.1.30

The organization uses data from clinical/service screening indicators and human resource screening indicators to assess and continuously improve staffing effectiveness.

Rationale for HR.1.30

Significant changes in nurse staffing level and the skill mix of nursing personnel in health care organizations raise questions about potential adverse effects on the quality and safety of patient care related to staffing effectiveness. The Joint Commission has developed a comprehensive approach to the management of staffing effectiveness that looks at staffing as more than just "numbers." The approach relies on data driven quality improvement principles and is objective and methodologically sound. Since the causes and consequences of diminished staffing effectiveness differ from organization to organization, the approach allows flexibility to reflect characteristics unique to individual health care settings.

Elements of Performance for HR.1.30

A 1. The organization identifies no fewer than two inpatient populations/settings for which data on staffing effectiveness are to be collected.

Note: *If the organization has only one population/setting, the organization may collect data for that single population/setting.*

A 2. The organization identifies the populations/settings (no less than two) based on assessment of relevant information or risk, including

- Knowledge about staffing issues likely to impact resident safety or quality of care
- Resident population served
- Type of setting

- Review of existing data (for example, incident logs, sentinel event data, performance improvement reports)
- Input from clinical staff who provide resident care

Note: *If the organization has only one population/setting, the organization need not apply these criteria.*

A 3. A minimum set of four indicators are selected for each of the identified inpatient populations/settings.

Note: *Organizations are free to choose the same set, the same set in part or completely different measure sets for each identified population/setting.*

A 4. The organization determines the indicators for each population/setting based on assessment of relevant information or risk, including the following:
- Knowledge about staffing issues likely to impact resident safety or quality of care
- Resident population served
- Type of setting
- Review of existing data (for example, incident logs, sentinel event data, performance improvement reports)
- Input from clinical staff who provide resident care

A 5. Of the four indicators required for each population/setting, two must be clinical/service indicators and two must be human resource indicators.

A 6. One of the human resource indicators and one of the clinical/service indicators must be selected from the Joint Commission's list of approved indicators.

Note: *Additional indicators may be selected from among the organization's own indicators.*

A 7. The human resource indicators for all identified populations/settings include all nursing staff (including registered nurses, licensed practical nurses, and nursing assistants or aides).

Note: *Decisions regarding stratification of data by discipline are left to the organization.*

A 8. When the organization chooses to include other practitioner groups (in addition to nursing staff in the human resource indicators for the identified populations/settings, this decision is based on the impact the absence of such care/service providers would be expected to have on resident outcomes.

A 9. The organization does the following:
- Defines the numerator and denominator for indicators chosen
- Standardizes the data element definitions for each indicator, including those indicators applied in more than one setting
- Determines acceptable ranges/parameters/trigger levels* for the indicators

---

* Acceptable ranges/parameters/trigger levels may be reflective of past performance, expert opinion, expert literature, or a combination of these. The ranges/parameters/trigger levels should be reasonable goals that are possible to attain. When desired ranges/parameters/trigger levels are not met, an investigation into the cause(s) is needed.

A 10. The organization does the following for each population/setting selected:
- Collects data for all indicators
- Analyzes data for all indicators
- Reviews all indicator data together when analyzing variation from desired performance for additional information that may assist in identifying any potential causes of variation
- Investigates to identify any staffing effectiveness issues when indicator data varies from expected
- Takes appropriate action in response to analyzed data

A 11. The organization reports at least annually to the leaders on the results of data analyses related to staffing effectiveness (*see* PI.1.10 and PI.2.20) and any actions taken to resolve identified problems.

List of Joint Commission Approved Subjects for Screening Indicators for Long Term Care

1. Prevalence of pressure ulcers (Clinical/Service)
2. Resident satisfaction (Clinical/Service)
3. Family satisfaction (Clinical/Service)
4. Prevalence of falls (Clinical/Service)
5. Resident complaints (Clinical/Service)
6. Injuries to residents (Clinical/Service)
7. Family complaints (Clinical/Service)
8. Restraint use (Clinical/Service)
9. Prevalence of unintended weight loss (Clinical/Service)
10. Elopements/wandering of residents (Clinical/Service)
11. Adverse drug events (Clinical/Service)
12. Prevalence of dehydration (Clinical/Service)
13. Pain assessment and management (that is, wait time to receive medications) (Clinical/Service)
14. Urinary tract infection rate (Clinical/Service)
15. Change in resident functioning (Clinical/Service)
16. Prevalence of malnutrition (Clinical/Service)
17. Activities of daily living (ADL) met or unmet (Clinical/Service)
18. Prevalence of urinary catheter use (Clinical/Service)
19. Average time in activities (Clinical/Service)
20. Antibiotic use (Clinical/Service)
21. Unexpected hospital admissions or emergency department visits (Clinical/Service)
22. Prevalence of untreated depression (Clinical/Service)
23. Prevalence of more than eight prescribed medications (Clinical/Service)
24. Pneumonia rate (Clinical/Service)
25. Unnecessary antipsychotic medication usage (Clinical/Service)

Chronic Care Measures

26. Residents whose need for more help with daily activities has increased (Clinical/Service) (National Quality Forum Measure)

27. Residents who lost too much weight (Clinical/Service) (National Quality Forum Measure)
28. Residents who experience moderate to severe pain during the seven-day assessment period (Clinical/Service) (National Quality Forum Measure)
29. Residents who were physically restrained during the seven-day assessment period (Clinical/Service) (National Quality Forum Measure)
30. Residents who spent most of their time in bed or in a chair in their room during the seven-day assessment period (Clinical/Service) (National Quality Forum Measure)
31. Residents with a decline in their ability to move about in their room or the adjacent corridor (Clinical/Service) (National Quality Forum Measure)
32. Residents with a urinary tract infection (Clinical/Service) (National Quality Forum Measure)
33. Residents with worsening of a depressed or anxious mood (Clinical/Service) (National Quality Forum Measure)

Chronic Care Measure Pairs

34. High-risk residents with pressure ulcers AND average-risk residents with pressure ulcers (Clinical/Service) (National Quality Forum Measure)
35. Residents who frequently lose control of the bowel or bladder (low-risk) AND residents who have a catheter in the bladder at any time during the 14-day assessment period (Clinical/Service) (National Quality Forum Measure)

Post-Acute Care Measures

36. Recently hospitalized residents with symptoms of delirium (Clinical/Service) (National Quality Forum Measure)
37. Recently hospitalized residents who experienced moderate to severe pain at any time during the seven-day assessment period (Clinical/Service) (National Quality Forum Measure)
38. Recently hospitalized residents with pressure ulcers (Clinical/Service) (National Quality Forum Measure)

Measures for All Nursing Home Residents

39. Pneumococcal polysaccharide vaccination of residents age 65 or older (Clinical/Service) (National Quality Forum Measure)
40. Influenza vaccination for all nursing home residents (Clinical/Service) (National Quality Forum Measure)
41. Staff vacancy rate (Human Resource)
42. Staff turnover rate (Human Resource)
43. Staff satisfaction (Human Resource)
44. Use of overtime (Human Resource)
45. Staff injury rate (Human Resource)
46. Nursing hours per resident day (registered nurse, licensed practical nurse, certified nursing assistant) compared to baseline such as actual versus planned or budgeted (Human Resource)
47. Staff training hours (Human Resource)
48. Agency usage/contract staff (Human Resource)
49. Understaffing as compared to organization's staffing plan (Human Resource)

50. Use of sick time (Human Resource)
51. Activity staff hours per resident day (Human Resource)
52. Number of dietary staff hours per resident day (Human Resource)
53. Number of housekeeping staff hours per resident day (Human Resource)
54. Average response time for consultation order (Human Resource)
55. Nurse staffing hours (Human Resource) (National Quality Forum Measure)

Note: *Additional information on nursing home care measures can be found at http://www.qualityforum.org.*

Standard HR.2.10

The organization provides initial orientation.

Rationale for HR.2.10

Orientation is a process in which initial job training and information is provided to staff and licensed independent practitioners. Staff and licensed independent practitioner orientation promotes safe and effective job performance. Some elements of orientation need to occur before staff and licensed independent practitioners provide care, treatment, and services. Other elements of orientation can occur when staff and licensed independent practitioners are providing care, treatment, and services.

Elements of Performance for HR.2.10

A 1. The organization determines what key elements of orientation should occur before staff and licensed independent practitioners provide care, treatment, and services.

C Ⓜ 2. The organization orients staff and licensed independent practitioners to the identified key elements prior to the provision of care, treatment, and services.

As appropriate, staff and licensed independent practitioner orientation addresses the following (EPs 3–7):

C Ⓜ 3. The organization's mission and goals

C Ⓜ 4. Organizationwide policies and procedures (including safety and infection control) and relevant unit, setting, or program-specific policies and procedures

C Ⓜ 5. Specific job duties and responsibilities and service, setting, or program-specific job duties and responsibilities related to safety and infection control

6. Not applicable

C Ⓜ 7. Cultural diversity and sensitivity

C Ⓜ 8. Staff orientation includes education about the rights of residents and ethical aspects of care, treatment, and services and the process used to address ethical issues

C Ⓜ 9. Staff orientation includes education about the effects of psychotropic medications as appropriate

Standard HR.2.20

Staff and licensed independent practitioners, as appropriate, can describe or demonstrate their roles and responsibilities relative to safety.

Rationale for HR.2.20

The human element is the most critical factor in any process, determining whether the right things are done correctly. The best policies and procedures for minimizing risks in the environment where care, treatment, and services are provided are meaningless if staff and licensed independent practitioners (if applicable) do not know and understand them well enough to perform them properly.

It is important that everyday precautions identified by the health care organization for minimizing various risks, including those related to resident safety and environmental safety,* are properly implemented. It is also important that the appropriate emergency procedures be instituted should an incident or failure occur in the environment.

Elements of Performance for HR.2.20

Staff and licensed independent practitioners, as appropriate, can describe or demonstrate the following (EPs 1–4):

C Ⓜ 1. Risks within the organization's environment

C Ⓜ 2. Actions to eliminate, minimize, or report risks

C Ⓜ 3. Procedures to follow in the event of an incident

C Ⓜ 4. Reporting processes for common problems, failures, and user errors

Standard HR.2.30

Ongoing education, including in-services, training, and other activities, maintains and improves staff competence.

Elements of Performance for HR.2.30

A 1. Staff training occurs when job responsibilities or duties change.

C Ⓜ 2. Staff participate in ongoing in-services, training, or other activities to increase knowledge of work-related issues.

C Ⓜ 3. Ongoing in-services and other education and training of staff are appropriate to the needs of the population(s) served and comply with law and regulation.

---

* The "Management of the Environment of Care" chapter of this book identifies risks associated with the following categories: safety, security, hazardous materials and wastes, emergency management, medical equipment, and utility management.

C Ⓜ 4. Ongoing in-services, training, or other staff activities emphasize specific job-related aspects of safety and infection prevention and control.

C Ⓜ 5. Ongoing in-services, training, or other staff education incorporate methods of team training, when appropriate.

C Ⓜ 6. Ongoing in-services, training, or other staff education reinforce the need and ways to report unanticipated adverse events.

C Ⓜ 7. Ongoing in-services or other staff education are offered in response to learning needs identified through performance improvement findings and other data analysis (that is, data from staff surveys, performance evaluations, or other needs assessments).

C Ⓜ 8. Ongoing staff education is documented.

9. Not applicable

A 10. Staff are educated, as appropriate to their responsibilities, about psychotropic medications including the following:
- The need for a medication in relation to the resident's documented diagnosis and condition
- The potential for drug–drug and drug–food interactions
- Adverse reactions to psychotropic medications
- The use of a medication for an appropriate duration
- The optimal dose
- Frequent monitoring of the medication's effectiveness
- Nonmedication interventions and alternatives developed through interdisciplinary team assessment
- Reduction and discontinuation of a medication

Standard HR.3.10

Staff competence to perform job responsibilities is assessed, demonstrated, and maintained.

Rationale for HR.3.10

Competence assessment is systematic and allows for a measurable assessment of the person's ability to perform required activities. Information used as part of competence assessment may include data from performance evaluations, performance improvement, and aggregate data on competence, as well as the assessment of learning needs.

Elements of Performance for HR.3.10

The competence assessment process for staff is based on the following (EPs 1–7):

A 1. The population(s) served.

A 2. The defined competencies to be required.

A 3. The competence assessment process for staff is based on the defined competencies to be assessed during orientation.

A 4. The defined competencies that need to be assessed and reassessed on an ongoing basis, based on techniques, procedures, technology, equipment, or skills needed to provide care, treatment, and services.

A 5. A defined time frame for how often competence assessments are performed for each person, minimally, once in the three-year accreditation cycle and in accordance with law and regulation.

A 6. The assessment methods (appropriate to determine the skill being assessed).

A 7. The use of qualified individuals to assess competence.

Note: *When there is no qualified individual in the organization that performs comparable care, treatment, and services, the organization may:*

- *Utilize qualified staff from other organizations to assist with the assessment of competence*

  or
- *Consult the appropriate professional organization guidelines with respect to expectations for competence and use these guidelines to assess competence*

C Ⓜ 8. The organization assesses and documents staff's ability to carry out assigned responsibilities safely, competently, and in a timely manner upon completion of orientation.

C Ⓜ 9. The organization assesses staff according to its competence assessment process.

A 10. When improvement activities lead to a determination that a person with performance problems is unable or unwilling to improve, the organization takes appropriate action (which may include modifying the person's job assignment).

Standard HR.3.20 Through HR.3.60

Not applicable

Standard HR.4.10

There is a process for ensuring the competence of all practitioners permitted by law and the organization to practice independently.

Elements of Performance for HR.4.10

1. Through 4. Not applicable

A 5. The organization has a defined process approved by the leaders for appointing and reappointing licensed independent practitioners.

A 6. At the time of initial granting of privileges, the organization verifies, by viewing a valid government-issued photo identification issued by a state or federal agency (e.g., drivers license or passport), that the individual being granted (clinical privileges) is the same individual identified in the credentialing documents.

Note: *Any licensed independent practitioner whose only role is to cover for another licensed independent practitioner(s) is exempt from this requirement.*

A 7. The credentialing process requires that the organization does the following:
- Verifies in writing current licensure, from the primary source at time of initial granting, renewal and revision of clinical privileges, and prior to licensure expiration
- Verifies in writing training (required by the organization to perform the clinical privileges) from the primary source at the time of initial granting and renewal and revision of clinical privileges
- Verifies in writing current competence from the primary source at time of initial granting of clinical privileges
- Obtains a statement from the applicant at the time of initial granting, renewal, or revision of clinical privileges that no health problems exist that could effect his or her ability to perform the privileges requested.*

Note: *Verification of current licensure with the primary source through a secure electronic communication or by telephone is acceptable, if this verification is documented. For additional information,* see *"primary source verification" in the Glossary.*

Note: *An external organization (for example, a credentials verification organization [CVO] or a Joint Commission–accredited health care organization functioning as a CVO) may be used to collect credentialing information. Both of these organizations must meet the CVO guidelines listed in the Glossary section of the accreditation manual.*

Note: *A primary source of verified information may designate to an agency the role of communicating credentials information. The delegated agency then becomes acceptable to be used as a primary source.*

A 8. All licensed independent practitioners that provide patient care possess a license, certification, or registration as required by law and regulation. (2)

9. Through 10. Not applicable

A 11. The governing body† does the following:
- Reviews recommendations made by the medical director
- Reviews documentation on which recommendations are based
- Reviews records of any hearings or appeals addressing adverse decisions
- Grants appropriate clinical privileges

---

* Organizations should consider the applicability of the Americans with Disabilities Act (ADA) to their credentialing and privileging activities, and, if applicable, review their policies and procedures. Federal entities are required to comply with the Rehabilitation Act of 1974.

† The organization administrator or a committee of two or more governing body members may substitute for a governing body.

12. Through 21. Not applicable

When the attending licensed independent practitioner designates a licensed independent practitioner (who is not privileged in the organization) to cover in his/her absence for a period of no more than 72 consecutive hours, the following requirements are met (EPs 22–25):

A 22. The medical director and the attending licensed independent practitioner determine that the covering licensed independent practitioner can perform those types of care, treatment, and services that are required

A 23. The organization verifies the current licensure of the covering licensed independent practitioner from the primary source prior to his or her provision of care, treatment and services

Note: *It may be more efficient to obtain a list of possible covering licensed independent practitioners ahead of time and verify licensure from the primary source in advance of the licensed independent practitioner actually covering for the attending.*

C Ⓜ 24. A documented review of orders issued by the covering licensed independent practitioner is conducted by the attending licensed independent practitioner upon return in the time frame defined by the organization

A 25. The modified process for credentialing and privileging can only be utilized for a covering licensed independent practitioner for up to 12 days* per calendar year but no more than 72 consecutive hours

Note: *If a licensed independent practitioner will be covering for more than 12 days per calendar year or more than 72 consecutive hours, this individual must undergo the full process for credentialing and privileging by the organization.*

Standard HR.4.20

Individuals permitted by law and the organization to practice independently are granted clinical privileges.

Elements of Performance for HR.4.20

A 1. Based on the scope of services provided, the organization establishes criteria for each privilege. These criteria include the following:

- Current licensure and/or certification as appropriate, verified with the primary source
- Successful completion of training specific to each requested privilege, verified with the primary source
- Peer† and or faculty recommendation
- Evidence of the ability to perform the requested privilege

* A day is considered as any portion of the day (whether it is 1 hour or 24 hours).

† *See* Glossary for definition of peer recommendation.

A 2. Before granting, renewing, or revising privileges, the medical director evaluates the following:
- Challenges to any licensure or registration
- Voluntary and involuntary relinquishment of any license or registration
- Voluntary and involuntary termination of medical staff membership at another organization
- Voluntary and involuntary limitation, reduction, or loss of clinical privileges
- Any evidence of an unusual pattern or an excessive number of professional liability actions resulting in a final judgment against the applicant
- Documentation as to the applicant's health status

A 3. The organization queries the National Practitioner Data Bank (NPDB) at the time of initial granting of privileges, as well as at least every two years thereafter for information on physicians and dentists granted clinical privileges.

C Ⓜ 4. Clinical privileges for licensed independent practitioners are delineated according to organization policy and based on the licensed independent practitioner's current credentials and competence, as well as the population(s) served and the types of care, treatment, and services provided in the organization.

A 5. The decision by leaders to appoint licensed independent practitioners is based on the credentials information obtained.

C Ⓜ 6. The licensed independent practitioner is notified in writing of the governing body's decision.

A 7. Individuals with clinical privileges practice within the scope of their privileges. ⚠3

Standard HR.4.30

The organization has a process for granting temporary clinical privileges, when appropriate.

Rationale for HR.4.30

There are two circumstances in which temporary clinical privileges may be granted. Each circumstance has different criteria for granting clinical privileges. The two circumstances are to meet the important needs of residents and for new applicants.

Elements of Performance for HR.4.30

A 1. Policies and procedures, rules, or regulations describe the process for granting temporary privileges for meeting the important needs of residents or for new applicants.

A 2. To grant temporary privileges to meet the important needs of residents, there must be verification (which can be done by telephone) of current licensure and current competence.

A 3. To grant temporary privileges for new applicants, there must be verification (which may be done by telephone) of the following:
- Current licensure
- Relevant education training or experience
- Current competence
- A query and evaluation of the NPDB for physicians or dentists

A 4. To grant temporary privileges for new applicants, the applicant has the following:
- A complete application
- No current or previously successful challenge to licensure or registration
- Not been subject to involuntary termination of professional or medical staff membership at another organization, when applicable to the discipline
- Not been subject to involuntary limitation, reduction, denial, or loss of clinical responsibilities privileges, when applicable to the discipline

A 5. The administrator or designee grants temporary privileges for meeting important resident needs and for new applicants upon recommendation of clinical leadership or the medical director.

A 6. Temporary privileges for new applicants are granted for no more than 120 days.

Standard HR.4.32

Not applicable

Standard HR.4.33

Not applicable

Standard HR.4.34

Not applicable

Standard HR.4.35

The organization may grant disaster privileges to volunteers eligible to be licensed independent practitioners.

Rationale for HR.4.35

When the disaster plan has been implemented (*see* Standard EC.4.10 for a description of emergency management planning requirements) and the immediate needs of the residents cannot be met, the organization may implement a modified credentialing and privileging process for eligible volunteer practitioners (*see* EPs 5–8). The usual process to credential and privilege practitioners would not allow a volunteer practitioner to provide immediate care, treatment, and services in the event of a disaster (refer to the Glossary for definitions of disaster and emergency) due to the length of time it would take to complete the process. A similar modified process for the assignment of disaster responsibilities for volunteers that are not independent practitioners exists at standard HR.1.25.

While this standard allows for a method to streamline the credentialing and privileging process, safeguards must be in place to assure that volunteer practitioners are competent to provide safe and adequate care, treatment, and services. Even in a disaster, the integrity of two parts of the usual credentialing and privileging process must be maintained:

1. Verification of licensure
2. Oversight of the care, treatment, and services provided

This option to grant disaster privileges to volunteer practitioners is made on a case-by-case basis in accordance with the needs of the organization and its residents, and on the qualifications of its volunteer practitioners.

There are a number of state and federal systems engaged in pre-event credentialing that may facilitate the implementation of disaster privileging of volunteers at the time of a disaster. Examples of such systems include the Medical Reserve Corps (MRC*) and the Emergency System for Advance Registration of Volunteer Health Professionals (ESAR-VHP†). It is expected that additional programs will emerge and evolve.

Elements of Performance for HR.4.35

A 1. Disaster privileges are granted only when the following two conditions are present: the emergency management plan has been activated, and the organization is unable to meet immediate resident needs.

A 2. The organization identifies in writing the individual(s) responsible for granting disaster privileges.

A 3. The organization describes in writing a mechanism (for example, direct observation, mentoring, and clinical record review) to oversee the professional performance of volunteer practitioners who receive disaster privileges.

* **MRC** Medical Reserve Corps units are comprised of locally-based medical and public health volunteers who can assist their communities during emergencies, such as an influenza epidemic, a chemical spill, or an act of terrorism. The MRC Program was formed in 2002, in cooperation with the White House's USA Freedom Corps, as one of the charter programs of Citizen Corps. Pre-identifying, training and organizing medical and public health professionals to strengthen their communities through volunteerism is at the core of the MRC concept. MRC volunteers offer their expertise throughout the year by supporting local public health initiatives, such as immunization and prevention activities. When an emergency community need occurs, MRC volunteers can work in coordination with existing local emergency response programs.

† **ESAR-VHP** The Emergency System for Advance Registration of Volunteer Health Professionals (ESAR-VHP) program, created by the Health Resources and Services Administration (HRSA), allows for the advance registration and credentialing of health care professionals needed to augment a hospital or other medical facility to meet increased resident/victim care and increased surge capacity needs.

A 4. The organization has a mechanism to identify the volunteer practitioners who have been granted disaster privileges.

A 5. In order for volunteers to be considered eligible to act as licensed independent practitioners, the organization obtains for each volunteer practitioner at a minimum a valid government-issued photo identification issued by a state or federal agency (for example, driver's license or passport) and at least one of the following:
- A current health care organization (such as a long term care, ambulatory care, or hospital) picture identification card that clearly identifies professional designation
- A current license to practice
- Primary source verification of the license
- Identification indicating that the individual is a member of a Disaster Medical Assistance Team (DMAT*), or MRC, ESAR-VHP, or other recognized state or federal organizations or groups
- Identification indicating that the individual has been granted authority to render resident care, treatment, and services in disaster circumstances (such authority having been granted by a federal, state, or municipal entity)
- Identification by current organization member(s) who possesses personal knowledge regarding the volunteer's ability to act as a licensed independent practitioner during a disaster

A 6. Primary source verification of licensure begins as soon as the immediate situation is under control, and is completed within 72 hours from the time the volunteer practitioner presents to the organization.

Note: *In the extraordinary circumstance that primary source verification cannot be completed in 72 hours (for example, no means of communication or a lack of resources), it is expected that it be done as soon as possible. In this extraordinary circumstance, there must be documentation of the following: why primary source verification could not be performed in the required time frame; evidence of a demonstrated ability to continue to provide adequate care, treatment, and services; and an attempt to rectify the situation as soon as possible. Primary source verification of licensure would not be required if the volunteer practitioner has not provided care, treatment, and services under the disaster privileges.*

A 7. The organization oversees the professional practice of volunteer licensed independent practitioners.

A 8. The organization makes a decision (based on information obtained regarding the professional practice of the volunteer) within 72 hours related to the continuation of the disaster privileges initially granted.

---

* **DMAT** A group of medical and support personnel designed to provide emergency medical care during a disaster or other unusual event. The DMAT is a component of the National Disaster Medical System (NDMS). The Department of Health and Human Services in partnership with other federal agencies such as Department of Defense, Department of Veterans Affairs, and the Federal Emergency Management Agency administer the program.

Standard HR.4.40

There are mechanisms, including a fair hearing and appeal process, for addressing adverse decisions regarding reappointment, denial, reduction, suspension, or revocation of clinical privileges that may relate to quality of care, treatment, and service issues.

Rationale for HR.4.40

Mechanisms for fair hearing and appeals processes are designed to allow the affected individual a fair opportunity to defend herself or himself regarding the adverse decision to an unbiased hearing committee, and an opportunity to appeal the decision of the committee to the governance function. The purpose of a fair hearing and appeal is to assure full consideration and reconsideration of quality and safety issues and, under the current structure of reporting to the NPDB, to allow practitioners an opportunity to defend themselves.

Elements of Performance for HR.4.40

The organization has developed a fair hearing and appeals process that does the following:

A 1. Is designed to provide a uniform and fair process

A 2. Has a mechanism to schedule a hearing of such requests

A 3. Has identified the procedures for the hearings to follow

A 4. Identifies or defines the composition of the hearing committee

A 5. Provides for a mechanism to appeal an adverse decision through the governance function

Standard HR.4.50

Clinical privileges and appointments/reappointments are reviewed and revised at least every two years.

Elements of Performance for HR.4.50

A 1. Policies and procedures or rules and regulations specify a period of no more than two years between appointments and reappointments and between granting, renewing, and revising clinical privileges.

C Ⓜ 2. Credential files for licensed independent practitioners contain substantive information and indicate that clinical privileges are reviewed or revised at least every two years and are revised as needed; in addition, appointments and reappointments are made for a period of no more than two years.

A 3. A reappraisal is conducted at the time of reappointment or renewal or revision of clinical privileges.

A 4. The reappraisal addresses current competence and includes the following:
- Confirmation of adherence to organization policies and procedures, rules, or regulations
- Relevant information from organization performance improvement activities when evaluating professional performance, judgment, and clinical or technical skills
- Any results of review of the individual's clinical performance
- Clinical performance in the organization that is outside acceptable standards

A 5. Credentials files contain clear evidence that the full range of privileges has been included in the reappraisal.

Standard HR.4.60 Through HR.5.40

Not applicable

Management of Information

Standard IM.1.10

The organization plans and designs information management processes to meet internal and external information needs.

Rationale for IM.1.10

Organizations vary in size, complexity, governance, structure, decision-making processes, and resources. Information management systems and processes vary accordingly. Only by first identifying the information needs can one then evaluate the extent to which they are planned for, and at what performance level the needs are being met. Planning for the management of information does not require a formal written information plan, but does require evidence of a planned approach that identifies the organization's information needs and supports its goals and objectives.

Elements of Performance for IM.1.10

A 1. The organization bases its information management processes on an assessment of internal and external information needs.
- The assessment identifies the flow of information throughout an organization, including information storage and feedback mechanisms.
- The assessment identifies the data and information needed: within and among departments, services, or programs; within and among the staff, the administration, and the governance for supporting relationships with outside services and contractors; with licensing, accrediting, and regulatory bodies; with purchasers, payers, and employers; for supporting informational needs between the organization and the residents; and for participating in research and databases.

A 2. To guide development of processes for managing information used internally and externally, the organization assesses its information management needs based on the following:
- Its mission
- Its goals
- Its services
- Staff
- Resident safety considerations
- Quality of care, treatment, and services
- Mode(s) of service delivery
- Resources
- Access to affordable technology
- Identification of barriers to effective communication among caregivers

A 3. The organization bases its management, staffing, and material resource allocations for information management on the scope and complexity of care, treatment, and services provided.

A 4. Identified staff participates in assessment, selection, integration, and use of information management systems for clinical/service and organization information.

A 5. The organization has an ongoing process to assess the needs of the organization, departments, and individuals for knowledge-based information.

A 6. The organization uses the assessment for knowledge-based information as a basis for planning.

Confidentiality and Security

Standard IM.2.10

Information privacy and confidentiality are maintained.

Rationale for IM.2.10

Confidentiality of data and information applies across all systems and to automated, paper, and verbal communications, as well as to clinical/service, financial, and business records and employee-specific information. The capture, storage, and retrieval processes for data and information are performed on a timely* basis without compromising the data and information's confidentiality. Protecting privacy and confidentiality of information is the responsibility of the whole organization. In achieving this responsibility, the organization provides safeguards for resident privacy and information confidentiality. These safeguards are consistent with available technology and legitimate needs for accessibility of the information by authorized individuals for the delivery of care, treatment, and services, effective functioning of the organization, research, and education.

* Defined by organization policy and based on the intended use of the information.

Elements of Performance for IM.2.10

A 1. The organization has a written policy(ies) for addressing the privacy* and confidentiality† of information, that is based on and consistent with law or regulation.

A 2. The organization's policy, including changes to the policy, has been communicated to staff.

A 3. The organization implements the policy.

A 4. The organization monitors compliance with the policy.

A 5. The organization improves privacy and confidentiality of information by monitoring information and developments in technology.

C Ⓜ 6. Individuals for whom identifiable health data and information are maintained or collected are made aware of how the data will be used and whether it will be disclosed.

A 7. Personal identifiers are removed to the extent possible for uses and disclosures of health information, consistent with maintaining the usefulness of the information.

C Ⓜ 8. Protected health information‡ is used for the purposes identified or as required by law or regulation and not further disclosed without resident authorization.

A 9. The organization preserves the privacy and confidentiality of data and information identified as sensitive.

Standard IM.2.20

Not applicable

Standard IM.2.30

Not applicable

Standard IM.3.10

The organization has processes in place to effectively manage information, including the capturing, reporting, processing, storing, retrieving, disseminating, and displaying of clinical/service and nonclinical data and information.

---

* **Privacy** An individual's right to limit the disclosure of personal information.

† **Confidentiality** The safekeeping of data/information so as to restrict access to individuals who have need, reason, and permission for such access.

‡ **Protected health information** Health information that contains information such that an individual person can be identified as the subject of that information.

Rationale for IM.3.10

Records resulting from data capture and report generation* are used for communication and continuity of the resident's care or financial and business operations over time. Records are also used for other purposes, including litigation and risk management activities, reimbursement, and statistics. Improved data capture and report generation systems enhance the value of the records. Potential benefits include improved resident care, quality and safety, improved efficiency, effectiveness and reduced costs in resident care, and financial and business operations. To maximize the benefits of data capture and report generation, these processes exhibit the following characteristics: unique ID, accuracy, completeness, timeliness,† interoperability,‡ retrievability,§ authentication and accountability,‖ auditability, confidentiality, and security.

The processing, storing, and retrieving functions are integral to electronic, computerized, and paper-based information systems in organizations. Important considerations for these functions include data elements, data accuracy, data confidentiality, data security, data integrity, permanence of storage (the time a medium safely stores information), ease of retrievability, aggregation of information, interoperability, clinical/service practice considerations, performance improvement, and decision support processing.

A goal for information storage is to be linked or centrally organized and accessible. This could include the organization having an index identifying where the information is stored and how to access it; or, as the organization moves to electronic systems, the organization creates information systems to be interoperable within the enterprise. As more organizations automate various processes and activities, it is important to share critical data among systems. As challenges of interoperability have arisen, standards organizations for the information technology field have stepped in to develop industry standards. It is important that the organization is aware of the standards development organizations and their recommendations.

Internally and externally generated data and information are accurately disseminated to users. Access to accurate information is required to deliver, improve, analyze, and advance resident care and the systems that support health care delivery. Information is accessed and disseminated through electronic information systems or paper-based records and reports. The use of information is considered in developing forms, screen displays, and standard or ad hoc reports.

---

* **Report generation** The process of analyzing, organizing, and presenting recorded information for authentication and inclusion in the resident's health care record or in financial or business records.

† **Timeliness** The time between the occurrence of an event and the availability of data about the event. Timeliness is related to the use of the data.

‡ **Interoperability** Enables authorized users to capture, share, and report information from any system, whether paper- or electronic-based.

§ **Retrievability** The capability of efficiently finding relevant information.

‖ **Accountability** All information is attributable to its source (person or device).

Elements of Performance for IM.3.10

A 1. Information technology industry standards or organization policies are used and address the following:
- Uniform data definitions
- Data capture
- Data display
- Data transmission

2. Standardize a list of abbreviations, acronyms, symbols, and dose designations that are not to be used throughout the organization.

Note: *The preceding requirement is not scored here. It is scored at NPSG.02.02.01.*

A 3. Minimum data sets, terminology, definitions, classifications, vocabulary, and nomenclature, including abbreviations, acronyms, symbols, and dose designations are standardized throughout the organization.

A 4. Quality control systems are used to monitor data content and collection activities.
- The method used provides for timely and economical data collection with the degree of accuracy, completeness, and discrimination necessary for their intended use
- The method used minimizes bias in the data and regularly assesses the data's reliability, validity, and accuracy
- Those responsible for collecting and reviewing the data are accountable for information accuracy and completeness

A 5. Storage and retrieval systems are designed to support organization needs for clinical/service and organization-specific information.
- Storage and retrieval systems are designed to balance the ability to retrieve data and information with the intended use for the data and information
- Storage and retrieval systems are designed to balance security and confidentiality issues with accessibility
- Systems for paper and electronic records are designed to reduce disruption or inaccessibility during such times as diminished staffing and scheduled and unscheduled downtimes of electronic information systems

A 6. Data and information are retained for sufficient time to comply with law or regulation.

A 7. Knowledgeable staff and tools are available for collecting, retrieving, and analyzing data and their transformation into information.

A 8. Data are organized and transformed into information in formats useful to decision makers.

A 9. Dissemination of data and information is timely* and accurate.

A 10. Data and information are disseminated in standard formats and methods to meet user needs and provide for retrievability and interpretation.

Standard IM.4.10

The information management system provides information for use in decision making.

Rationale for IM.4.10

Information management supports timely and effective decision making at all organization levels. The information management processes support managerial and operational decisions, performance improvement activities, and resident care, treatment, and service decisions. Clinical and strategic decision making depends on information from multiple sources, including the resident record, knowledge-based information, comparative data/information, and aggregate data/information.

Elements of Performance for IM.4.10

A 1. The organization has the ability to collect and aggregate data and information to support care, treatment, and service delivery and operations, including the following:
- Individual care, treatment, and services and care, treatment, and service delivery
- Decision making
- Management and operations
- Analysis of trends
- Performance comparisons over time throughout the organization and with other organizations
- Performance improvement
- Infection control
- Resident safety

A 2. To support clinical decision making, information found in the resident record is:
- Readily accessible
- Accurate
- Complete
- Organized for retrieval of data
- Timely*

A 3. Comparative performance data and information are used for decision making, when available.

Standard IM.5.10

Knowledge-based information resources are readily available, current, and authoritative.

* **Timely** Defined by organization policy and based on the intended use of the information.

Rationale for IM.5.10

Organization practitioners and staff have access to knowledge-based information* to do the following:

- Acquire and maintain the knowledge and skills needed to maintain and improve competence
- Assist with clinical/service and management decision making
- Provide appropriate information and education to residents and families
- Support performance improvement and resident safety activities
- Support the institution's educational and research needs

Elements of Performance for IM.5.10

1. Not applicable

A 2. The organization provides access to knowledge-based information resources† needed by staff in any of the following forms: print, electronic, Internet, or audio.

A 3. Knowledge-based information resources are available to clinical/service staff, through electronic means, after-hours access to an in-house collection, or other methods.

A 4. The organization has a process for providing access to knowledge-based information resources when electronic systems are unavailable.

Standards IM.6.10 Through IM.6.40

Not applicable

Standard IM.6.50

Designated qualified staff accept and transcribe verbal or telephone orders from authorized individuals.

Rationale for IM.6.50

Processes for receiving, transcribing, and authenticating verbal or telephone orders are established to protect the quality of resident care, treatment, and services.

Elements of Performance for IM.6.50

A 1. Qualified personnel are identified, as defined by organization policy and in accordance with law or regulation, and authorized to receive and record verbal or telephone orders.

---

* **Knowledge-based information** A collection of stored facts, models, and information that can be used for designing and redesigning processes and for problem solving. In the context of this manual, knowledge-based information is found in the clinical, scientific, and management literature.

† Examples of knowledge-based information resources include current texts; periodicals; indexes; abstracts; reports; documents; databases; directories; discussion lists; successful practices; equipment and maintenance user manuals; standards; protocols; practice guidelines; clinical trials and other resources.

C Ⓜ 2. Verbal or telephone orders are dated and identifies the names of the individuals who gave, received, and implemented the order.

A 3. When required by law or regulation, verbal or telephone orders are authenticated within the specified time frame.

4. For verbal or telephone orders or for telephonic reporting of critical test results, verify the complete order or test result by having the person receiving the information record and "read-back" the complete order or test result.

Note: *The preceding requirement is not scored here. It is scored at NPSG.02.01.01.*

Standards IM.6.60 Through IM.6.120

Not applicable

Standard IM.6.130

Clinical record documentation includes the provision of education and its effectiveness.

Element of Performance for IM.6.130

C Ⓜ 1. The provision of and the resident's response to education are documented in the clinical record.

Standards IM.6.140 Through IM.6.280

Not applicable

2009 SLTC

Glossary (GL)

GL

Glossary

abuse Intentional maltreatment of an individual which may cause injury, either physical or psychological. *See also* neglect.

mental abuse Includes humiliation, harassment, and threats of punishment or deprivation.

physical abuse Includes hitting, slapping, pinching, or kicking. Also includes controlling behavior through corporal punishment.

sexual abuse Includes sexual harassment, sexual coercion, and sexual assault.

accountability *See* information management.

accreditation Determination by the Joint Commission's accrediting body that an eligible health care organization complies with applicable Joint Commission standards. *See also* accreditation decisions.

accreditation committee The committee of The Joint Commission's Board of Commissioners responsible for oversight of its accreditation process.

accreditation cycle A period of accreditation at the conclusion of which, accreditation expires unless a full survey is performed.

accreditation decisions Categories of accreditation that an organization can achieve based on a Joint Commission survey. These decision categories are:

Accredited The organization is in compliance with all standards at the time of the on-site survey or has successfully addressed all requirements for improvement in an Evidence of Standards Compliance (*see* definition) report within 45 days following the posting of the Accreditation Survey Findings Report.

Provisional Accreditation The organization fails to successfully address all requirements for improvement in an Evidence of Standards Compliance (*see* definition) report within 45 days following the posting of the Accreditation Survey Findings Report.

Conditional Accreditation The organization is not in substantial compliance with the applicable standards, as usually evidenced by a count of the number of standards identified as not compliant at the time of survey, which is between 1½ and 3 standard deviations above the mean number of not compliant standards for organizations in that accreditation program. The organization must remedy identified problem areas through preparation and submission of ESC and subsequently undergo an on-site, follow-up survey.

Preliminary Denial of Accreditation There is a justification to deny accreditation to the organization as usually evidenced by a count of the number of not compliant standards at the time of survey, which is at least three standard deviations above the mean number of standards identified as not compliant for organizations in that accreditation program. The decision is subject to review and appeal prior to the determination to deny accreditation; the appeal process may also result in a decision other than Denial of Accreditation.

Denial of Accreditation The organization has been denied accreditation. All review and appeal opportunities have been exhausted.

Preliminary Accreditation The organization demonstrates compliance with selected standards in the first of two surveys conducted under the Early Survey Policy Option 1 (*see* definition).

accreditation process A continuous process whereby health care organizations are required to demonstrate to the Joint Commission that they are providing safe, high-quality care, as determined by compliance with Joint Commission standards, National Patient Safety Goals recommendations, and performance measurement requirements. Key components of this process are an on-site evaluation of an organization by Joint Commission surveyors, a Periodic Performance Review (PPR), and quarterly submission of performance measurement data to the Joint Commission, as applicable.

accreditation survey findings Findings from an on-site evaluation conducted by the Joint Commission's surveyors that results in an organization's accreditation decision.

Accreditation Survey Findings Report A report of an organization's survey findings; the report includes requirements for improvement (*see* definition), and supplemental findings (*see* definition), as appropriate.

activity services Structured activities designed to help an individual develop or maintain creative, physical, and social skills through participation in recreation, art, dance, drama, social, or other activities.

acuity The degree of psychosocial risk of health treatment or the degree of dependency or functional status of the resident.

administration **1.** The fiscal and general management of an organization, as distinct from the direct provision of services. **2.** *See* medication management, administration.

admitting privileges Authority issued to admit individuals to a health care organization. Individuals with admitting privileges may practice only within the scope of the clinical privileges granted by the organization's governing body.

advance directive A document or documentation allowing a person to give directions about future medical care or to designate another person(s) to make medical decisions if the individual loses decision-making capacity. Advance directives may include living wills, durable powers of attorney, do-not-resuscitate (DNR) orders, right to die, or similar documents listed in the Patient Self-Determination Act that express the resident's preferences.

advanced practice registered nurse A registered nurse who has gained additional knowledge and skills through successful completion of an organized program of nursing education that prepares nurses for advanced practice roles and has been certified by the Board of Nursing to engage in the practice of advanced practice nursing.

When standards reference the term "licensed independent practitioner," this language is not to be construed to limit the authority of a licensed independent practitioner to delegate tasks to other qualified health care personnel (for example, physician assistants and advanced practice registered nurses) to the extent authorized by state law or a state's regulatory mechanism or federal guidelines and organizational policy.

adverse drug event A resident injury resulting from a medication, either because of a pharmacological reaction to a normal dose, or because of a preventable adverse reaction to a drug resulting from an error.

adverse drug reaction (ADR) Unintended, undesirable, or unexpected effects of prescribed medications or of medication errors that require discontinuing a medication or modifying the dose; require initial or prolonged hospitalization; result in disability; require treatment with a prescription medication; result in cognitive deterioration or impairment; are life threatening; result in death; or result in congenital anomalies.

advocate A person who represents the rights and interests of another individual as though they were the person's own, to realize the rights to which the individual is entitled, obtain needed services, and remove barriers to meeting the individual's needs. *See also* surrogate decision maker.

analyzing *See* information management.

anesthesia and sedation The administration to an individual, in any setting, for any purpose, by any route, medication to induce a partial or total loss of sensation for the purpose of conducting an operative or other procedure. Definitions of four levels of sedation and anesthesia include the following:

minimal sedation (anxiolysis) A drug-induced state during which residents respond normally to verbal commands. Although cognitive function and coordination may be impaired, ventilatory and cardiovascular functions are unaffected.

moderate sedation/analgesia (conscious sedation) A drug-induced depression of consciousness during which residents respond purposefully to verbal commands, either alone or accompanied by light tactile stimulation. Reflex withdrawal from a painful stimulus is not considered a purposeful response. No interventions are required to maintain a patent airway, and spontaneous ventilation is adequate. Cardiovascular function is usually maintained.

deep sedation/analgesia A drug-induced depression of consciousness during which residents cannot be easily aroused, but respond purposefully following repeated or painful stimulation. The ability to independently maintain ventilatory function may be impaired. Residents may require assistance in maintaining a patent airway and spontaneous ventilation may be inadequate. Cardiovascular function is usually maintained.

anesthesia Consists of general anesthesia and spinal or major regional anesthesia. It does *not* include local anesthesia. General anesthesia is a drug-induced loss of consciousness during which residents are not arousable, even by painful stimulation. The ability to independently maintain ventilatory function is often impaired. Residents often require assistance in maintaining a patent airway, and positive pressure ventilation may be required because of depressed spontaneous ventilation or drug-induced depression of neuromuscular function.

Cardiovascular function may be impaired.

anesthetic gases Any gas delivered throught the respiratory system as a component of general anesthesia or sedation. This may include inhalation anesthetics distributed in liquid form that when vaporized produce an anesthetic gas (for example, isoflurane, sevoflurane) or nonliquid compresssed gases (for example, nitrous oxide). Oxygen is not included in this definition.

anesthetizing location Any area used for the administration of anesthetic agents.

appeal process The process afforded to an organization that receives a Preliminary Denial of Accreditation (*see* definition), which includes the organization having a right to make a presentation to a Review Hearing Panel (*see* definition) before the Accreditation Committee takes final action to deny accreditation.

assessment **1.** For purposes of resident assessment, the process established by an organization for obtaining appropriate and necessary information about each individual seeking entry into a health care setting or service. The information is used to match an individual's need with the appropriate setting, care level, and intervention. **2.** For purposes of performance improvement, the systematic collection and review of resident-specific data.

auditability *See* information management.

authenticate To verify that an entry is complete, accurate, and final.

authentication *See* information management.

behavioral health A broad array of mental health, chemical dependency, habilitation, and rehabilitation services provided in settings such as inpatient, day treatment, residential, and outpatient.

best practices Clinical, scientific, or professional practices that are recognized by a majority of professionals in a particular field. These practices are typically evidence based and consensus driven.

biologicals Medicines made from living organisms and their products, including serums, vaccines, antigens, and antitoxins.

blood component A fraction of separated whole blood, for example, red blood cells, plasma, platelets, and granulocytes.

blood derivative A pooled blood product, such as albumin, gamma globulin, or Rh immune globulin whose use is considered significantly lower in risk than that of blood or blood components.

blood transfusion services Services relating to transfusing and infusing individuals with blood, blood components, or blood derivatives.

blood usage measurement An activity that entails measuring, assessing, and improving the ordering, distributing, handling, dispensing, administering, and monitoring of blood and blood components.

business occupancy *See* occupancy.

bylaws A governance framework that establishes the roles and responsibilities of a body and its members.

capture *See* information management.

care plan A written plan, based on data gathered during assessment, that identifies care needs, describes the strategy for providing services to meet those needs, documents treatment goals and objectives, outlines the criteria for terminating specified interventions, and documents the progress in meeting goals and objectives. The format of the plan in some organizations may be guided by resident-specific policies and procedures, protocols, practice guidelines, clinical paths, care maps, or a combination thereof. The care plan may include care, treatment, habilitation, and rehabilitation.

care planning (or planning of care) Individualized planning and provision of services that addresses the needs, safety, and well-being of the resident. The plan, which formulates strategies, goals, and objectives, may include narratives, policies and procedures, protocols, practice guidelines, clinical paths, care maps, or a combination of these.

chemical restraint *See* restraint.

CLIA '88 The Clinical Laboratory Improvement Amendments of 1988.

clinical or consultant pharmacist services The provision of professional care and services by a legally qualified pharmacist. This includes the assessment of the appropriateness of medication orders, the ongoing evaluation and review of the resident's medication regimen and pharmaceutical care plan, ongoing monitoring of medication effects in individual residents, provision of drug information, oversight of the medication management process to improve resident safety, and other cognitive medication- related services.

clinical privileges Authorization granted by the appropriate authority (for example, the governing body) to a practitioner to provide specific care, treatment, or services in an organization within well-defined limits, based on the following factors, as applicable: license, education, training, experience, competence, health status, and judgment.

clinical record *See* record.

clinical record services The activities designed to ensure the accuracy, completeness, timeliness, accessibility, and safe, secure, and confidential storage of individuals' medical records.

clinical service groups (CSGs) Groups of residents in distinct, clinical populations for which data are collected. Tracer residents are selected according to CSGs.

community The individuals, families, groups, agencies, facilities, or institutions within the geographic area served by a health care organization.

competence or competency A determination of an individual's skills, knowledge, and ability to meet defined expectations.

complex organization An organization that provides for more than one level of care (for example, acute, subacute, chronic) and type (for example, pediatric, dental, behavioral) of health care service, usually in more than one type of setting (for example, hospital, behavioral, home). An example is an organization that provides acute care, long term care, and home care services.

complex organization survey A Joint Commission survey in which standards from more than one accreditation manual are used in assessing compliance. This type of survey may include using specialist surveyors appropriate to the standards selected for survey.

compliance with a standard (see definition) Meeting the requirements of a standard through compliance with its element(s) of performance (EPs).

component A health care delivery entity (for example, service, program, related entity) that meets survey eligibility criteria under one of the Joint Commission accreditation programs. Multiple components comprise a complex organization.

confidentiality An individual's right, within the law, to personal and informational privacy, including his or her health care records. *See also* information management.

consultation **1.** Provision of professional advice or services. **2.** For purposes of Joint Commission accreditation, advice that is given to staff members of surveyed organizations relating to compliance with standards that are the subject of the survey.

consultation report **1.** A written opinion by a consultant that reflects, when appropriate, an examination of the individual and the individual's medical record(s). **2.** Information given verbally by a consultant to a care provider that reflects, when appropriate, an examination of the individual. The individual's care provider usually documents those opinions in the clinical/case record.

continuing care Care provided over time; in various settings, programs, or services; spanning the illness-to-wellness continuum.

continuing education Education beyond initial professional preparation that is relevant to the type of care delivered in an organization, that provides current knowledge relevant to an individual's field of practice or service responsibilities, and that may be related to findings from performance-improvement activities.

continuity The degree to which the care of individuals is coordinated among practitioners, among organizations, and over time.

continuum of care Matching the individual's ongoing needs with the appropriate level and type of care, treatment, or service within an organization or across multiple organizations.

contract A formal agreement for care, treatment, or services with any organization, agency, or individual that specifies the services, personnel, products, or space provided by, to, or on behalf of the organization and specifies the consideration to be expended in exchange. The agreement is approved by the governing body or comparable entity.

contracted services Services provided through a written agreement with another organization, agency, or individual. The agreement specifies the services or personnel to be provided on behalf of the applicant organization and the fees to provide these services or personnel.

contractual agreement An agreement with any organization, group, agency, or individual for services or personnel to be provided by, to, or on behalf of the organization. Such agreements are defined in written form, such as in a contract, letter of agreement, or memorandum of understanding.

control chart A graphic display of data in the order they occur with statistically determined upper and lower limits of expected common-cause variation. A control chart is used to identify special causes of variation, to monitor a process for maintenance, and to determine if process changes have had the desired effect.

control limit In statistics, an expected limit of common-cause variation, sometimes referred to as either an upper or a lower limit. Variation beyond a control limit is evidence that special causes are affecting a process. Control limits are calculated from process data and are not to be confused with engineering specifications or tolerance limits. Control limits are typically plotted on a control chart.

coordination of care The process of coordinating care, treatment, or services provided by a health care organization, including referral to appropriate community resources and liaison with others (such as the individual's physician, other health care organizations, or community services involved in care, treatment, or services) to meet the ongoing identified needs of individuals, to ensure implementation of the plan of care, and to avoid unnecessary duplication of services.

credentialing The process of obtaining, verifying, and assessing the qualifications of a health care practitioner to provide resident care services in or for a health care organization.

credentials Documented evidence of licensure, education, training, experience, or other qualifications.

Credentials Verification Organization (CVO) Any organization that bases its decision in part on information obtained from a CVO should have confidence in the completeness, accuracy, and timeliness of that information. To achieve this level of confidence, the organization should evaluate the agency providing the information initially and then periodically as appropriate. The principles that guide such an evaluation include the following:

- The agency makes known to the user the data and information it can provide
- The agency provides documentation to the user describing how its data collection, information development, and verification process(es) are performed
- The user is given sufficient, clear information on database functions, including any limitations of information available from the agency (practitioners not included in the database), the time frame for agency responses to requests for information, and a summary overview of quality control processes related to data integrity, security, transmission accuracy, and technical specifications
- The user and agency agree on the format for transmitting credentials information about an individual from the CVO
- The user can easily discern what information transmitted by the CVO is from a primary source and what is not
- For information transmitted by the agency that can go out of date (licensure, board certification), the CVO provides the date the information was last updated from the primary source
- The CVO certifies that the information transmitted to the user accurately represents the information obtained by it
- The user can discern whether the information transmitted by the CVO from a primary source is all the primary source information in the CVO's possession pertinent to a given item or, if not, where additional information can be obtained.

- The user can engage the CVO's quality control processes when necessary to resolve concerns about transmission errors, inconsistencies, or other data issues that may be identified from time to time
- The user has a formal arrangement with the CVO for communicating changes in credentialing information

criteria **1.** Expected level(s) of achievement, or specifications against which performance or quality may be compared. **2.** For purposes of eligibility for a Joint Commission survey, the conditions necessary for health care organizations and networks to be surveyed for accreditation by the Joint Commission.

critical results Test results that are abnormal to a degree that it may indicate a life threatening situation. (also known as critical values)

critical test A test or exam that always requires rapid communication of results, whether those results are normal or abnormal.

data *See* information management.

decentralized laboratory testing *See* point-of-care testing.

delineation of clinical privileges The listing of the specific clinical privileges an organization's staff member is permitted to perform in the organization.

dementia A deterioration of intellectual function associated with pathological changes in the brain that causes changes in behavior and personality. Dementia does not include loss of intellectual functioning caused by clouding consciousness, as in delirium, nor that caused by depression or other functional mental disorders.

dental services Services provided by a dentist, or a qualified individual under the supervision of a dentist, to improve or maintain the health of an individual's teeth, oral cavity, and associated structures.

dentist An individual who has received the degree of either doctor of dental surgery or doctor of dental medicine and who is licensed to practice dentistry.

designated equivalent sources Selected agencies that have been determined to maintain a specific item(s) of credential(s) information that is identical to the information at the primary source. Designated equivalent sources include but are not limited to the following:

- The American Medical Association (AMA) Physician Masterfile for verification of a physician's United States or Puerto Rican medical school graduation and residency completion
- The American Board of Medical Specialities (ABMS) for verification of a physician's board certification
- The Educational Commission for Foreign Medical Graduates (ECFMG) for verification of a physician's graduation from a foreign medical school
- The American Osteopathic Association (AOA) Physician Database for predoctoral education accredited by the AOA Bureau of Professional Education, postdoctoral education approved by the AOA Council on Postdoctoral Training, and Osteopathic Specialty Board Certification
- The Federation of State Medical Boards (FSMB) for all actions against a physician's medical license
- The American Academy of Physician Assistants (AAPA) Profile for physician assistant education and National Certification Commission (NCCPA) certification

dietetic services The delivery of care pertaining to the provision of nutrition and food service to individuals.

director of nursing A registered professional nurse who is responsible for the full-time, direct supervision of nursing services and who is currently licensed by the state in which he or she practices. Attributes of this position may be further defined in regulatory statutes.

disaster *See* emergency.

disaster plan *See* emergency management plan.

discharge The point at which an individual's active involvement with an organization or program is terminated and the organization or program no longer maintains active responsibility for the care of the individual.

discharge planning A formalized process in a health care organization through which the need for a program of continuing and follow-up care is ascertained and, if warranted, initiated for each resident.

disinfection The use of a chemical procedure that eliminates virtually all recognized pathogenic microorganisms but not necessarily all microbial forms (e.g., bacterial endospores) on inanimate objects.

dispensing *See* medication management; pharmacy services.

drug *See* medication.

drug administration *See* medication management.

drug allergies A state of hypersensitivity induced by exposure to a particular drug antigen resulting in harmful immunologic reactions on subsequent drug exposures, such as a penicillin drug allergy. *See* medication.

drug dispensing *See* medication management.

e-App The electronic version of an organization's application for accreditation.

Early Survey Policy A policy that provides two options to organizations undergoing their initial Joint Commission survey. Under both options, the organization undergoes two surveys. Under the first option, the first survey is limited in scope and successful completion results in Preliminary Accreditation (*see* definition). Under the second option, the first survey is a full survey, and successful completion can lead to the organization being Accredited (*see* definition). The second survey in both options is required and will address all standards.

effectiveness The degree to which care is provided in the correct manner, given the current state of knowledge, to achieve the desired or projected outcome(s) for the individual.

efficacy The degree to which the care of the individual has been shown to accomplish the desired or projected outcome(s).

efficiency The relationship between the outcomes (results of care) and the resources used to deliver care.

elements of performance (EPs) The specific performance expectations and/or structures or processes that must be in place for an organization to provide safe, high-quality care, treatment, and services.

emergency **1.** An unexpected or sudden occasion, as in emergency surgery needed to prevent death or serious disability. **2.** A natural or man-made event that significantly disrupts the environment of care (for example, damage to the organization's building[s] and grounds due to severe winds, storms, or earthquakes); that significantly disrupts care, treatment, or services (for example, loss of utilities such as power, water, or telephones due to floods, civil disturbances, accidents, or emergencies in the organization or its community); or that results in sudden, significantly changed or increased demands for the organization's services (for example, a bioterrorist attack, building collapse, or plane crash in the organization's community). Some emergencies are called *disasters* or *potential injury creating events (PICEs)*.

emergency, life-threatening A situation (e.g., major trauma, neck injury) in which an individual requires resuscitation or other support to sustain life.

emergency management plan The organization's written document describing the process it would implement for managing the consequences of natural disasters or other emergencies that could disrupt the organization's ability to provide care, treatment, and services. The plan identifies specific procedures that describe mitigation, preparedness, response and recovery strategies, actions, and responsibilities. *See also* emergency, mitigation activities, preparedness activities.

encryption *See* information management.

endemic infection *See* infection, endemic infection.

enteral nutrition *See* nutrition, enteral nutrition.

entry The process by which an individual comes into a setting, including screening and/or assessment by the organization or the practitioner to determine the capacity of the organization or practitioner to provide the care, treatment, or services required to meet the individual's needs.

environmental tours Activities routinely used by the organization to determine the presence of unsafe conditions and whether the organization's current processes for managing environmental safety risks are being practiced correctly and effectively.

epidemic infection *See* infection, epidemic infection.

equipment management Activities selected and implemented by the organization to assess and control the clinical and physical risks of fixed and portable equipment used for diagnosis, treatment, monitoring, and care.

evidenced-based Based on empirical evidence or in the absence of empirical evidence, expert consensus (such as consensus statements promoted by professional societies).

Evidence of Standards Compliance (ESC) report A report submitted by a surveyed organization within 45 days of its survey, which details the action(s) that it took to bring itself into compliance with a standard or clarifies why the organization believes that it was in compliance with the standard for which it received a requirement for improvement. An ESC must address compliance at the element of performance (EP) level and include a measure of success (MOS) (*see* definition) for all appropriate EP corrections.

exploitation Taking unjust advantage of another for one's own advantage or benefit.

failure modes and effect analysis *See* risk assessment, proactive.

family The person(s) who plays a significant role in an individual's life. This may include a person(s) not legally related to the individual. This person(s) is often referred to as a surrogate decision maker if authorized to make care decisions for the individual should he or she lose decision-making capacity. *See also* guardian; surrogate decision maker.

fire rated

fire rated Material that has undergone a test and is fire protection rated or fire resistance rated.

Fire Resistance Rating The time, in minutes or hours, that materials or assemblies have withstood a fire exposure as determined by the tests, or methods based on tests, prescribed by the NFPA.

Fire Protection Rating The designation indicating the duration of the fire test exposure to which a fire door assembly or fire window assembly was exposed and for which it meant all the acceptance criteria as determined in accordance with NFPA 252, Standard Methods of Fire Tests of Door Assemblies, or NFPA 257, Standard on Fire Test for Window and Glass Block Assemblies, respectively.

fire safety management Activities selected and implemented by the organization to assess and control the risks of fire, smoke, and other byproducts of combustion that could occur during the organization's provision of care, treatment, or services.

fire watch The assignment of a person or persons to an area for the express purpose of protecting occupants from fire or similar emergencies. Examples of this protection include:

- notifying the fire department, the building occupants, or both of an emergency
- preventing a fire from occurring
- extinguishing small fires

foot pound A unit of work done by a force of one pound acting through a distance of one foot in the direction of the force.

formulary A list of medications and associated information related to medication use.

free text *See* information management.

governance The individual(s), group, or agency that has ultimate authority and responsibility for establishing policy, main-taining quality of care, and providing for organization management and planning. Other names for this group include the board, board of trustees, board of governors, and board of commissioners.

guardian A parent, trustee, conservator, committee, or other individual or agency empowered by law to act on behalf of or be responsible for an individual. *See also* family; surrogate decision maker.

hazard vulnerability analysis The identification of potential emergencies and the direct and indirect effects these emergencies may have on the health care organization's operations and the demand for its services.

hazardous condition Any set of circumstances (exclusive of the disease, disorder, or condition for which the resident is undergoing care, treatment, or services) defined by the organization that significantly increases the likelihood of a serious adverse outcome.

hazardous materials and waste Materials whose handling, use, and storage are guided or defined by local, state, or federal regulation (for example, the Occupational Safety and Health Administration's Regulations for Bloodborne Pathogens regarding the disposal of blood and blood-soaked items; the Nuclear Regulatory Commission's regulations for the handling and disposal of radioactive waste), hazardous vapors (for example, gluteraldehyde, ethylene oxide, nitrous oxide), and hazardous energy sources (for example, ionizing or nonionizing radiation, lasers, microwave, ultrasound). Although the Joint Commission considers infectious waste as falling into this category of materials, federal regulations do not define infectious or medical waste as hazardous waste.

hazardous materials and waste management Activities selected and implemented by the organization to assess and control occupational and environmental hazards of materials and waste that require special handling. *See* hazardous materials and waste.

health care–associated infection An infection acquired concomitantly by an individual who is receiving or who has received care, treatment, or services by a health care organization. The infection may or may not be a result of care.

health care occupancy *See* occupancy.

hospice An organized program that consists of services provided and coordinated by an interdisciplinary team to meet the needs of residents who are diagnosed with a terminal illness and have a limited life span. The program specializes in palliative management of pain and other physical symptoms, meeting the psychosocial and spiritual needs of the resident and the resident family or other primary care person(s), utilization of volunteers, and provision of bereavement care to survivors. This includes, but is not limited to, all programs licensed as hospices, and Medicare-certified hospice programs. All services provided by the hospice (e.g., pharmacy and home medical equipment services) and care provided in all settings (inpatient, nursing home, etc.) are included.

human subject research The use of individuals in the systematic study, observation, or evaluation of factors on preventing, assessing, treating, and understanding an illness. The term applies to all behavioral and medical experimental research that involves human beings as experimental subjects.

indicator A measure used to determine, over time, an organization's performance of functions, processes, and outcomes.

infection The transmission of a pathogenic microorganism to a host, with subsequent invasion and multiplication, with or without resulting symptoms of disease.

endemic infection The usual level or presence of an agent or disease in a defined population during a defined period.

epidemic infection A higher-than-expected level of infection by a common agent in a defined population during a defined period.

infection control program An organized system of services designed to meet the needs of the organization or individual in relation to the surveillance, prevention, and control of infection.

information management Terms applicable to information management functions:

- **accountability** All information is attributable to its source (person or device).
- **analyzing** The process that interprets data and transforms it into information.
- **auditability** The ability to do a methodical examination and verification of all information activities such as entering and accessing.
- **authentication** The validation of correctness for both the information itself and the person who is the author or user of the information.
- **capture** The process of recording representations of human thought, perceptions, or actions, as well as device- generated data or information that is gathered and/or computed about a resident as part of a health care encounter or about other matters in a health care organization.
- **confidentiality** The safekeeping of data/information so as to restrict access to individuals who have need, reason, and permission for such access.
- **data** Uninterpreted observations or facts.
- **electronic health information** A computerized format of the health care information in paper records that is used for the same range of purposes as paper records, namely to familiarize readers with the resident's status; to document care, treatment, and services; to plan for discharge; to document the need for care, treatment, and services; to assess the quality of care, treatment, and services; to determine reimbursement rates; to justify reimbursement claims; to pursue clinical or epidemiological research; and to measure outcomes of the care, treatment, and service process.
- **encryption** The process of transforming plain text (readable) into cipher text that is unreadable without a special software key.
- **free text** Free-flowing, nonstructured type of speaking, writing, or inputting information.
- **integrity** In the context of data security, data integrity means the protection of data from accidental or unauthorized intentional change.
- **interactive text** A more complex version of structured text, as it interactively prompts and provides feedback to the person using it. Typically, it uses a higher level of computer intelligence that interacts with the person who records information.
- **interoperability** Enables authorized users to capture, share, and report information from any system, whether paper based or electronic based.
- **knowledge-based information** A collection of stored facts, models, and information that can be used for designing and redesigning processes and for problem solving. In the context of the manual, knowledge-based information is found in the clinical, scientific, and management literature.
- **nonrepudiation** The inability to dispute a document's content or authorship.
- **privacy** An individual's right to limit the disclosure of personal information.
- **processing** The manipulation of data and information by editing and updating.

- **protected health information** Health information that contains information such that an individual person can be identified as the subject of that information.
- **report generation** The process of analyzing, organizing, and presenting recorded information for authentication and inclusion in the resident's health care record or in financial or business records.
- **retrievability** The capability of efficiently finding relevant information.
- **security** The protection of data from intentional or unintentional destruction, modification, or disclosure.
- **structured text** A process that requires authors to put specific information into specific fields with passive guidance by the information system. In paper-based systems, a form encourages a practitioner to fill in fields or boxes. Electronic systems use the same principle for templates or macros, which are guides used to create standardized information documentation. The purpose is to produce data of more consistent quality, make information more usable for decision support, make information more complete and more easily retrievable, and save documentation time.
- **timeliness** The time between the occurrence of an event and the availability of data about the event. Timeliness is related to the use of data.
- **transmission** The sending of data and information from one location to another.

informed consent Agreement or permission accompanied by full notice about what is being consented to. A resident must be apprised of the nature, risks, and alternatives of a medical procedure or treatment before the physician or other health care professional begins any such course. After receiving this information, the resident then either consents to or refuses such a procedure or treatment.

initial survey An accreditation survey of a health care organization not previously accredited by the Joint Commission, or an accreditation survey of an organization performed without reference to any prior survey findings.

integrity *See* information management.

interactive text *See* information management.

interdisciplinary Communication; discussion; planning; evaluation; and care, treatment, and service activities that occur formally and informally between and among team members who are representatives of multiple disciplines.

interim life safety measures A series of 11 administrative actions intended to temporarily compensate for significant hazards posed by existing National Fire Protection Association 101® 2000 *Life Safety Code®* (*LSC*) deficiencies or construction activities. *See also Life Safety Code®*; fire safety management.

interoperability *See* information management.

interpretation services Interpretation services provide for the communication needs of patients who have limited English proficiency or are deaf/hard of hearing. An interpreter is a person who renders a message spoken or signed in one language into one or more languages. Unlike translation, which works only with written text, interpretation works only with spoken/signed language.

intravenous (IV) admixture The preparation of a pharmaceutical product which requires the measured addition of a medication to a 50ml, or greater, bag or bottle of IV fluid (for example, IV, IM, IT, SC, and so on). It does not include the drawing-up of medications into a syringe for immediate use (i.e., reconstitution), or the assembly and activation of an IV system that does not involve the measurement of the additive.

invasive procedures Invasive procedures involve the puncture or incision of the skin, insertion of an instrument, or insertion of foreign material into the body. Invasive procedures may be performed for diagnostic or treatment-related purposes.

investigational medication A medication or placebo used as part of a research protocol or clinical trial.

involuntary seclusion An individual's separation from other individuals or from the individual's room against his or her will or the will of his or her legal representative.

Joint Commission on Accreditation of Healthcare Organizations An independent, not-for-profit organization dedicated to improving the quality of care in organized health care settings. Founded in 1951, its members represent the American College of Physicians–American Society of Internal Medicine, the American College of Surgeons, the American Dental Association, the American Hospital Association, the American Medical Association, the public, and the nursing profession. The Joint Commission engages in issues and activities concerning the advancement of health care safety and quality, including public policy initiatives, standards development, and accreditation and certification programs.

knowledge-based information *See* information management.

laboratory *See* pathology and clinical laboratory services.

leader An individual who sets expectations, develops plans, and implements procedures to assess and improve the quality of the organization's governance, management, clinical, and support functions and processes. Leaders include (when applicable to the organization's structure) the owners, members of the governing body, the chief executive officer, director of nursing, medical director, and other senior managers, and the leaders of the licensed independent practitioners.

licensed independent practitioner Any practitioner permitted by law and by the organization to provide care and services, without direction or supervision, within the scope of the practitioner's license and consistent with individually granted clinical privileges. When standards reference the term "licensed independent practitioner," this language is not to be construed to limit the authority of a licensed independent practitioner to delegate tasks to other qualified health care personnel (for example, physician assistants and advanced practice registered nurses) to the extent authorized by state law or a state's regulatory mechanism or federal guidelines and organizational policy.

licensure A legal right that is granted by a government agency in compliance with a statute governing an occupation (such as medicine, nursing, psychiatry, or clinical social work) or the operation of an activity (such as in a long term care or residential treatment center).

***Life Safety Code®* (*LSC*)** A set of standards for the construction and operation of buildings, intended to provide a reasonable degree of safety to life during fires; prepared, published, and periodically revised by the National Fire Protection Association and adopted by the Joint Commission to evaluate health care organizations under its life-safety management program. *See also* fire safety management; interim life safety measures; occupancy.

life support equipment Any device used for the purpose of sustaining life and whose failure to perform its primary function, when used according to manufacturer's instructions and clinical protocol, leads to resident death in the absence of immediate intervention (examples include ventilators, anesthesia machines, and heart-lung bypass machines).

long term care The health and personal care services provided to chronically ill, aged, physically disabled, or developmentally disabled persons in an institution or in the place of residence. These persons are not in an acute phase of illness, but require convalescent, physical, supportive, and/or restorative services on a long-term basis.

long term care facility An organization that provides nursing care and related services for individuals who require medical, nursing, rehabilitation, or subacute care services. Such a facility may be certified for participation in the Medicare and/or Medicaid program as a skilled nursing facility or a nursing facility.

long term care pharmacy services Services that include the procurement, preparation, dispensing, and distribution of pharmaceutical products to residents of a nursing home or other long term care facility.

look-alike / sound-alike drugs Similar drug names, either written or spoken, which may lead to potentially harmful medication errors when confused for each other.

loss of protective reflexes An inability to handle secretions without aspiration or to maintain a patent airway independently.

management of information *See* information management.

means of egress A continuous and unobstructed way of travel from any point in a building or structure to a public way consisting of three separate and distinct parts: the exit access; the exit; and the exit discharge.

measure of success (MOS) A numerical or quantifiable measure usually related to an audit that determines whether an action was effective and sustained due four months after Evidence of Standards Compliance report (*see* definition) approval.

measurement The systematic process of data collection, repeated over time or at a single point in time.

medical equipment Fixed and portable equipment used for the diagnosis, treatment, monitoring, and direct care of individuals. *See also* equipment management.

medical history A component of the medical record consisting of an account of an individual's history, obtained whenever possible from the individual, and including at least the following information: chief complaint, details of the present illness or care needs, relevant past history, and relevant inventory by body systems.

medical record *See* record.

medical staff The body of all licensed independent practitioners and other practitioners privileged through the medical staff process who are subject to the medical staff bylaws. This body may include others, such as retired practitioners who no longer practice in the organization but who wish to continue their membership in the body. The medical staff includes both members of the organized medical staff and non-members of the organized medical staff who are privileged to provide medical level care.

medication Any prescription medications; sample medications; herbal remedies; vitamins; nutriceuticals; over-the-counter drugs; vaccines; diagnostic and contrast agents used on or administered to persons to diagnose, treat, or prevent disease or other abnormal conditions; radioactive medications; respiratory therapy treatments; parenteral nutrition; blood derivatives; intravenous solutions (plain, with electrolytes and/or drugs); and any product designated by the Food and Drug Administration (FDA) as a drug. This definition of medication does not include enteral nutrition solutions (which are considered food products), oxygen, and other medical gases.

medication error Any preventable event that may cause inappropriate medication use or jeopardize resident safety. *See also* adverse drug reaction; sentinel event.

medication history A delineation of the drugs used by an individual (both past and present), including prescribed and unprescribed drugs and alcohol, along with any unusual reactions to those drugs. *See* medication.

medication management The process an organization uses to provide medication therapy to individuals served by the organization. The steps in the medication management process include:

- **selection** Safe and appropriate selection of medications available for prescribing, storage, and/or use in the organization.
- **procurement** The task of obtaining selected medications from a source outside the organization. It does not include obtaining a medication from the organization's own pharmacy, which is considered part of the ordering and dispensing processes.
- **storage** The task of appropriately maintaining a supply of medications on the organization's premises.
- **secure** In locked containers, in a locked room, or under constant surveillance.
- **prescribing or ordering** Synonymous terms for when a licensed independent practitioner transmits a legal order or prescription to the organization directing the preparing, dispensing, and administering of a specific medication to a specific resident. It does not include requisitions for medication supplies.• **transcribing** The process by which an order from a licensed independent practitioner is documented either in writing or electronically.
- **preparing** The compounding, manipulation, or other activity needed to get a medication ready

for administration exactly as ordered by the licensed independent practitioner.

- **dispensing** Providing, furnishing, or otherwise making available a supply of medications to the individual for whom it was ordered or their representative by a licensed pharmacy according to a specific prescription or medication order, or by a licensed independent practitioner authorized by law to dispense. Dispensing does not involve providing an individual with a dose of medication previously dispensed by the pharmacy.
- **administration** The provision of a prescribed and prepared dose of an identified medication to the individual for whom it was ordered to achieve its pharmacological effect. This includes directly introducing the medication into or onto the individual's body.
- **self-administration** Independent use by a resident of a medication, including medications that may be held by the organization for independent use by the resident.
- **monitoring** The ongoing evaluation of an individual to whom a medication was administered, to ascertain the effectiveness and efficacy of the medication therapy and prevent the occurrence of any serious adverse outcomes.

medication-management measurement The measurement, assessment, and improvement of the prescribing or ordering, preparing and dispensing, administering, and monitoring of medications.

medication reconciliation The process of identifying the name, dosage, route, and frequency for every medication currently being taken and ordering medication based on reference to this list.

mental abuse *See* abuse, mental abuse.

minimum data set (MDS) A core set of screening, clinical and functional status elements, including common definitions and coding categories, that forms the foundation of the comprehensive assessment for all residents of long term care facilities certified to participate in Medicare or Medicaid. The items in the MDS standardize communication about resident problems and conditions within facilities, between facilities, and between facilities and outside agencies.

mission statement A written expression that sets forth the purpose of an organization or one of its components. The generation of a mission statement usually precedes the formation of goals and objectives.

mitigation activities Those activities an organization undertakes in attempting to lessen the severity and impact of a potential emergency. *See* emergency.

multidisciplinary team A group of clinical staff members composed of representatives from a range of professions, disciplines, or service areas.

near miss Used to describe any process variation that did not affect an outcome, but for which a recurrence carries a significant chance of a serious adverse outcome. Such a near miss falls within the scope of the definition of a sentinel event, but outside the scope of those sentinel events that are subject to review by the Joint Commission under its Sentinel Event Policy.

neglect The absence of minimal services or resources to meet basic needs. Neglect includes withholding or inadequately providing food and hydration (without physician, resident, or surrogate approval), clothing, medical care, and good hygiene. It may also include placing the individual in unsafe or unsupervised conditions. *See also* abuse.

network An entity offering comprehensive or specialty services that provides, or provides for, integrated health care services to a defined population of individuals. Networks are characterized by a centralized structure that coordinates and integrates services provided by components and practitioners participating in the network.

nonrepudiation *See* information management.

nursing The health profession dealing with nursing care and services as (1) defined by the Code of Ethics for Nurses with Interpretive Statements, Nursing's Social Policy Statement, Nurses' Bill of Rights, Scope and Standards of Nursing Practice of the American Nurses Association, and specialty nursing organizations; and (2) defined by relevant state, commonwealth, or territory nurse practice acts and other applicable laws and regulations.

nursing care Professional processes of assessment, diagnosis, planning, implementation, and evaluation based on the art and science of nursing to promote health, its recovery, or a peaceful and dignified death. This includes, but is not limited to, assisting individuals, families, communities, and/or populations in understanding health needs and carrying out therapeutic plans and activities.

nursing home A health care organization with inpatient beds and an organized professional staff that provides continuous nursing and other health-related, psychosocial, and personal services to residents who are not in an acute phase of illness, but who require continued care on an inpatient basis.

nursing services One or more defined units or departments within a health care organization with accountability for the delivery of quality nursing care to individuals, families, communities, and/or populations. Personnel, fiscal, capital, and intellectual resources focus on resident safety via interdisciplinary collaboration, integrated data and information management, and communication within all planning, implementation, and evaluation activities.

nursing staff Personnel within a health care organization who are accountable for providing and assisting in the provision of nursing care. Such personnel must include registered nurses (RNs), and may include others such as advanced practice registered nurses (APRNs), licensed practical or vocational nurses (LPNs/LVNs), and nursing assistants or other designated unlicensed assistive personnel.

nutriceuticals Nutritional supplements formulated in a pharmaceutical dosage form and used with the intention of deriving medical or health benefits, including preventing and treating disease. Such products range from isolated nutrients, dietary supplements, and diets to genetically engineered "designer" foods, herbal products, and processed foods such as cereals, soups, and beverages.

nutrition The sum of the processes by which one takes in and uses nutrients.

enteral nutrition Nutrition provided via the gastrointestinal tract. Enteral nutrition encompasses both oral (delivered through the mouth) and tube (provided through a tube or catheter that delivers nutrients distal to the mouth) routes.

parenteral nutrition Nutrients that are provided intravenously, bypassing the digestive tract, which may contain protein, sugar, fat, and added vitamins and minerals as needed by the resident. Related terms are total parenteral nutrition (TPN), partial parenteral nutrition (PPN), and hyperalimentation (HA).*

nutrition assessment A comprehensive process for defining an individual's nutrition and hydration status using medical, nutrition and medication intake histories, physical examination, anthropomorphic measurements, and laboratory data.

nutrition care Interventions and counseling to promote appropriate nutrition and fluid intake, based on nutrition and hydration assessment and information about food, other sources of nutrients, and meal preparation consistent with the individual's cultural background and socioeconomic status. Nutrition therapy, a component of medical treatment, includes enteral and parenteral nutrition. *See also* nutrition.

nutrition screening A process used to indicate the need for a nutritional assessment to determine whether a resident is malnourished or at risk for malnourishment.

occupancy

ambulatory health care occupancy An occupancy used to provide services or treatment to four or more residents at the same time that either (1) renders them incapable of providing their own means of self-preservation in an emergency or (2) provides outpatient surgical treatment requiring general anesthesia.

business occupancy An occupancy used to provide outpatient care, treatment, or services that do not meet the criteria in the ambulatory health care occupancy definition (for example, three or fewer residents at the same time who are either rendered incapable of self-preservation in an emergency or are undergoing general anesthesia).

health care occupancy An occupancy used for purposes such as medical or other care, treatment, or services provided to persons suffering from physical or mental illness, disease or infirmity; and for the care of infants, convalescents, or infirm aged persons. Health care occupancies provide sleeping facilities for four or more occupants and are occupied by persons who are mostly incapable of self-preservation because of age, physical or mental disability, or because of security measures not under the occupant's control. Health care occupancies include hospitals, nursing homes, and limited care facilities.

residential occupancy An occupancy in which sleeping accommodations are provided for normal residential purposes and include all buildings designed to provide sleeping accommodations.

operative and other high-risk procedures Surgical or other procedures that put the resident at risk of death or disability. This does not include use of medications that place residents at risk.

organization's strengths Areas in which an organization's performance is exemplary, as evidenced by the implementation of innovative approaches to meeting Joint Commission standards. An organization will not be cited for having a strength if the organization has a related not compliant standard and/or partially compliant element of performance (EP).

organized medical staff The governance structure of the medical staff, including the medical staff bylaws and rules and regulations to which the medical staff is subject. This structure is approved by the governing body of the organization. Long term care organizations do not necessarily have organized medical staffs.

parenteral nutrition *See* nutrition, parenteral nutrition.

parenteral product A sterile pharmaceutical preparation introduced into the body through a route other than the digestive tract, as by subcutaneous, intramuscular, or intravenous injection or infusion.

pathology and clinical laboratory services The services that provide information on diagnosis, prevention, or treatment of disease or the assessment of health, through the examination of the structural and functional changes in tissues and organs of the body that cause or are caused by disease. It also includes the biological, microbiological, serological, chemical, immunohematological, hematological, or other examination of materials derived from the human body.

patient An individual who receives care, treatment, or services. For hospice providers, the patient and family are considered a single unit of care. Synonyms used by various health care fields include client, resident, customer, patient and family unit, consumer, and health care consumer. *See also* resident.

patient identifiers Information directly associated with an individual that reliably identifies the individual as the person for whom the service or treatment is intended. Acceptable identifiers may be the individual's name, an assigned identification number, telephone number, or other person-specific identifier.

peer recommendation Information submitted by an individual(s) in the same professional discipline as the applicant reflecting their perception of the practitioner's clinical practice, ability to work, as part of a team, and ethical behavior or the documented peer evaluation of practitioner specific data collected from various sources for the purpose of evaluating current competence.*

performance improvement The continuous study and adaptation of a health care organization's functions and processes to increase the probability of achieving desired outcomes and to better meet the needs of individuals and other users of services.

performance measurement system A method of gauging organization performance that facilitates improvement through the collection of data and information and the dissemination of process and/or outcome measures over time.

Periodic Performance Review (PPR) An additional requirement of the accreditation process whereby an organization reviews its compliance with all applicable Joint Commission standards, completes and submits to the Joint Commission a plan of action (*see* definition) for any standard not in full compliance, including the identification of a measure of success (MOS) (*see* definition), and chooses to engage in a telephone discussion with a member of the Standards Interpretation Group staff to determine the acceptability of the plan of action. The PPR encourages organizations to be in continuous compliance with Joint Commission standards. At the time of the next full survey, surveyors validate that the MOS were implemented and effective.

pharmaceutical care and services Services provided directly or through written contract with another organization that include procuring, preparing, dispensing, and/or distributing pharmaceutical products and the ongoing monitoring of the recipient to identify, prevent, and resolve medication-related problems.

pharmacist An individual who has a degree in pharmacy and is licensed and registered to prepare, preserve, compound, and dispense drugs and chemicals.

pharmacist, consultant An individual who has a degree in pharmacy and is licensed and registered in accordance with pharmacy law and regulation. This individual provides services to a long term care facility, including conducting retrospective drug-regimen reviews (DRRs) of all residents' medications on at least a monthly basis; providing written recommendations (interventions) for medication order changes, as appropriate, based on the DRR; assessing medication use; consulting with the long term care facility on various drug-utilization management techniques such as formulary management, therapeutic interchange, generic substitution, drug-use evaluation, and disease management; and participating in a long term care facility's continuous quality improvement programs and on other resident care–oriented committees (for example, infection control).

pharmacy A licensed location where drugs are stored and dispensed.

pharmacy services The provision of pharmaceutical care and services involving the preparation and dispensing of medications, and medication-related devices and supplies by a licensed pharmacy, with or without the provision of clinical or consultant pharmacist services.

physical abuse *See* abuse.

physical rehabilitation services The professional and technical care provided by rehabilitation professionals that assists physically disabled persons to attain, increase, or maintain functional capacity.

physical restraint *See* restraint.

physician A doctor of medicine or doctor of osteopathy who, by virtue of education, training, and demonstrated competence, is granted clinical privileges by the organization to perform a specific diagnostic or therapeutic procedure(s) and who is fully licensed to practice medicine.

physician assistant An individual who practices medicine with supervision by licensed physicians, providing residents with services ranging from primary medicine to specialized surgical care. The scope of practice is determined by state law, the supervising physician's delegation of responsibilities, the individual's education and experience, and the specialty and setting in which the individual works. When standards reference the term "licensed independent practitioner," this language is not to be construed to limit the authority of a licensed independent practitioner to delegate tasks to other qualified health care personnel (for example, physician assistants and advanced practice registered nurses) to the extent authorized by state law or a state's regulatory mechanism or federal guidelines and organizational policy.

physician licensure The process by which a legal jurisdiction, such as a state, grants permission to a physician to practice medicine after finding that he or she has met acceptable qualification standards. Licensure also involves ongoing regulation of physicians by the legal jurisdiction, including the authority to revoke or otherwise restrict a physician's license to practice.

plan A detailed method, formulated beforehand, that identifies needs, lists strategies to meet those needs, and sets goals and objectives. The format of the plan may include narratives, policies and procedures, protocols, practice guidelines, clinical paths, care maps, or a combination of these.

plan for improvement For purposes of Joint Commission accreditation, an organization's written statement that details the procedures to be taken and timeframes to correct existing *Life Safety Code®* (*LSC*) deficiencies. *See also* Statement of Conditions™ (SOC); interim life safety measures; *Life Safety Code®*.

Plan of Action A plan detailing the action(s) that an organization will take to come into compliance with a Joint Commission standard. A plan of action must be completed for each element of performance (EP) (*see* definition) associated with a not compliant standard. A measure of success (MOS) (*see* definition) must also be included in the plan of action as indicated in the accreditation manual.

podiatrist An individual who has received the degree of doctor of podiatry medicine and who is licensed to practice podiatry.

point-of-care testing Analytical testing performed at sites outside the traditional laboratory environment, usually at or near where care is delivered to individuals. Testing may range from simple waived procedures, such as fecal occult blood, to more sophisticated chemical analyzers. The testing may be under the control of the main laboratory, the direction of another specialized laboratory (such as for arterial blood gas), or the nursing service. Testing may be categorized as waived, moderate, or high complexity under CLIA '88. Also called alternate site testing, decentralized laboratory testing, and distributed site testing.

policies and procedures The formal, approved description of how a governance, management, or clinical care process is defined, organized, and carried out.

practice guidelines Tools that describe processes found by clinical trials or by consensus opinion of experts to be the most effective in evaluating and/or treating a resident who has a specific symptom, condition, or diagnosis, or describe a specific procedure. Synonyms include practice parameter, protocol, preferred practice pattern, and guideline.

preadmission procedures An organization's process for obtaining appropriate and necessary information for each individual seeking admission into a health care setting or service. The information is used to match the individual need with the level of care required and to the appropriate setting.

Preliminary Denial of Accreditation *See* accreditation decisions.

preparedness activities Those activities an organization undertakes to build capacity and identify resources that may be used if an emergency occurs. *See* emergency.

prescribing or ordering *See* medication management.

primary source The original source or an approved agent of that source of a specific credential that can verify the accuracy of a qualification reported by an individual health care practitioner. Examples include medical school, graduate education, state medical board, and federal and state licensing boards.

primary source verification Verification of an individual health care practitioner's reported qualifications by the original source or an approved agent of that source. Methods for conducting primary source verification of credentials include direct correspondence, documented telephone verification or secure electronic verification from the original qualification source, or reports from credentials verification organizations that meet the 10 Joint Commission requirements. *See* the notes for HR.1.20 EP 3.

priority focus areas (PFAs) Processes, systems, or structures in a health care organization that significantly impact the quality and safety of care. The PFAs are:

- Assessment and Care/Services
- Communication
- Credentialed Practitioners
- Equipment Use
- Infection Control
- Information Management
- Medication Management
- Organizational Structure
- Orientation and Training
- Patient Safety
- Physical Environment
- Quality Improvement Expertise and Activity
- Rights and Ethics
- Staffing

primary PFA Every standard is linked to one or more PFAs. When a surveyor has findings under a standard, he or she determines which of the linked PFAs is most related to the specific finding—this becomes the *primary* PFA. For example, a finding under standard HR.1.10 may be assigned a primary PFA of Staffing. The organization's accreditation report is organized by PFA.

secondary PFAs The additional PFAs that are also related to a specific finding, in addition to the primary PFA. For example, a finding under standard HR.1.10 may be assigned a secondary PFA of Orientation and Training. The organization's accreditation report also lists the secondary PFAs.

Priority Focus Process (PFP) The process for standardizing the priorities for sampling during an organization's survey based on information collected about the organization prior to survey. The process also helps to focus the survey on areas that are critical to that organization's resident safety and quality-of-care processes. Examples of such information may include, but are not limited to, data from the organization's e-App (*see* definition); past survey finding data process; complaint and sentinel event information; data collected from external sources, such as MedPar data; performance measurement data; and previous survey results.

Priority Focus Tool (PFT) An automated tool that supports the Priority Focus Process (PFP) through the use of algorithms, or sets of rules, to transform a health care organization's data into information that guides the survey process.

privacy *See* information management.

privileging The process whereby a specific scope and content of resident care services (that is, clinical privileges) are authorized for a health care practitioner by a health care organization, based on evaluation of the individual's credentials and performance. *See* licensed independent practitioner.

processing *See* information management.

program An organized system of services designed to address the needs of an organization or individual.

protected health information *See* information management.

Provisional Accreditation *See* accreditation decisions.

psychoactive *See* psychotropic/psychopharmacologic medication.

psychotropic/psychopharmacologic medication Any medication whose intended purpose is to alter perception, mental status, or behavior. These include, but are not limited to, those drugs that produce drug dependence. Some examples of drug classes that are considered psychotropic/ psychopharmacologic medications include, but are not limited to, hypnotics, antipsychotics, long- and short-acting benzodiazepines, sedatives/anxiolytics, and antidepressants.

Public Information Policy A Joint Commission policy governing the disclosure of specific information about the performance of a health care organization or network, as well as accreditation-related information that remains confidential. This policy covers the Joint Commission's Quality Reports, information publicly disclosed on request, complaint information, aggregate performance data, data released to government agencies, and the Joint Commission's right to clarify information that an accredited organization releases about its accreditation status.

qualified individual An individual or staff member who is qualified to provide care, treatment, or services by virtue of the following: education, training, experience, competence, registration, certification or applicable licensure, or law or regulation. Examples of qualified individuals include: activities coordinator, administrator, audiologist, child psychiatrist, clinical chaplain, creative arts therapist, dietetic services supervisor, dietitian, registered dietitian, health information administrator, health information technician, licensed practical nurse (LPN), medical radiation physician, medical technologist, music therapist, occupational therapist, occupational therapy assistant, physiatrist, physical therapist assistant, physical therapist, psychiatric nurse, psychologist, radiologic technologist, recreational therapist, recreational therapist assistant or technician, respiratory care technician, respiratory therapist, respiratory therapy technician, social work assistant, social worker, and speech-language pathologist.

quality control A process that consists of measuring performance, comparing performance against goals, and acting on the differences when performance falls short of defined goals.

quality of care The degree to which health services for individuals and populations increase the likelihood of desired health outcomes and are consistent with current professional knowledge. Dimensions of performance include the following: resident perspective issues; safety of the care environment; and accessibility, appropriateness, continuity, effectiveness, efficacy, efficiency, and timeliness of care.

Quality Report A report that is available to the public that provides information about an organization's accreditation decision and the effective date for the decision, any special quality awards the organization received, the accreditation services included in the organization's accreditation award, any disease-specific care certification(s) and the effective date of each certification received by the organization, the implementation of National Patient Safety Goals by the organization, the organization's performance against National Quality Improvement Goals and the organization's performance in relation to Patient Experience of Care measures.

range orders Orders in which the dose or dosing interval varies over a prescribed range, depending on the situation or individual's status.

rationale for a standard Background, justification, or additional information about a standard. A rationale is *not* scored. Not every standard has a rationale.

read-back A method to ensure understanding of information being communicated, often used between members of a caregiving team. The process involves the receiver of a verbal or telephone order writing down the complete order or test result or entering it into a computer, then reading it back, and receiving confirmation from the individual who gave the order or test result.

reassessment Ongoing data collection, which begins on initial assessment, comparing the most recent data with the data collected at earlier assessments.

record **1.** The account compiled by physicians and other health care professionals of a variety of resident health information, such as assessment findings, treatment details, and progress notes. **2.** (data source) Data obtained from the records or documentation maintained on a resident in any health care setting (for example, hospital, home care, long term care, practitioner office). Includes automated and paper medical record systems.

referral The sending of an individual (1) from one clinician to another clinician or specialist, (2) from one setting or service to another, or (3) by one physician (the referring physician) to another physician(s) or other resource, either for consultation or care.

registered nurse (RN) An individual who is qualified by an approved post-secondary program or baccalaureate or higher degree in nursing and licensed by the state, commonwealth, or territory to practice professional nursing.

report generation *See* information management.

reprocessing All operations performed to render a contaminated reusable or single-use device resident ready. The steps may include cleaning and disinfection/sterilization. The manufacturer of reusable devices and single-use devices that are marketed as non-sterile should provide validated reprocessing instructions in the labeling.

requirement for improvement A recommendation that is required to be addressed in the organization's Evidence of Standards Compliance (ESC, *see* definition) report and needs to be addressed in order for the organization to retain its accreditation decision. Failure to adequately address a requirement for improvement after two opportunities will result in a recommendation to place the organization in Conditional Accreditation (*see* definition).

resident The recipient of care from a long term care provider or assisted living community.

resident tracer The process used by the Joint Commission of evaluating a resident's total care experience within a health care organization.

residential occupancy *See* occupancy.

respiratory care services Delivery of care to provide ventilatory support and associated services for individuals.

restorative services Goal-directed interventions that assist or promote a resident's ability to attain his or her maximum functional potential.

restraint Any method (chemical or physical) of restricting a resident's freedom of movement, including seclusion, physical activity, or normal access to his or her body that (1) is not a usual and customary part of a medical diagnostic or treatment procedure to which the resident or his or her legal representative has consented; (2) is not indicated to treat the resident's medical condition or symptoms; or (3) does not promote the resident's independent functioning.

chemical restraint The inappropriate use of a sedating psychotropic drug to manage or control behavior.

physical restraint Any method of physically restricting a person's freedom of movement, physical activity, or normal access to his or her body.

resuscitative services Personnel, supplies, and processes used to resuscitate an individual.

retrievability *See* information management.

Review Hearing Panel A panel of three individuals, including one member of the Joint Commission Accreditation Committee, which hears a presentation on the facts of the case by an organization in Preliminary Denial of Accreditation, should the organization desire such a presentation.

risk assessment, proactive An assessment that examines a process in detail including sequencing of events; assesses actual and potential risk, failure, or points of vulnerability; and, through a logical process, prioritizes areas for improvement based on the actual or potential resident care impact (criticality).

risk-management activities Clinical and administrative activities that organizations undertake to identify, evaluate, and reduce the risk of injury to residents, staff, and visitors and the risk of loss to the organization itself.

root cause analysis A process for identifying the basic or causal factor(s) that underlie variation in performance, including the occurrence or possible occurrence of a sentinel event.

run chart A display of data in which data points are plotted as they occur over time (for example, observed weights over time) to detect trends or other patterns and variation occurring over time. Run charts, as opposed to tabular frequency displays, are capable of time-order analytic studies.

safety The degree to which the risk of an intervention (for example, use of a drug or a procedure) and risk in the care environment are reduced for a resident and other persons, including health care practitioners.

safety management Activities selected and implemented by the organization to assess and control the impact of environmental risk, and to improve general environmental safety.

scope of care or services The activities performed by governance, managerial, clinical, or support staff.

security *See* information management.

security management A component of an organization's management of the environment of care program that maintains and improves the general security of the care environment.

self-administration *See* medication management, administration.

sentinel event An unexpected occurrence involving death or serious physical or psychological injury, or the risk thereof. Serious injury specifically includes loss of limb or function. The phrase *or the risk thereof* includes any process variation for which a recurrence carries a significant chance of a serious adverse outcome.

sexual abuse *See* abuse.

Shared Visions–New Pathways® A Joint Commission initiative to progressively sharpen the focus of the accreditation process on care systems critical to the safety and quality of resident care.

skilled nursing/complex medical care Typically provided in a skilled nursing facility or unit, a program or service that provides goal directed, time limited, skilled nursing or skilled rehabilitative services that are coordinated by an interdisciplinary team, and are generally reimbursed by Medicare, Medicaid, or third party insurance. Typical residents/patients are those who had an acute illness, injury, or exacerbation of a disease process. It is goal-oriented treatment rendered immediately after, or instead of, acute hospitalization to treat one or more specific, active, complex medical conditions or to administer one or more technically complex treatments in the context of an individual's underlying long-term conditions and overall situation.

social work services Services to assist clients and their families in addressing social, emotional, and economic stresses associated with illness or injury. Such services are provided by a qualified social worker or a social work assistant under the supervision of a qualified social worker. These services can be provided directly or through contract with another organization or individual.

staff As appropriate to their roles and responsibilities, all people who provide care, treatment, and services in the organization, including those receiving pay (e.g., permanent, temporary, and part-time personnel, as well as contract employees), volunteers, and health profession students. The definition of staff does not include licensed independent practitioners who are not paid staff.

staffing effectiveness The number, competence, and skill mix of staff as related to the provision of needed services.

standard A statement that defines the performance expectations, structures, or processes that must be in place for an organization to provide safe, high-quality care, treatment, and services.

Statement of Conditions™ (SOC) A proactive document that helps an organization to do a critical self-assessment of its current level of compliance and describe how to resolve any *Life Safety Code*® (*LSC*) deficiencies. The SOC was created to be a "living, ongoing" management tool that should be used in a management process that continually identifies, assesses, and resolves *LSC* deficiencies.

sterilization The use of a physical or chemical procedure to destroy all microbial life, including highly resistant bacterial endospores.

subacute care *See* skilled nursing/complex medical care.

supplemental finding A recommendation that is not required to be addressed in an organization's Evidence of Standards Compliance (ESC) report (*see* definition), but should be addressed by the organization internally. A supplemental finding is also factored into an organization's Priority Focus Process (PFP) at its next survey.

surrogate decision maker Someone appointed to act on behalf of another. Surrogates make decisions only when an individual is without capacity or has given permission to involve others. *See also* advocate; family.

survey A key component in the accreditation process, whereby a surveyor(s) conducts an on-site evaluation of an organization's compliance with Joint Commission standards.

full survey A survey that assesses an organization's compliance with all applicable Joint Commission standards.

initial survey A survey of a health care organization not previously accredited by the Joint Commission, or a survey of an organization performed without reference to any prior survey findings.

surveyor For purposes of Joint Commission accreditation, a nurse or administrator with experience in the field of long term care who meets the Joint Commission's surveyor selection criteria, evaluates standards compliance, and provides education and consultation regarding standards compliance to surveyed long term care organizations.

system A set of interrelated parts that work together toward a common goal.

system tracer A session during an on-site survey devoted to evaluating high-priority safety and quality-of-care issues on a systemwide basis throughout the organization. Examples of such issues may include infection control, medication management, staffing effectiveness, and the use of data.

systems analysis The evaluation of how well a health care organization's systems function.

threshold for Conditional Accreditation At least two but not more than three standard deviations above the mean number of not compliant standards; the threshold for Conditional Accreditation is one rule for receiving Conditional Accreditation.

threshold for Preliminary Denial of Accreditation At least three standard deviations above the mean number of not compliant standards; the threshold for Preliminary Denial of Accreditation is one rule for receiving Preliminary Denial of Accreditation.

timeliness *See* information management.

titrating orders Orders in which the dose is either progressively increased or decreased in response to the individual's status.

total parenteral nutrition *See* nutrition, parenteral nutrition.

tracer methodology A tool used by a process surveyor(s) during an on-site survey to analyze an organization's systems, with particular attention to identified priority focus areas (PFAs), by following individual residents, residents, or clients through the organization's health care process in the sequence experienced by the patients, residents, or clients. Depending on the health care setting, this may require surveyors to visit multiple care units, departments, or areas within an organization or a single care unit to trace the care rendered to a patient, resident, or client.

transfer The formal shifting of responsibility for the care of an individual (1) from one care unit to another, (2) from one clinical service to another, (3) from one licensed independent practitioner to another, or (4) from one organization to another.

transfer agreement A written understanding that provides for the reciprocal transfer of individuals between health care organizations.

translation services Translation services provide *translation* of written documents into other languages. A translator is a person who converts the written text of one language into the written text of one or more languages. Unlike interpretation, which works with spoken/signed language, translation works only with written text.*

transmission *See* information management.

unit dose Medication to be given to a particular patient at a specific time packaged in the exact dosage required for that time.

urgent A degree of severity of illness or injury that is less severe than immediately life-threatening (emergency), but requiring care more quickly than elective care.

urgent/immediate care services Those services sought for conditions that are considered less critical than those that need to be seen in an emergency center, but are not scheduled with the individual's primary care provider or the provider's designee.

utilities management Activities selected and implemented by the organization to assess and control the risks of utility systems of buildings that support the provision of care, treatment, or services. Included are those activities that ensure the operational reliability of such systems and those activities for responding to a failure of such systems.

utility systems Building systems for life support; surveillance, prevention, and control of infection; environment support; and equipment support. These can include electrical distribution; emergency power; vertical and horizontal transport; heating, ventilating, and air conditioning; plumbing, boiler, and steam; piped gases; vacuum systems; or communication systems including data-exchange systems.

utilization management The examination and evaluation of the appropriateness of the utilization of an organization's resources. Also referred to as a utilization review.

waived testing Tests that meet the Clinical Laboratory Improvement

Amendments of 1988 (CLIA '88) requirements for waived tests; are cleared by the Food and Drug Administration for home use; employ methodologies that are so simple and accurate as to render the likelihood of erroneous results negligible; or pose no risk of harm to a resident if the test is performed incorrectly.

written Information that is documented in hardcopy or electronic formats.

2009
SLTC
Index
(IX)

XI

Index

H

I

J

M